Dental Clinical Procedures using Artificial Intelligence

Arthur Rodriguez Gonzalez Cortes
Editor

Dental Clinical Procedures using Artificial Intelligence

Springer

Editor
Arthur Rodriguez Gonzalez Cortes
Department of Dental Surgery
Faculty of Dental Surgery
University of Malta
Msida, Malta

ISBN 978-3-032-24894-7 ISBN 978-3-032-24895-4 (eBook)
https://doi.org/10.1007/978-3-032-24895-4

This Springer imprint is published by the registered company Springer Nature Switzerland AG
The registered company address is: Gewerbestrasse 11, 6330 Cham, Switzerland

This book is dedicated to my family, with whom I have learned and for whom I will always be there to transmit the value of love, empathy, care, and dedication.

Prof. Arthur Cortes

Foreword

I was delighted to be invited to write the foreword to this book. My son Arthur also invited his brother Thomaz to contribute to a chapter, which made this task particularly meaningful to me.

In 2015, Arthur was completing his postdoctoral studies at Harvard University, while Thomaz was finishing his MBA at the Massachusetts Institute of Technology. Working in such different fields, I never imagined that they could be together, years later, in a single project. Artificial Intelligence (AI) made it possible since they were going to different, but not parallel paths.

Having worked as a dentist for more than 50 years, I began my career at a time when creativity and inventiveness were indispensable. The techniques available then made us almost artisans, relying on limited materials and a narrow range of instruments. With minimal image technology, surgical procedures were performed almost blindly, often depending on the operator's skill and experience.

Over the decades, we have witnessed an extraordinary transformation. We have come a long way to reach digital technology, which has brought us fantastic tools and precision that once seemed unimaginable, and has revolutionized dentistry. Procedures such as implant placement and bone grafting are now inseparable from the use of digital surgical guides.

Digital technology, as Arthur showed us in his previous book *Digital Dentistry* has taken over the entire dental field, making it hard to work without it. Yet some colleagues did not embrace these innovations and, as a result, were left behind.

Artificial Intelligence is now triggering a new leap in dentistry.

In every field of dentistry, clinicians depend profoundly on researchers, whose studies illuminate the mechanisms and best applications of emerging technologies. AI has been blending concepts and results, expanding its scope of action across many fields. In dentistry, in a very short time, AI will be present in virtually all areas—from endodontics to restorative dentistry, from the study and interpretation of images to surgical and prosthetic planning in implantology. It is easy to imagine using it in orthodontics and prosthodontics, from planning to final results. Through these advances, dentists will be able to provide increasingly individualized treatments and therapies, tailored precisely to each patient's needs.

The idea of creating a machine capable of reasoning is not new. Arthur, an excellent chess player, was deeply impressed when he was very young, by the story of IBM's Deep Blue, a chess computer developed in 1977 to challenge world champions. Deep Blue learned to select optimal moves in response to those of its human opponent. In the historic series of six games, the computer won two, the champion won one, and three ended in draws. This marked a symbolic moment in the dialogue between human intellect and computational reasoning. Arthur, even in his YouTube channel, Understanding Dentistry, has been using AI for some time now.

Artificial intelligence learns through both success and error, refining algorithms and building a foundation of accumulated knowledge. In this respect, AI behaves much like a human being developing skills from experience and self-improvement. When faced again with a similar challenge, AI responds with greater precision. This continuous learning process explains why the term intelligence is so appropriate, as it mirrors the natural evolution of human understanding.

Let us therefore allow Arthur, Thomaz, and their colleagues, with this book, to guide us on this remarkable journey towards the future of dentistry working with AI, making it easy to navigate through this period of technological change, learning how to deal with the challenges, and enjoying the benefits that AI offers to follow the principles of dentistry.

We can be sure that this future has already begun, just as we can be certain that the future will always be tomorrow.

Private Practice
São Paulo, Brazil

Djalma Nogueira Cortes

Acknowledgments

The editor would also like to thank all contributors that have dedicated their time as chapter co-authors of this book. All their efforts are highly appreciated.

The editor would also like to thank the companies Zirkonzahn (Gais, Italy), 3Shape A/S (Copenhagen, Denmark), Trinckle 3D GmbH (Berlin, Germany), Diagnocat Ltd. (San Francisco, CA, USA), and the international planning center Beyond Digital Solutions (BDS3D, Curitiba, Brazil) for encouraging this book.

This book is intended to show our experience using artificial intelligence in dental clinical procedures. The comments on software steps, functionalities, advantage, and drawbacks are based on the experience of the authors, assessed at the time of writing this book. For detailed updated information on the artificial intelligence (AI) platforms, please visit their websites, as the AI tools and techniques are constantly updated by the developers. Details of techniques and case studies are provided along with scientific evidence and explanations. We hope that our experience and the knowledge in this book may benefit all readers in some way.

Introduction: Review of Basic Concepts of Digital Dentistry and Artificial Intelligence

Digital workflow in Dentistry has widely been known as the advent of digital technologies such as Computer-Aided Design and Computer-Aided Manufacturing (CAD-CAM) to enhance oral diagnosis and the predictability of dental treatments. In this process, digital impressions of the dental arches and occlusal registrations are taken by means of intraoral or desktop scanners and exported as *Standard Tessellation Language* (STL) files. These can be superimposed to facial 3D scans or photographs for esthetic analyses. Further 3D images from cone beam computed tomography (CBCT) can also be obtained in the Digital Imaging and Communications in Medicine (DICOM) file format and added to the project if bone data is needed for diagnosis or surgical planning. The resulting group of files is then imported into an implant planning or a CAD software program to enable the design of restorations, surgical guides, orthodontic appliances, and so forth. Any designed object will also be exported as an independent STL file, to be fabricated using either subtractive (milling) or additive (3D printing) manufacturing methods. Such workflow has led to the rise of new dental research projects, techniques and clinical business models, ranging from clinics that outsource digital tasks to fully integrated in-house laboratories, each with specific equipment needs and financial considerations. It is also noteworthy that these digital methods are still intended to be used as enhancing tools to apply the same fundamental principles of clinical dentistry considered in conventional and analog workflows [1].

The modern field of study developed from the digital techniques has been called Digital Dentistry (Table 1). Its ongoing development has eventually led to the creation of technological methods using artificial intelligence (AI), which refers to the ability of a machine to execute tasks that require the human intelligence, such as visual perception and clinical decision-making procedures. Among the main AI techniques used in dentistry are machine learning and deep learning models. Nevertheless, as discussed in the further chapters of this book, the successful implementation of these AI tools depends on the basic and clinical knowledge of the dental clinician, who is the ultimate responsible for all clinical decisions.

Table 1 Review of important concepts of Digital Dentistry

Concepts	Meaning
Pixel values	Numbers from pixels relative to their grayscale levels on radiographs
DICOM	Digital Imaging and Communications in Medicine. A standard file extension of 3D imaging methods such as CBCT and MRI
STL	The most used file extension for 3D objects such as intraoral scans
PLY and OBJ	Additional file extensions of 3D objects including color information
Mesh	Structure of the surface geometry of STL files made of linked triangles
Intraoral scan	A 3D digital impression performed by intraoral scanners
Threshold	Value used in imaging processing to segment an image
Virtual patient	3D digital model of the patient from combined 3D images, aligned in the same coordinates
Accuracy	Ability of a method to correctly outline/identify/measure a structure

AI and Its Relationship with Dentistry

Imagine a hypothetical world where dentistry is as advanced as it can be today. All clinics have the most complex instruments, 3D scanners, digital workflows, and AI systems used for diagnosis and treatment. Yet in this imaginary world, something as simple as a toothbrush has never been invented. Even basic oral hygiene would therefore require a visit to the dentist. Dental healthcare would then be solely dependent on third parties, expensive, and limited to trained professionals.

For many years, AI techniques looked similar. Powerful tools existed but using them required deep technical expertise. Building AI solutions meant custom data pipelines, model training, and specialized teams.

The emergence of general-purpose models known as Large Language Models (LLMs) changed this situation. These "General Pre-trained Transformers," such as ChatGPT (Open AI), Gemini (Google), and Copilot (Microsoft) made it significantly easier to leverage machine intelligence to a wide array of tasks. This could be comparable to the invention of brushing teeth in our hypothetical world. LLMs provide a general and reusable form of intelligence that anyone can use. With natural language as the interface, users can build AI-driven workflows, generate structured outputs, and solve practical problems without developing models from scratch.

Nevertheless, just as brushing teeth does not replace dentists, LLMs do not replace specialized AI models. In fact, one could argue that even brushing teeth in the wrong manner does not improve dental hygiene. On the other hand, a simple toothbrush does improve access and largely increases the baseline of the value created by dental hygiene. With the current state of AI, such technology has evolved from a rare and complex procedure to a daily tool that many people can use. From Christopher Strachey's checkers-playing AI in 1951 [2], the technology has become present across industries and professions, as well as in our daily lives.

The Flow of AI: From Data to Value Creation

The value from AI is only created when a clear and complete flow is followed. Technical sophistication alone is not sufficient. In practice, five steps are required for an AI system to move from data to solving real-world problems.

The first step is the data source. Every AI application starts with data that serves as its input. This may include images, text, signals, or structured records. If the data is incomplete, biased, or poorly defined, the AI system cannot perform reliably, regardless of how advanced the model may be [3]. Furthermore, some data may be input for model creation or training, while other portions of data may be input directly from the user at each utilization of the model. As an example, when one asks ChatGPT to summarize a text, the user inputs the text to be summarized at the model utilization, while OpenAI has trained its GPT-4 on many billions of words coming from a diverse range of sources.

The second step is insight. This is what the AI system produces from the data. Such insight can take many forms, such as a prediction, a numerical score, a classification, or a summary of complex information. At this stage, the output exists only as information—i.e., simply by itself, it has no practical effect.

The third step is action. A given AI output becomes useful only when it leads to a concrete action, decision, or change. This may involve for example alerting a clinician, modifying a treatment plan, prioritizing cases, or automating a task. Without action, even highly accurate insights remain futile.

The fourth step is value. Effective AI applications address a clearly defined problem and generate measurable benefits. These benefits may include improved accuracy, time savings, cost reduction, or better outcomes. While many AI systems are technically impressive, not all of them solve a real underlying problem in a meaningful way. Such value can come in many forms: a dentist, for instance, may automate a task to save time, may cross-check treatment plans to reduce risk and increase the probability of success or even may have the radiological images searched by specialized AI to find earlier (and often imperceptible to humans) signs of a potentially grave condition.

The fifth step and most overlooked step is sustainability. An AI system must remain reliable over time—even more so in health-related applications. Although LLMs have reduced the effort required to build AI applications, they do not eliminate maintenance challenges. Complex systems that rely on multiple data pipelines and models are harder to manage. Even off-the-shelf models such as LLMs are non-deterministic; this means that changes in data, infrastructure, or model behavior can alter results, even when the same input is provided. Consider a hypothetical scenario of a model that was trained in thousands of images from a given MRI machine; after a year of usage, the doctor using it starts inputting imagery from a completely new machine, with distinct traces of color, resolution, and other technical characteristics. The precision of the insight of the model may or may not be severely reduced—a risk that must never remain unmanaged by a thorough clinician.

As one can infer from the value creation flow described, it is vital to clarify roles and responsibilities of those who interact with AI systems. In simplified view, AI applications typically involve two distinct groups of individuals. The first is composed of builders, who are responsible for designing, implementing, and maintaining the AI system. They define how data is processed, how models behave, and how outputs are delivered. In a dental context, a builder may be a software engineer or data scientist who develops an AI system for radiograph analysis using Python and machine learning frameworks. The other group are the users who interact on a recurrent basis and benefit from the AI system. These individuals do not necessarily need to have deep understanding of how the model is built although thorough conceptual understanding is highly advised. On the aforementioned example, the dentist is the user of the AI application built by the software engineer to analyze radiographic imagery. The dentist focuses on clinical decisions, while part of the technical complexity of the application (e.g., the python code and the multiple libraries used) remain transparent to such usage.

While such distinction enables faster technological advancement, it may also bring risks of usage and sustainability. The first step to mitigate those is to have builders that understand users and the value they intend to create with the new tooling, as well as users with thorough conceptual knowledge of what was built.

For this reason, knowledge about how AI works is also important for dental users. In this context, recent systematic reviews described important AI concepts for the dental professional, as shown in Table 2 [4, 5]:

Table 2 Review of important concepts about AI for the dental professional

Concept	Explanation/meaning	Application examples/purpose
Artificial Intelligence (AI)	**Systems capable of performing tasks that normally require human intelligence, including perception, reasoning, learning, and decision-making**	**AI-assisted diagnosis in dentistry; automated medical decision support; intelligent software systems**
Data Science	An interdisciplinary field focused on extracting knowledge from data through statistics, analysis, engineering, and visualization	Analysis of large dental patient datasets to identify outcome trends or risk factors
AI Algorithms	Formal sets of rules and procedures that define how AI systems process data and produce outputs	Algorithms that analyze radiographs to detect anomalies or measure anatomical structures
Machine Learning (ML)	**A subfield of AI in which models learn patterns directly from data rather than being explicitly programmed**	**Predicting caries presence, treatment success, or implant failure risk**
Supervised Learning	Learning from labeled data to perform classification or prediction tasks	Predictive detection of caries from annotated radiographs; outcome prediction models

Table 2 (continued)

Concept	Explanation/meaning	Application examples/purpose
Unsupervised Learning	Learning from unlabeled data to discover patterns or structure within datasets	Clustering patients by periodontal risk; identifying hidden patterns in clinical data
Semi-Supervised Learning	Learning approach that combines limited labeled data with large volumes of unlabeled data	Improving radiograph classification when expert annotations are scarce
Reinforcement Learning	Learning through interaction with an environment using reward signals to guide decisions	Optimization of appointment scheduling; adaptive treatment planning strategies
Neural Networks (NNs)	**Computational models inspired by biological neurons, capable of learning complex nonlinear relationships**	**Modeling complex relationships between clinical variables and outcomes**
Artificial Neural Networks (ANN)	General purpose multi-layer neural networks applicable to structured data, signals, and images	Predicting treatment outcomes; estimating working length from radiographic data
Deep Learning (DL)	Neural networks with many layers that learn hierarchical representations directly from raw data	Automated detection of caries, bone loss, and anatomical landmarks in radiographs
Convolutional Neural Networks (CNN)	Deep learning architectures specialized for visual data and spatial pattern recognition	Image-based analysis of bitewings, panoramic radiographs, and CBCT scans
Recurrent Neural Networks (RNN)	Neural networks designed for sequential or temporal data	Analysis of time series data such as patient-monitoring signals
Transformer Models	Neural architectures based on attention mechanisms that model long range dependencies	Language understanding systems; multimodal AI combining text and images
Large Language Models (LLMs)	Large-scale transformer models trained on vast text corpora to understand and generate natural language	Automated dental reports; clinical note summarization; patient communication; literature review support
Dimensionality Reduction Methods	**Techniques that reduce data complexity while preserving relevant information**	**Feature reduction in radiomics; visualization of high dimensional clinical data**
Clustering Methods	**Techniques that group data points based on similarity without predefined labels**	**Patient stratification by disease risk; discovery of disease subtypes**

Bold Letters: Category related to the concepts presented below

Training and Application

ML models are trained on large datasets. To prevent "overfitting" (when a model performs well on training data but poorly on new data), a technique called data augmentation (e.g., rotating and resizing images) can be used to increase the sample size. An AI model's performance is entirely dependent on the quality of the data it learns from and the rigor of its training process. For dental applications, this process typically follows three important stages. The first is data collection and preparation. The foundation of any effective AI model is a high-quality, comprehensive, and standardized dataset. Raw data such as thousands of radiographs or images must be meticulously cleaned and processed. This involves removing redundant features, managing missing information, and ensuring the data is representative of the diverse patient populations that could benefit from the method. The next stage is the model training. The most common training strategy in healthcare is supervised learning. In this process, the algorithm is fed a "training set" of data that has already been labeled with the correct outcomes by human experts. For example, a model designed to detect caries would be trained on thousands of radiographs where a radiologist has already marked which images contain caries and which do not. The algorithm learns to associate specific visual patterns with the "caries" label. Then, the final stage of the model validation and testing occurs. After initial training, the model's internal parameters are fine-tuned using a separate "validation set" to improve its performance. Finally, to measure its actual effectiveness, the model is evaluated on a "test set" of new unseen data that was not used in the training or validation steps. This final test demonstrates how accurate the model can generalize its knowledge to predict clinical outcomes in a real-world scenario.

This rigorous training process enables AI models to perform a wide array of specialized tasks across the dental field. Furthermore, trained algorithms are also becoming available for the dental clinician as AI tools available in dental commercial AI-driven software programs, such as Second Opinion (Pearl) and Diagnocat (Diagnocat Ltd.). These are AI-driven diagnostic platforms that can detect several common pathologies and alterations on radiographs [5]. The alterations detected include but are not limited to caries, bone loss, marginal discrepancies in restorations, and periodontal calculus. Among the main features of AI in dentistry discussed in this book are:

- Automated classification and morphological assessment of teeth, as well as identification of patient demographic features and anatomical landmarks (further discussed in Chap. 1).
- Automated caries detection on radiographic images (further discussed in Chap. 2).
- Automated pathology diagnosis and classification (further discussed in Chap. 3).
- Periodontal Assessment (further discussed in Chap. 4).
- Automated dental reports with generative AI (further discussed in Chap. 5).
- Automated improvement of digital impressions and virtual patients (further discussed in Chap. 6).
- Automated tissue segmentation for dental treatment planning (further discussed in Chap. 7).
- Automated cephalometric measurements for orthodontic analyses (further discussed in Chap. 8).
- Automated steps of image-guided surgical planning (further discussed in Chap. 9).
- Automated Design of Restorations and Prostheses, as well prediction of their clinical outcomes (further discussed in Chap. 10).

This book should also be used by the dental clinician to review the ethical and regulatory considerations as well as the risks and limitations of the implementation of AI in the clinical practice [6], as further discussed in Chap. 5. With adequate knowledge of ethical standards for implementation, AI has the potential to lead to a novel standard of care in modern dentistry. As a supportive partner, AI could allow the dental community to optimize the available clinical workflows and could potentially improve diagnostic accuracy, optimize treatment outcomes, and ultimately elevate the quality and accessibility of care for patients, which is a very important and relevant aspect from a public health perspective.

A Provocation: Machine Learning and Its Multiple Facets

Despite not being the entire focus of this book, and with the deliberate intent to instigate intellectual curiosity on the reader and AI user, this introduction finishes by describing and illustrating 12 families of ML Models (Table 3). As one will notice, all the progress and endless possibilities derived from LLMs made accessible to public in late 2022 are comprised within a subset of one of the 12 model families listed (Table 3, item 10A). All others are extensively used underneath the technology of our daily lives, from watches that can perform electrocardiograms

Table 3 Types of AI models and applications

Name	Description	Model examples	Application examples
Linear and Generalized Linear Models	Models that learn linear relationships between inputs and outputs, optionally using link functions	Linear Regression, Logistic Regression, Ridge, Lasso	Predicting implant failure risk; estimating treatment duration; appointment no-show prediction
Instance-Based Models	Models that make predictions by comparing new cases to stored examples rather than learning explicit parameters	k-NN, Radius Neighbors	Finding similar orthodontic cases; case-based treatment recommendations
Probabilistic Graphical Models	Models that explicitly represent uncertainty and conditional dependencies using probability theory	Naive Bayes, Bayesian Networks, HMMs	Caries risk assessment; disease progression modeling; diagnostic decision support
Decision Tree Models	Rule-based models that partition data hierarchically into interpretable decisions	Decision Trees, CART	Chairside decision support (restore vs. monitor); treatment eligibility screening
Ensemble Methods (Non-neural)	Models that combine multiple base learners to improve accuracy and robustness	Random Forests, XGBoost, LightGBM	Radiograph-based caries detection from handcrafted features; outcome prediction models

Table 12.1 (continued)

Name	Description	Model examples	Application examples
Support Vector Methods	Margin-based models that learn optimal decision boundaries, often using kernels	SVM, SVR	Classification of normal vs. pathological radiographs; biomedical signal analysis
Clustering Models	Unsupervised models that group data based on similarity without labeled outcomes	k-Means, DBSCAN, GMM	Patient stratification by periodontal risk; discovery of disease subtypes
Dimensionality Reduction and Manifold Learning	Models that compress high-dimensional data while preserving relevant structure	PCA, ICA, t-SNE, UMAP	Feature reduction in radiomics; visualization of patient populations; noise reduction
Shallow Neural Networks	Neural models with limited depth that learn nonlinear input–output mappings	Perceptron, Shallow MLP	Predicting working length from radiographs; basic clinical outcome prediction
Deep Learning Models	Multi-layer neural networks that learn hierarchical representations from raw data	CNNs, RNNs, Deep Autoencoders, Transformers	Automated caries detection; bone loss measurement on CBCT; cephalometric landmark detection
Large Language Models (LLMs)	Transformer-based deep learning models trained on massive text corpora to model and generate human language	OpenAI's ChatGPT, Google Gemini, Microsoft Copilot	Automated dental reports; clinical note summarization; patient communication; literature review assistance
Reinforcement Learning Models	Models that learn optimal actions through interaction with an environment and reward feedback	Q-Learning, Policy Gradients	Appointment scheduling optimization; adaptive treatment planning; robotics research
Evolutionary and Genetic Algorithms	Population-based optimization models inspired by biological evolution	Genetic Algorithms, Genetic Programming	Implant placement optimization; prosthesis design; ML hyperparameter optimization

and detect atrial fibrillation to complex computer games. It is suggested that there is still limitless opportunity to build on such important techniques to advance healthcare, dental treatments, and quality of life.

Thomaz Rodriguez Gonzalez Cortes
Arthur Rodriguez Gonzalez Cortes

References

1. Cortes ARG. Digital dentistry: a step-by-step guide and case atlas. Hoboken, NJ: Wiley; 2022. https://doi.org/10.1002/9781119852025.
2. Hodges A. Alan Turing: the logical and physical basis of computing. IEEE Ann Hist Comput. 1992;14(3):18–26.
3. Cross JL, Choma MA, Onofrey JA. Bias in medical AI: implications for clinical decision-making. PLOS Digit Health. 2024;3(11):e0000651.
4. Ghaffari M, Zhu Y, Shrestha A. A review of advancements of artificial intelligence in dentistry. Dentist Rev. 2024;4:100081. https://doi.org/10.1016/j.dentre.2024.100081.
5. Sitaras S, Tsolakis IA, Gelsini M, Tsolakis AI, Schwendicke F, Wolf TG, Perlea P. Applications of artificial intelligence in dental medicine: a critical review. Int Dent J. 2025;75(2):474–86. https://doi.org/10.1016/j.identj.2024.11.009.
6. Lal A, Nooruddin A, Umer F. Concerns regarding deployment of AI-based applications in dentistry—a review. BDJ Open. 2025;11(1):27. https://doi.org/10.1038/s41405-025-00319-7.

Contents

Editor and Contributors

About the Editor

Arthur Rodriguez Gonzalez Cortes Prof. Arthur Cortes is a researcher on artificial intelligence, digital dentistry, and radiology. He completed a postdoctoral fellowship on radiology at Harvard University, and he is a fellow, speaker, and study club director of the International Team for Implantology (ITI). He has been teaching and clinically performing dentistry for more than 15 years. Prof. Cortes is a member of several professional associations and has transferred knowledge with his YouTube channel: Understanding Dentistry, for which even the soundtracks are made by him as his hobby is playing his musical instruments and record his own songs. Besides his role of editor, Prof. Arthur Cortes is also an author contributing to all chapters of this book.

Contributors

Malek Abu-Gharbieh Institut für Werkzeugmaschinen und Fabrikbetrieb, Berlin, Germany

Rafik Akhmad Charité University, Berlin, Germany

Ana Paula Ayres University of São Paulo, São Paulo, Brazil

Otavio Henrique Pinhata-Baptista Military Hospital of São Paulo Area (HMASP), São Paulo, Brazil

Shizhu Bai State Key Laboratory of Oral & Maxillofacial Reconstruction and Regeneration, Xi'an, China
National Clinical Research Center for Oral Diseases, Xi'an, China
Digital Center, School of Stomatology, The Fourth Military Medical University, Xi'an, China

Adam Bartolo Faculty of Dental Surgery, University of Malta, Msida, Malta

Adriana Bartolo BroadStreet Dental Centre, Hamrun, Malta

Florian Beuer Charité University, Berlin, Germany

Shaban Burgoa GoBeyond Dental Courses, Houston, TX, USA

Nicholas Busuttil Dougall Faculty of Dental Surgery, University of Malta, Msida, Malta

Clifford Camilleri Master of Oral Implantology, Goethe University Frankfurt a.M., Frankfurt am Main, Germany

Arthur Rodriguez Gonzalez Cortes Faculty of Dental Surgery, University of Malta, Msida, Malta

Thomaz Rodriguez Gonzalez Cortes McKinsey & Company, São Paulo, Brazil

Angelica de Moura e Costa MAC Radiology Institute, Curitiba, Brazil

Alan Jony de Moura e Costa GoBeyond Dental Courses, Houston, TX, USA

Laura Althea Cuschieri Faculty of Dental Surgery, University of Malta, Msida, Malta

Mauricio Pesce Gomes da Costa Doc Digital Institute, São Paulo, Brazil

Hossam Dawa CESPU University, Porto, Portugal

Lisya Vizotto de Barros University of São Paulo, São Paulo, Brazil

José Lincoln de Queirós Jr. ClickDent, Brasilia, Brazil

Sergio Candido Dias Private Practice, São Paulo, Brazil

Vinicius Dutra Department of Oral Pathology, Medicine, and Radiology, Indiana University, School of Dentistry, Indianapolis, IN, USA

Jesus Torres Garcia-Denche Complutense University of Madrid, Madrid, Spain

Laura Godoy Ruíz Complutense University of Madrid, Madrid, Spain

Thomas Martin Grixti Private Practice, Msida, Malta

Virgilio Gutierrez GoBeyond Dental Courses, Houston, TX, USA

Ji Yong Han Seoul National University, Seoul, South Korea

Min Suk Heo Seoul National University, Seoul, South Korea

Reinhilde Jacobs OMFS-IMPATH Research Group, Department of Imaging and Pathology, Faculty of Medicine, KU Leuven, Leuven, Belgium
Department of Oral and Maxillofacial Surgery, University Hospitals Leuven, Leuven, Belgium
Department of Dental Medicine, Karolinska Institute, Stockholm, Sweden

Gino Kopp Kopp Dental Institute, Curitiba, Brazil

Fernanda Kopp Kopp Dental Institute, Curitiba, Brazil

Pierre Lahoud Division of Periodontology and Oral Microbiology, Department of Oral Health Sciences, Faculty of Medicine, KU Leuven, Leuven, Belgium
OMFS-IMPATH Research Group, Department of Imaging and Pathology, Faculty of Medicine, KU Leuven, Leuven, Belgium
Department of Conservative Dentistry, Periodontology and Digital Dentistry, LMU University Hospital, LMU Munich, Munich, Germany

Fernando Antonio Reis Laurino São Paulo State University—UNESP, São Paulo, Brazil

Jiani Liu State Key Laboratory of Oral & Maxillofacial Reconstruction and Regeneration, Xi'an, China
National Clinical Research Center for Oral Diseases, Xi'an, China
Digital Center, School of Stomatology, The Fourth Military Medical University, Xi'an, China

Roberto Adrian Markarian Clínica Implart, São Paulo, Brazil

Bruno B. R. Matias University of São Paulo, São Paulo, Brazil

Juliana No-Cortes Faculty of Dental Surgery, University of Malta, Msida, Malta

Claudio Mendes Pannuti University of São Paulo, São Paulo, Brazil

David Peñarrocha-Oltra University of Valencia, Valencia, Spain

Miguel Peñarrocha-Diago University of Valencia, Valencia, Spain

Tatiana Cursino Pereira São Paulo State University—UNESP, São Paulo, Brazil

Jorge Alonso Perez-Barquero University of Valencia, Valencia, Spain

Lucas Rodrigues Pinheiro Private Practice, São Paulo, Brazil

Mariana Balcewicz Pozza GoBeyond Institute, Curitiba, Brazil

Guillermo Pradies Complutense University of Madrid, Madrid, Spain

Giuseppe Alexandre Romito University of São Paulo, São Paulo, Brazil

Guilherme Saavedra São Paulo State University—UNESP, São Paulo, Brazil

Andreas Dominik Schwitalla Charité University, Berlin, Germany

Newton Sesma University of São Paulo, São Paulo, Brazil

Faleh Tamimi McGill University, Montreal, Canada

Marcelo Lucchesi Teixeira University of São Paulo, São Paulo, Brazil

Alexandre Domingues Teixeira-Neto GoBeyond Dental Institute, Curitiba, Brazil

Thi Ngoc Trang Tran Faculty of Dental Surgery, University of Malta, Msida, Malta

Rui Xie State Key Laboratory of Oral & Maxillofacial Reconstruction and Regeneration, Xi'an, China
National Clinical Research Center for Oral Diseases, Xi'an, China
Digital Center, School of Stomatology, The Fourth Military Medical University, Xi'an, China

Baoluo Xing Gao Afonso X el Sabio University, Madrid, Spain
Complutense University of Madrid, Madrid, Spain

Part I

Oral Diagnosis

Anatomical Assessment of the Jaws with Artificial Intelligence

1

Adam Bartolo and Arthur Rodriguez Gonzalez Cortes

Applications of artificial intelligence (AI) in medicine and dentistry are rapidly expanding, with dental imaging emerging as a particularly promising domain. Conventional interpretation of routine radiographic imaging modalities such as panoramic, periapical, and cephalometric radiographs can be labor-intensive, time-consuming, and subject to observer variability. These challenges have led to the creation and development of digital technological solutions to improve workflow efficiency, enhance diagnostic accuracy, and optimize patient care. Deep learning models can be used as tools to address these needs by automating complex imaging analysis, identifying subtle patterns, as well as providing quantitative and reproducible anatomical measurements [1]. It is important to note, however, that the quality and resolution of the dental and radiographic images may significantly influence the accuracy of the AI systems, as it also commonly affects the diagnostic accuracy of dental professionals [2], and the execution of digital workflows in dentistry [3].

AI-assisted anatomical assessments can be divided into two main groups. The first group comprises AI-powered tools designed to identify patient-level features such as age, sex, and craniofacial growth stage. The second group includes applications of AI in identifying, measuring, and classifying a wide range of anatomical structures and prosthetic elements within the oral and maxillofacial complex.

Several of the articles in the literature reviewed below are diagnostic studies. To better understand these, it is important to get familiar with scientific terms such as diagnostic accuracy, sensitivity, and specificity. Diagnostic accuracy is considered the ability of a diagnostic test to correctly identify or rule out a given disease or alteration. Diagnostic sensitivity is the separate ability of this test to correctly identify those with a disease (true positives), while specificity is the ability to

A. Bartolo · A. R. G. Cortes (✉)
Faculty of Dental Surgery, University of Malta, Msida, Malta
e-mail: adam.bartolo@um.edu.mt; arthur.nogueira@um.edu.mt

A. R. G. Cortes (ed.), *Dental Clinical Procedures using Artificial Intelligence*,
https://doi.org/10.1007/978-3-032-24895-4_1

correctly identify those without a disease (true negatives). Another important concept is the precision, which refers to the closeness of agreement between repeated measurements. This, in turn, could include intraobserver reliability and interobserver reproducibility.

1.1 AI-Powered Identification of Patient Features

The accurate assessment of patient-specific features is a requirement to make a diagnosis and perform treatment planning in several dental specialties. In orthodontics and pediatric dentistry, determining a patient's growth stage is critical for timing clinical interventions. In forensic dentistry, estimating age and sex from dental records is essential for human identification. Traditionally, these assessments rely on manual qualitative evaluations of specific indicators on radiographs. Recent research demonstrates that AI models can automate and enhance these processes, learning to extract discriminative features from routine radiographs to provide objective, quantitative, and efficient assessments.

1.1.1 Age and Sex Estimation

AI models have shown promising results in automating the estimation of chronological age and sex from panoramic radiographs. A study performed in 2025 developed a multitask deep learning model based on the EfficientNetB0 architecture to analyze a dataset of panoramic radiographs from a Thai population aged 7–23 years [4]. For age estimation, the model achieved an overall root mean square error (RMSE) of 1.67 years and a mean absolute error (MAE) of 1.15 years. The accuracy was notably higher in the younger cohort (7–14 years), with an RMSE of just 0.95 years. In contrast, a worse performance was observed for the older cohort (15–23 years), which presented a RMSE increased to 1.87 years. Such disparity is attributed to the reduced dental developmental activity in late adolescence, which provides fewer distinct morphological features for the model to analyze. Nonetheless, for sex recognition, the same model demonstrated strong performance, with an overall accuracy of 87.8% and an area under the curve (AUC) of 0.94. These findings suggest a high degree of reliability.

Complementing these findings, another study proposed a two-stage deep learning approach for automated dental age calculation [5]. Their method used first the Scaled-YOLOv4 model to detect dental germs on panoramic radiographs. Then, the EfficientNetV2 M model was employed to classify the developmental stage of the germs assessed. This fully automated workflow yielded a mean absolute error of just 0.261 years, which is favorable when compared to the calculations of human experts. While both studies demonstrated sub-year accuracy, the specialized two-stage approach of the aforementioned study [5], which first isolates dental germs before classification, achieved a significantly lower mean absolute error compared to the end-to-end model used by the previously mentioned study performed in 2025

(0.261 years vs. 1.15 years) [4], suggesting that task-specific workflows may yield higher precision.

1.1.2 Craniofacial Growth and Maturation Assessment

Determining the stage of craniofacial growth, particularly the pubertal growth spurt, is essential for effective orthodontic treatment planning. AI can be applied to automate this assessment on lateral cephalograms, which has the advantage of eliminating the subjectivity of conventional methods. The application of such methods in orthodontics is also discussed further in Chap. 8.

The group of Zhang and collaborators introduced CDSNet, a novel deep learning model for assessing patient growth stages by analyzing features from the cervical vertebrae, dentition, and frontal sinus simultaneously [6]. This multi-region approach proved highly effective, with an accuracy of 90.99%. This represented a significant improvement (approximately 26%) when compared to the conventional cervical vertebral maturation (CVM) method, which relies solely on vertebral morphology. The use of an explainability module (Grad-CAM) confirmed that the whole decision-making process involved the three anatomical regions targeted by the study, validating its novel approach.

Another study used an Inception-v3 convolutional neural network (CNN) model to detect pubertal growth spurts by analyzing CVM stages on lateral cephalometric radiographs [7]. A key finding from this research was the trade-off between diagnostic granularity and model accuracy. When using the original six-stage CVM classification, the model achieved a total success rate of 39% on cropped images. Furthermore, by simplifying the task to a clinical three-stage classification (i.e., identifying stages as pre-spurt, spurt, or post-spurt), the success rate improved significantly to 62%. This suggests that while highly detailed classifications are clinically valuable, AI models could potentially perform more reliably when focused on broader and clinically relevant categories.

The findings of these studies collectively suggest that the capacity of AI to automate the identification of important clinical and demographic patient features is reliable, leading to faster and more objective methods than the conventional ones.

1.2 AI-Driven Identification and Classification of Anatomical and Prosthetic Structures

One of the most important AI-driven tools in modern dentistry is the automated identification of anatomical structures. This enables automated classification and linear measurements from teeth, retained roots, dental implants, grafts, and lesions to important anatomical landmarks, such as the maxillary sinus, nasal fossa, nasopalatine canal, submandibular fossa, mandibular canal, and the mental foramen.

The shape of every structure identified with AI can also be completely outlined and even exported as a separate region of interest of a diagnostic image. Such process is called anatomical segmentation, and it can be volumetrically performed if the images analyzed are 3D. However, since segmentation methods and tools are commonly used in surgical and treatment planning, this topic will be fully discussed further in Chap. 7.

Accurately identifying and segmenting anatomical structures, pathologies, and dental devices in radiographs are foundational tasks for most cases requiring detailed diagnosis and treatment planning. Since the conventional methods are repetitive and time-consuming, several medical and dental research projects and studies have focused on the development of AI-driven automated segmentation methods [1]. As discussed further in this book, AI with deep learning excels at visual recognition tasks, offering the potential to streamline workflows, improve consistency, and provide quantitative data for clinical analysis across a wide range of related applications.

1.2.1 Tooth Identification and Segmentation

Hundreds of millions of dental images are captured and interpreted manually by dental clinicians around the globe. The sheer scale of this task underscores the transformative potential of automation in dental imaging and radiographic interpretation to ensure efficiency and quality of dental healthcare. Accurate tooth identification is very important in dental treatments for several reasons, such as providing the necessary foundation for precise diagnosis as well as enabling a clear communication among practitioners (Fig. 1.1), and effective treatment planning (Fig. 1.2). Furthermore, incorrect tooth identification may lead to severe malpractice, such as wrong-site tooth extraction, which stands as one of the most common reasons for compensation claims filed against oral and maxillofacial surgeons [8]. Furthermore, reliable tooth identification can serve as a tool for estimating age [9] and identifying humans in archaeological and forensic settings [10].

Despite a good opportunity for automation, tooth identification can be affected by several factors acting as challenges for algorithm development and system validation. While the theoretical basis for identification relies on tooth position, morphology, and arrangement relative to the adjacent teeth, factors such as morphological variations, dynamic dentition stages, anatomical anomalies, pathologies, dental restorations, and appliances can pose challenges to the accuracy of the tooth identification process (Fig. 1.3).

A primary challenge is the dynamic nature of human dentition, possessing two distinct sets of teeth over a lifetime. The properties and shapes of these teeth are in a constant state of flux, changing significantly as an individual grows, develops, and matures. Primary teeth, which erupt during infancy, are eventually replaced by permanent teeth in a transitional phase that begins after the age of 5. This life cycle means that at any given time, the dentition of a patient may be in one of several different stages, with possible significant variations in tooth type,

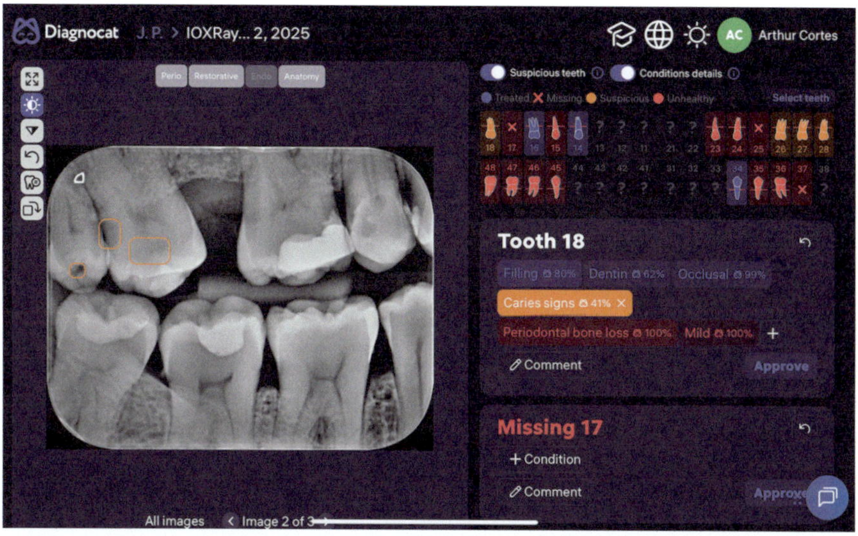

Fig. 1.1 AI-driven analysis of a bitewing radiography with the Diagnocat software. Note that the presence of tooth 18 (right maxillary third molar, in the FDI notation) and the absence of tooth 17 were identified correctly, despite the presence of a fourth upper distomolar

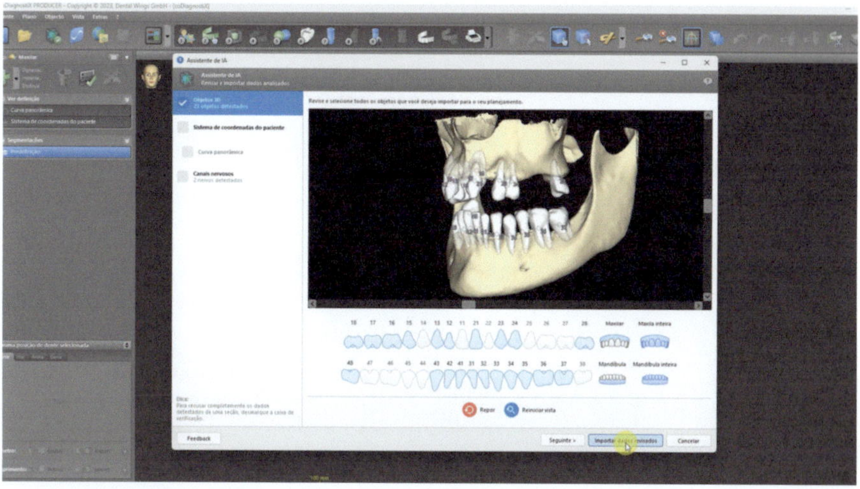

Fig. 1.2 Screenshot of the AI assistant tool of the implant planning software coDiagnostiX (Dental Wings), showing automated teeth identification

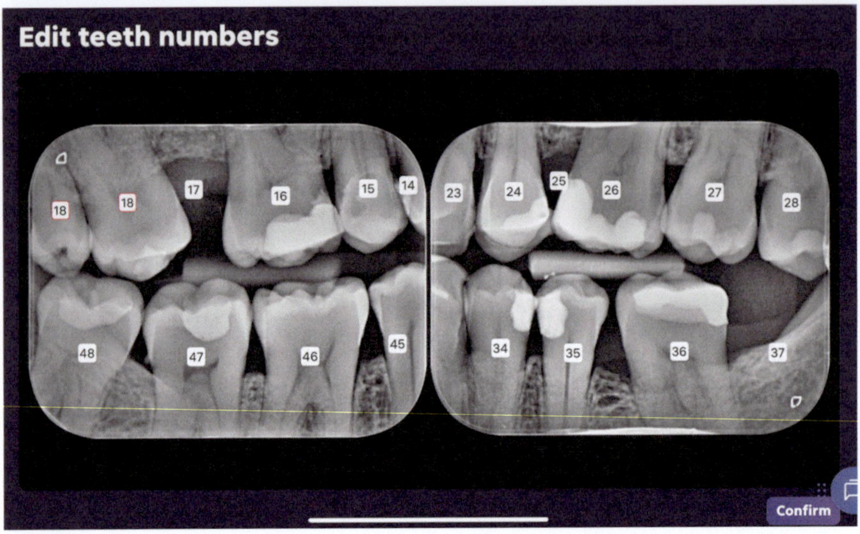

Fig. 1.3 Screenshot of the Diagnocat 2.0 (Diagnocat Ltd., San Francisco, CA, USA) software tool to edit or correct automated teeth numbers. Note that the fourth molar presenting microdontia was identified as a second tooth 18

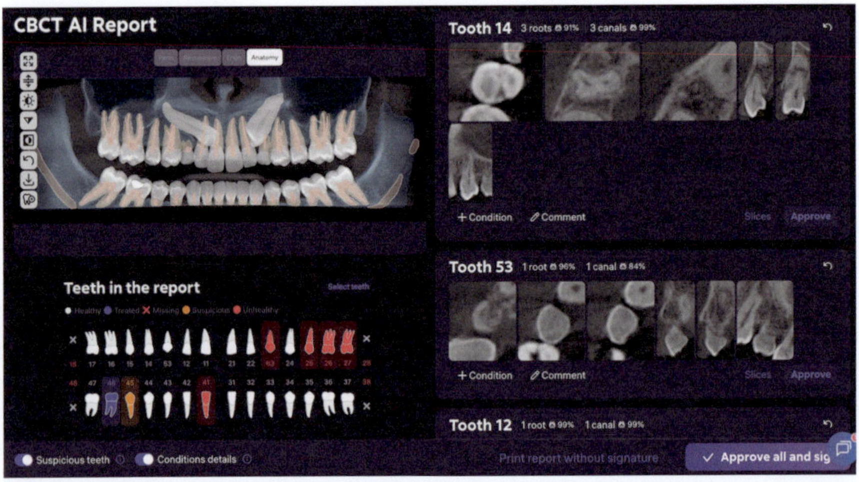

Fig. 1.4 CBCT analysis with the Diagnocat software. Note that the maxillary impacted canines were outlined but not numbered and did not show in the report, although the maxillary deciduous canines were identified correctly

morphology, position, and arrangement. This natural dynamism presents a substantial obstacle for automated systems that require consistent patterns for accurate identification (Fig. 1.4).

The challenge of dynamic dentitions was described in a study by Chen and collaborators [11]. They utilized a faster R-CNN (region-based convolutional neural network) to detect and number teeth on periapical radiographs. However, the system exhibited failures directly related to foundational complexities. The model did not apply to mixed or primary dentition and failed in complex cases with anatomical anomalies. This inability to handle pediatric patients highlights a significant gap between the capabilities of AI algorithms and the requirements of a dental clinical tool for general purposes.

Furthermore, the standard pattern of human dentition can also be disrupted by congenital conditions and pathological issues, which may also complicate the task of automated tooth identification. Among these conditions are tooth number anomalies such as supernumerary teeth (Fig. 1.5), retained primary teeth, and hypodontia (congenitally missing teeth). These alterations could break the expected sequence and arrangement of the dental arch, invalidating the positional and adjacency-based

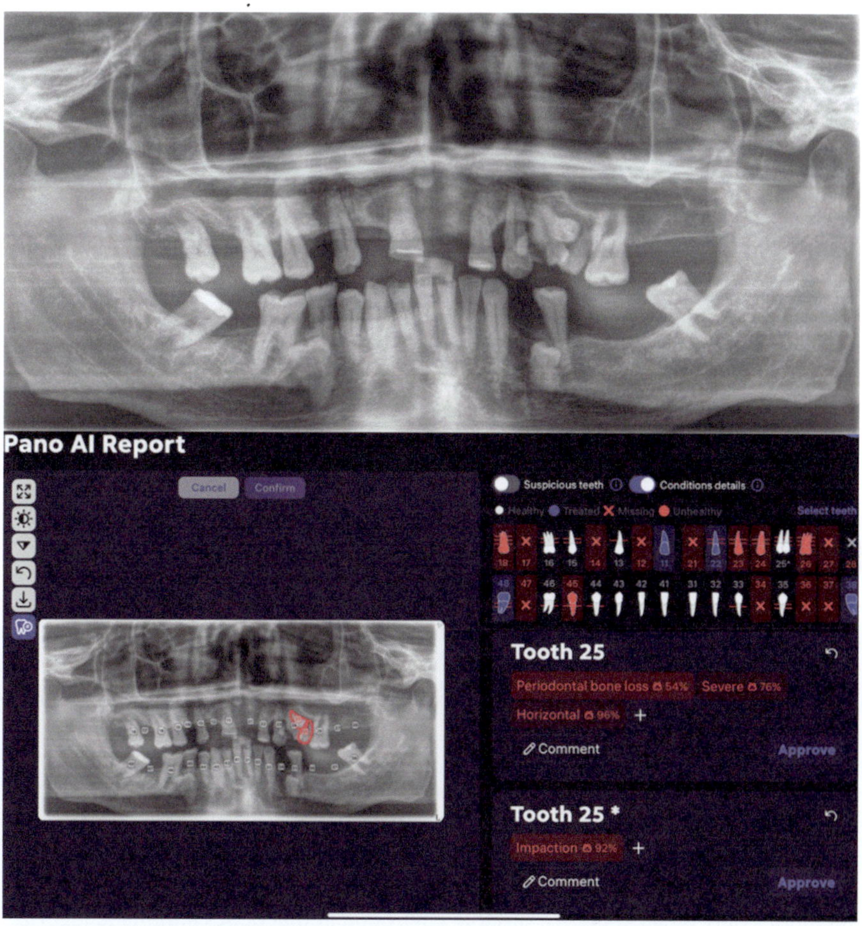

Fig. 1.5 Panoramic radiographic analysis with the Diagnocat software. Note that the impacted supernumerary tooth was outlined, identified, and named as tooth 25*

heuristics that several identification algorithms rely upon [12]. The loss of teeth due to disease or trauma also creates gaps and disrupts the regular adjacent arrangement, removing key reference points for identification algorithms. Finally, common issues such as caries, embedded or impacted teeth, and misshapen teeth can fundamentally alter the morphological features that automated systems use to classify and identify specific teeth.

Furthermore, iatrogenic factors (i.e., conditions caused by dental interventions) introduce artificial structures that can confound automated interpretation systems. The presence of dental restorations, prosthetic devices, and orthodontic appliances adds a layer of complexity by introducing material shapes not found in clinical and radiographic examinations of the natural dentition. In this context, an algorithm trained to recognize the radiographic density (i.e., pixel values) and morphology of natural enamel and dentin may fail to correctly interpret a tooth that has been significantly altered by a crown, bridge, or orthodontic bracket.

Another common additional limitation that emerges from past studies on AI methods is small datasets for training and constrained settings, where actual complexities commonly found in the clinical routine were scarce or absent [11, 13–15]. Furthermore, these approaches have mostly focused on specific tasks related to teeth identification, rather than providing a comprehensive solution.

The work of Lin and collaborators exemplifies a region-specific approach [13]. Their system employed local thresholding, contour extraction, and a support vector machine to segment and number teeth on bitewing radiographs. While proof of concept was valid, its practical utility was constrained as the method was limited to molar and premolar sites, rendering it incapable of analyzing a full dentition. Moreover, the method performance may be affected by inadequate image quality and teeth morphology alterations, which is a challenge for common clinical situations with anatomical variations or imaging artifacts.

In another study, the inability to account for tooth loss was the primary weakness of the shape template-based system proposed [14]. This system used a template--fitting technique on panoramic radiographs to match predefined shapes of permanent teeth to the main radiographic image. However, the results were unstable on radiographs with missing teeth. This fragility demonstrates the limitations of rigid, template-based models in a variable biological system.

To address this challenge with 3D imaging, a study by Cui and collaborators developed a sophisticated method combining an edge-enhancing algorithm with a 3D region proposal network to be used with CBCT images [15]. This system achieved satisfactory results in cases with common teeth configurations, which represents progress in the field. Nevertheless, cases with complex and uncommon teeth distribution showed worsen results. This suggests that even advanced techniques may struggle to overcome the fundamental challenges posed by the dental variations seen routinely in dental clinics. The combination of dynamic dentition stages, frequent disruption from anatomical anomalies, and the introduction of iatrogenic alterations may create a highly variable environment that defies simplistic algorithmic solutions. As the documented failures of previous academic studies underscore, systems developed in constrained settings using idealized datasets are also not viable for widespread clinical or forensic use, in which patient safety and accurate human identification are very important priorities.

Based on the studies mentioned above, there is a need for further developments of automated dental identification systems. It is suggested that the next generation of AI technology should be architected for resilience, designed not on idealized models but on principles of anatomical variability, and trained on datasets that include the complexities inherent to human dentition.

On the other hand, recent studies have shown promising results with robust AI models. Xu et al. developed a two-stage deep learning framework for this task on panoramic radiographs. Their AI algorithm first uses a U-Net architecture model to extract the region of interest (ROI) containing the entire alveolar ridge. Then another model named Hybrid Task Cascade (HTC) is used for the final segmentation and tooth numbering. This algorithm was trained on a large, heterogeneous dataset of over 6000 images covering primary, mixed, and permanent dentitions and achieved outstanding performance, with precision and recall exceeding 97% for both segmentation and numbering and a mean intersection-over-union (mIoU) of 92.5%. Another study focusing specifically on the challenging mixed dentition stage utilized the YOLOv8 architecture on periapical radiographs to perform tooth numbering, reporting a high accuracy of 89% [16].

A major challenge in developing such models is the need for large and meticulously annotated datasets. To address this issue, another research group introduced a self-supervised learning framework based on the DINOv2 Vision Transformer. This approach first pretrained the model on 74,292 unlabeled periapical radiographs, allowing it to learn the intrinsic features of dental anatomy without human guidance. The model was then fine-tuned on only 229 labeled images. Despite the limited labeled data, this framework achieved highly accurate segmentation of teeth, pulp chambers, restorations, caries, and periapical lesions, significantly outperforming fully supervised models such as the U-Net. This finding demonstrates the transformative potential of self-supervised learning to reduce the reliance on time-consuming expert annotation, which is a primary challenge in the development of medical AI [17].

1.2.2 Dental Prosthesis and Restoration Detection

Identifying existing restorations and prostheses is essential for clinical assessment and automated reporting (Fig. 1.6). A research study developed a faster R-CNN model to detect seven different types of dental restorations on panoramic radiographs [18]. The model demonstrated strong performance and high precision across most categories included (appliance, bridge, endodontic filling, crown filling, implant, single crown, and retainer).

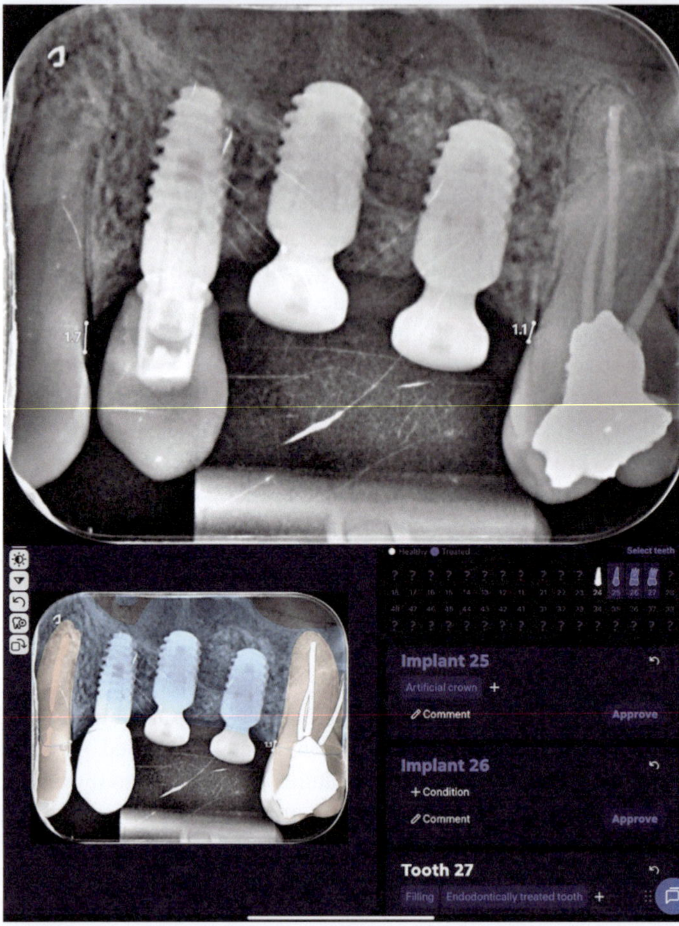

Fig. 1.6 Screenshot of the Diagnocat software. Note the correct identification of implants, prosthetic crown, restoration, and endodontic treatment

1.2.3 Inferior Alveolar Nerve (IAN) and Mandibular Canal Analysis

Evaluating the proximity of the mandibular third molar to the inferior alveolar nerve (IAN) is critical for predicting the risk of nerve injury during extraction. Although nerves are not visible on radiographs, several software tools to locate the mandibular canal are called terms such as "nerve mapping." A scoping review found that AI, particularly CNN-based models, plays a crucial role in automating this assessment [19]. The U-Net architecture has been widely employed for the segmentation of the mandibular canal on both panoramic radiographs and cone-beam computed tomography (CBCT) images. These models have demonstrated high segmentation accuracy, achieving Dice coefficients ranging from 0.80 to 0.94, providing clinicians with a reliable tool for preoperative risk assessment.

Considering the importance of respecting the mandibular canal and mental foramen limits, most of the implant planning software programs have incorporated an AI tool for automated identification and segmentation of the mandibular canal (Figs. 1.7 and 1.8). AI-driven software programs dedicated to diagnosis and treatment planning also identify and outline these anatomical structures. Of note, the Diagnocat software is able to include such segmentation as part of the "3D model" tool (Fig. 1.9), which will be discussed further in Chaps. 6 and 7. One challenge for the segmentation, however, may be the presence of anatomical variations, such as a bifurcated mandibular canal, which should be diagnosed appropriately by an oral radiologist using a robust DICOM viewer software (Fig. 1.10).

1.2.4 Root Canal Morphology

One of the AI applications useful in the field of endodontics is the automated root canal morphology. A comprehensive literature review outlined several related functions of AI models that have been successfully applied [20]. Among the most important ones are general analyses of root and canal morphology, detection of specific anatomical variations such as C-shaped root canals, segmentation of the pulp cavity, endodontic treatments, and detection of periapical lesions. The latter will be further discussed in Chap. 3.

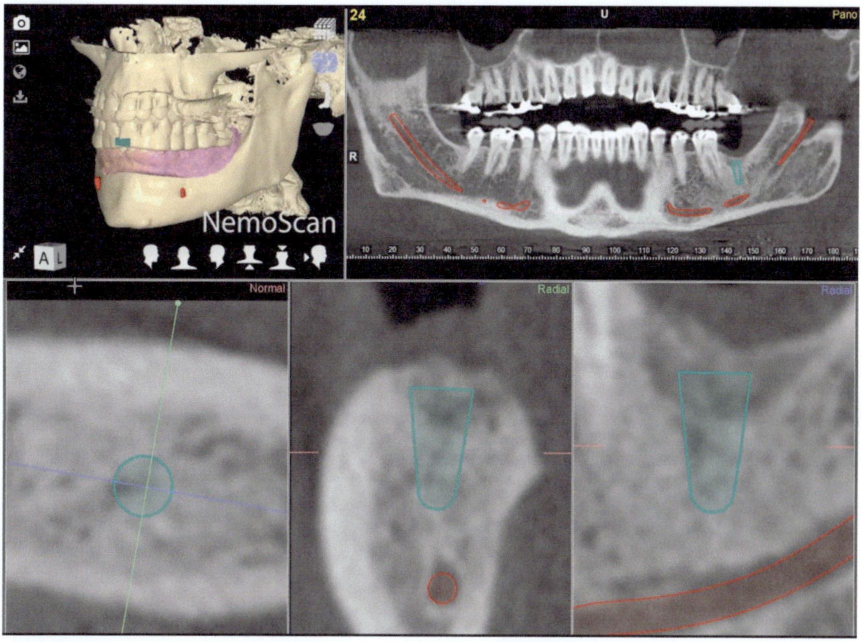

Fig. 1.7 Screenshot of the Nemoscan software (Nemotec). Note the automated identification and outline of both mandibular canals and mental foramens in red color

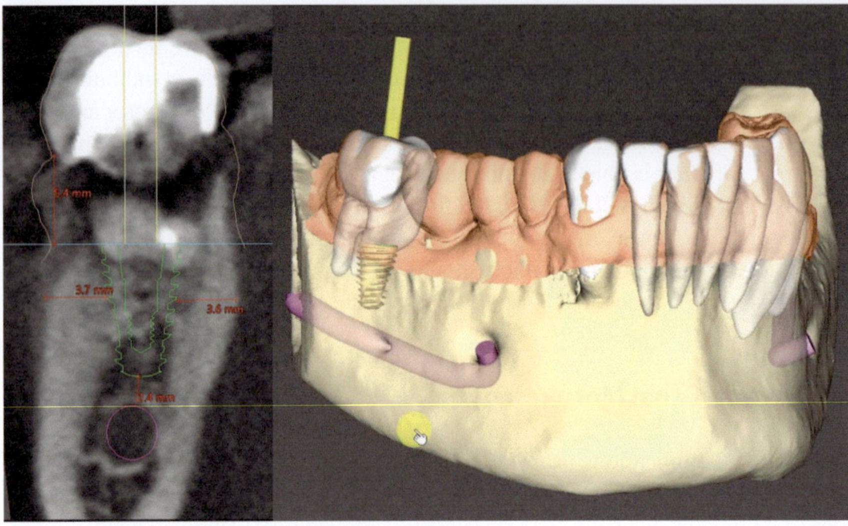

Fig. 1.8 Automated identification and outline of the mandibular canal and mental foramen (pink color) with the coDiagnostiX software for virtual implant planning

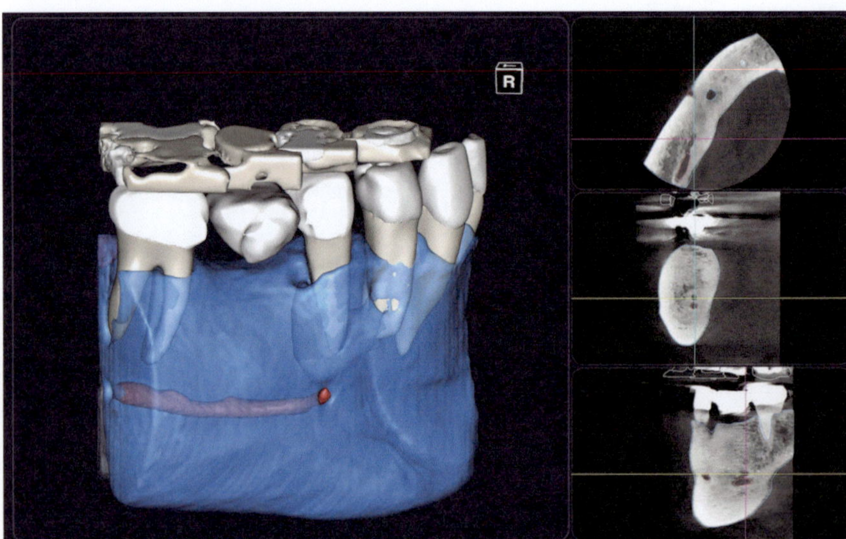

Fig. 1.9 Automated identification and outline of the right mandibular canal and mental foramen (red color) with the Diagnocat software. Note the bifurcation of the mandibular canal on the 2D planes, which was not included in the segmentation

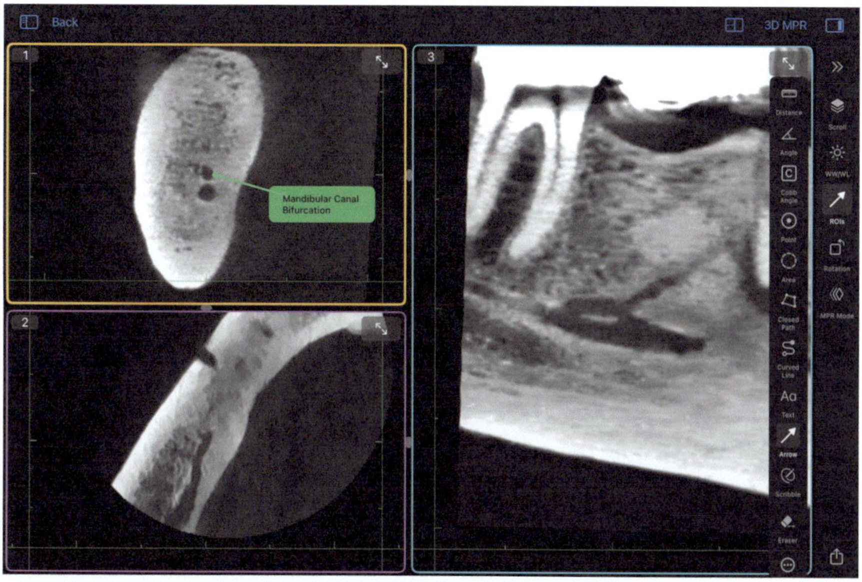

Fig. 1.10 Analysis of the CBCT scan of Fig. 1.9 with a DICOM viewer (Falcon MD, iCAT Solutions Ltd.), showing the bifurcation of the mandibular canal

Another previous study presented a deep learning model developed to detect on CBCT scans and segment automatically unobturated fourth canals (i.e., mesial buccal 2) in maxillary molars that had undergone endodontic treatment [21]. A total of 58 CBCT were used, achieving an accuracy of 0.90. Despite the satisfactory diagnostic performance, the authors of this study also reported that the segmentation was considerably affected by artifacts on the images.

The number of roots and number of canals can usually be identified and recorded by several commercial AI-driven dental software programs. However, it is important to assess the ability of the software to outline the correct shapes of treated and untreated root canals (Fig. 1.11). This task is easier when the CBCT used has high resolution (e.g., small voxel size and field-of-view) and with software programs that perform full assessments on 3D images, such as the Diagnocat, which can also detect anatomical variations such as supernumerary roots of anterior teeth (Fig. 1.12).

1.2.5 Analysis of the Airways and Other Relevant Structures

AI is also being used for three-dimensional analysis of adjacent anatomical structures, such as the oral and nasopharyngeal airways. A study utilized AI-powered software (Nemofab, Nemotec) for the automatic segmentation and volumetric analysis of the upper airways from CT scans of patients without dentofacial deformities [22]. The analysis revealed significant correlations between airway volume and the

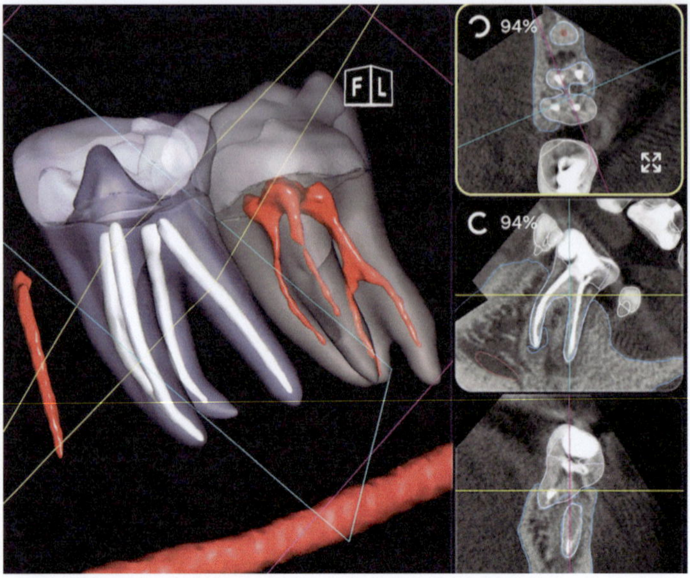

Fig. 1.11 Automated CBCT segmentation of treated (tooth 36) and untreated root canals (tooth 37), as well as the mandibular canal (red color) with the Diagnocat software

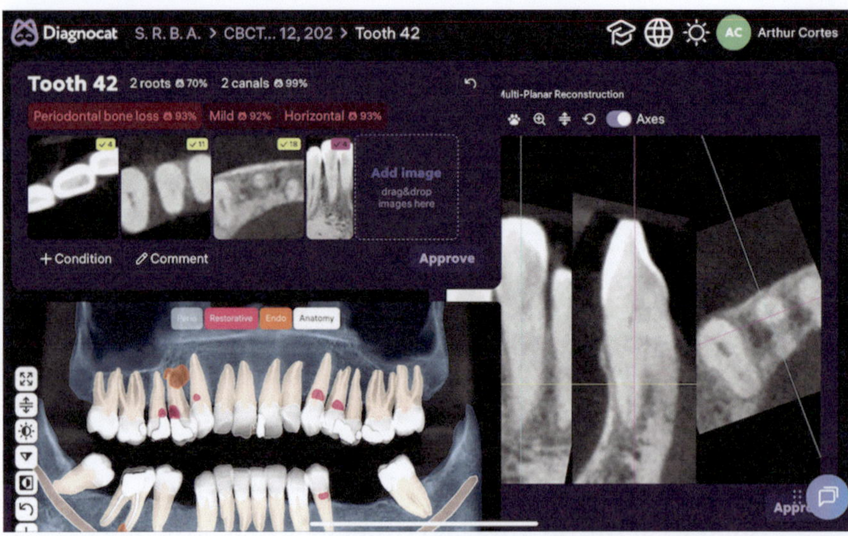

Fig. 1.12 CBCT analysis of tooth 42 with the Diagnocat software. Note that the software correctly detected the presence of two roots and two root canals despite the classification as a mandibular lateral incisor

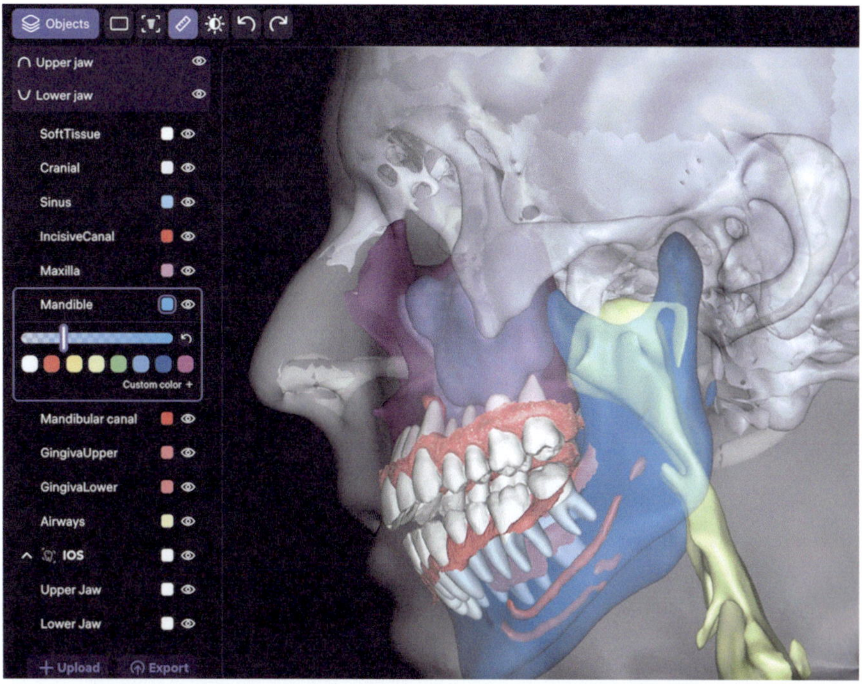

Fig. 1.13 Automated segmentation of the oropharyngeal and nasopharyngeal airways (yellow color), maxilla (purple), and mandible (blue) with the Diagnocat software

following demographic and anatomical factors: younger individuals, particularly males, tended to have greater airway volumes; a neck circumference below 40 cm was associated with a 28.04% reduction in airway volume; and a low minimum axial area (<110 mm^2) was correlated with a significant decrease in the total airway volume.

The Diagnocat software was also tested by a study and confirmed accurate to perform volumetric airway measurements, as compared with qualified human dental professionals [23]. Due to the presence of scientific evidence, this was one of the main software programs chosen to assess and illustrate the clinical case analyses of this book (Fig. 1.13). Figure 1.14 shows a similar AI-powered segmentation tool of the Nemoscan software (Nemotec).

To perform these analyses, one needs to upload the original DICOM files from a CBCT scan to import into the Diagnocat AI system, which is built upon a deep convolutional neural network. This system operates by means of a sophisticated pipeline of pretrained fully convolutional networks. These networks, based on a 3D U-Net architecture, perform what is described as "voxel-perfect segmentations" of important structures such as teeth, jaws, nasopalatine and mandibular canals, and the maxillary sinuses (Figs. 1.15 and 1.16) [24]. This detailed segmentation also

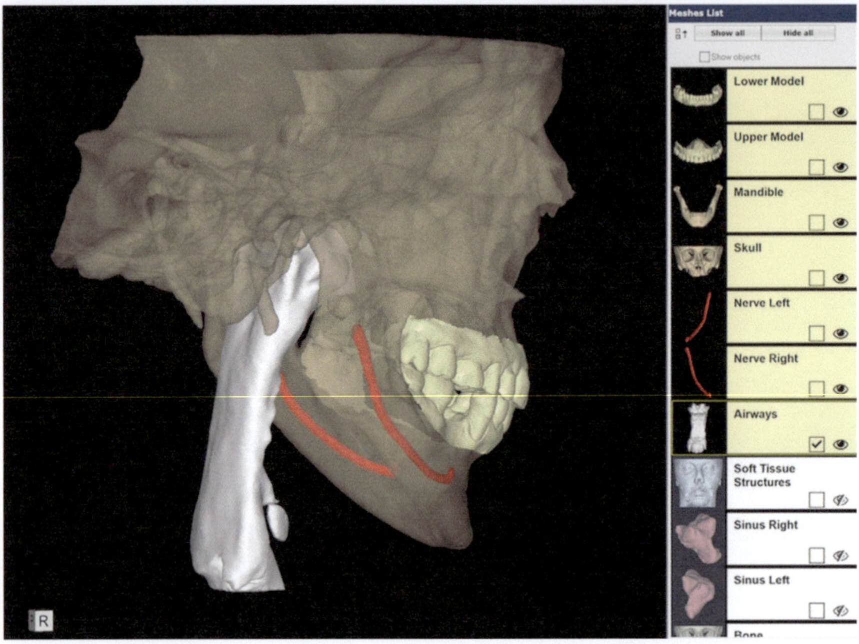

Fig. 1.14 Automated segmentation of the airways (white) with the Nemoscan software

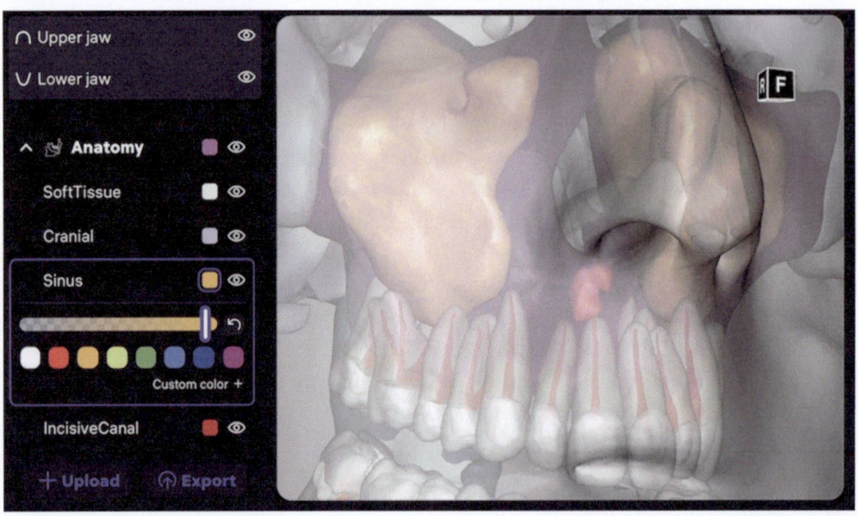

Fig. 1.15 Automated segmentation of the maxillary sinuses (orange), nasopalatine canal (red), and soft tissue contours such as the nose with the Diagnocat software. Note that each tooth mesh from the CBCT was made transparent to assess the morphology of the root canals

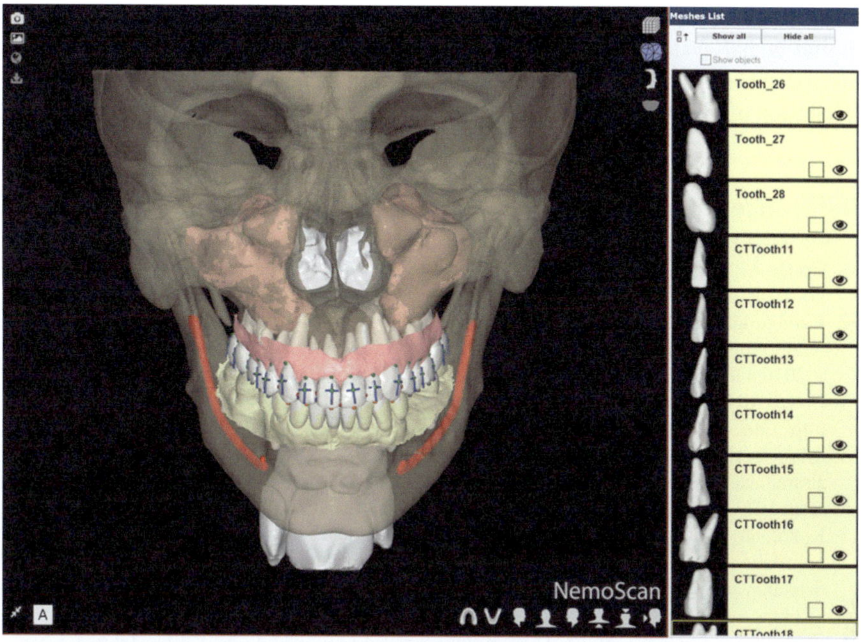

Fig. 1.16 Automated segmentation of the maxillary sinuses (red) and teeth from CBCT and intraoral scans to form the virtual patient on the Nemoscan software

allows the system to identify missing tooth locations and subsequently generate an automated implant planning report, complete with bone measurements for potential implant size and placement, as further discussed in Chaps. 7 and 9.

1.3 Conclusion

This review of recent literature suggests that AI deep learning architectures such as CNNs, U-Net, and Transformers possess significant potential across a diverse spectrum of applications in dental radiographic analysis. Studies on AI models are consistently achieving high levels of accuracy, from patient characterization including age and growth stage estimation to the granular segmentation of teeth, pathologies, and prosthetic devices. Therefore, these tools have potential to enhance diagnostic precision, improve workflow efficiency, and provide objective, quantitative data to support clinical decision-making by the dental professional responsible for the treatment.

Nonetheless, it has also been noted that the potential of the integration of AI in digital dental systems can only be fully explored after addressing the limitations discussed herein and in Chap. 5 to ensure ethical standards along with adequate collaboration between AI software developers and dental clinicians.

References

1. Cortes ARG. Artificial intelligence in planning oral rehabilitations: current status. Appl Sci. 2024;14:4093. https://doi.org/10.3390/app14104093.
2. Kamburoğlu K, Kursun S. A comparison of the diagnostic accuracy of CBCT images of different voxel resolutions used to detect simulated small internal resorption cavities. Int Endod J. 2010;43(9):798–807. https://doi.org/10.1111/j.1365-2591.2010.01749.x.
3. Cortes ARG. Digital dentistry: a step-by-step guide and case atlas. Hoboken, NJ: Wiley; 2022. https://doi.org/10.1002/9781119852025.
4. Sributsayakarn N, Intharah T, Hirunchavarod N, Pornprasertsuk-Damrongsri S, Jiraratanasopha V. Automated age and sex estimation from dental panoramic radiographs. Int Dent J. 2025;75(6):103967. https://doi.org/10.1016/j.identj.2025.103967.
5. Kokomoto K, Kariya R, Muranaka A, Okawa R, Nakano K, Nozaki K. Automatic dental age calculation from panoramic radiographs using deep learning: a two-stage approach with object detection and image classification. BMC Oral Health. 2024;24(1):143. https://doi.org/10.1186/s12903-024-03928-0.
6. Zhang Y, Lu Z, Zhou J, Sun Y, Yi W, Wang J, Du T, Li D, Zhao X, Xu Y, Li C, Qi K. CDSNet: an automated method for assessing growth stages from various anatomical regions in lateral cephalograms based on deep learning. J World Fed Orthod. 2025;14(3):154–60. https://doi.org/10.1016/j.ejwf.2024.09.007.
7. Nogueira-Reis F, Cascante-Sequeira D, Farias-Gomes A, de Macedo MMG, Watanabe RN, Santiago AG, Tabchoury CPM, Freitas DQ. Determination of the pubertal growth spurt by artificial intelligence analysis of cervical vertebrae maturation in lateral cephalometric radiographs. Oral Surg Oral Med Oral Pathol Oral Radiol. 2024;138(2):306–15. https://doi.org/10.1016/j.oooo.2024.02.017.
8. Lee JS, Curley AW, Smith RA. Institute of Medicine. Prevention of wrong-site tooth extraction: clinical guidelines. J Oral Maxillofac Surg. 2007;65(9):1793–9. https://doi.org/10.1016/j.joms.2007.04.012.
9. Demirjian A, Goldstein H, Tanner JM. A new system of dental age assessment. Hum Biol. 1973;45(2):211–27.
10. Nomir O, Abdel-Mottaleb M. Human identification from dental X-ray images based on the shape and appearance of the teeth. IEEE Trans Inf Forensics Secur. 2007;2(2):188–97. https://doi.org/10.1109/TIFS.2007.897245.
11. Chen H, Zhang K, Lyu P, Li H, Zhang L, Wu J, Lee CH. A deep learning approach to automatic teeth detection and numbering based on object detection in dental periapical films. Sci Rep. 2019;9(1):3840. https://doi.org/10.1038/s41598-019-40414-y.
12. Laganà G, Venza N, Borzabadi-Farahani A, Fabi F, Danesi C, Cozza P. Dental anomalies: prevalence and associations between them in a large sample of non-orthodontic subjects, a cross-sectional study. BMC Oral Health. 2017;17(1):62. https://doi.org/10.1186/s12903-017-0352-y.
13. Lin PL, Lai YH, Huang PW. An effective classification and numbering system for dental bitewing radiographs using teeth region and contour information. Pattern Recognit. 2010;43:1380–92.
14. Wirtz A, Mirashi SG, Wesarg S. Automatic teeth segmentation in panoramic X-ray images using a coupled shape model in combination with a neural network. In: Frangi A, Schnabel J, Davatzikos C, Alberola-López C, Fichtinger G, editors. Medical image computing and computer assisted intervention—MICCAI 2018, Lecture notes in computer science, vol. 11073. Cham: Springer; 2018. https://doi.org/10.1007/978-3-030-00937-3_81.

15. Cui Z, Li C, Wang W. ToothNet: automatic tooth instance segmentation and identification from cone beam CT images. In: IEEE/CVF Conference on Computer Vision and Pattern Recognition (CVPR), Long Beach, CA, USA; 2019. p. 6361–70. https://doi.org/10.1109/CVPR.2019.00653.
16. Yücetürk B, Güner Z. Deep learning approach for tooth numbering and restoration detection on pediatric periapical radiographs in mixed dentition. Clin Oral Investig. 2025;29(11):495. https://doi.org/10.1007/s00784-025-06542-8.
17. Hu M, Zhang Q, Wei Z, Jia P, Yuan M, Yu H, Yin X, Peng J. Self-supervised learning enhances periapical films segmentation with limited labeled data. J Dent. 2025;163:106150. https://doi.org/10.1016/j.jdent.2025.106150.
18. Benvenuto M, Bologna M, Fortunati A, Perazzo C, Cellina M, Cè M, Rubiu G, Martini I, Sala D, Di Palma L, Fazzini D, Alba S, Papa S, Alì M. Detection of dental restorations and prosthesis devices in panoramic dental X-ray using fast region-based convolutional neural network. Dentomaxillofac Radiol. 2025;2025:twaf079. https://doi.org/10.1093/dmfr/twaf079.
19. Ahn S, Kim M, Kim J, Park W. Application of deep learning in evaluating the anatomical relationship between the mandibular third molar and inferior alveolar nerve: a scoping review. Med Oral Patol Oral Cir Bucal. 2025;2025:27584. https://doi.org/10.4317/medoral.27584.
20. Mohammad-Rahimi H, Sohrabniya F, Ourang SA, Dianat O, Aminoshariae A, Nagendrababu V, Dummer PMH, Duncan HF, Nosrat A. Artificial intelligence in endodontics: data preparation, clinical applications, ethical considerations, limitations, and future directions. Int Endod J. 2024;57(11):1566–95. https://doi.org/10.1111/iej.14128.
21. Albitar L, Zhao T, Huang C, Mahdian M. Artificial intelligence (AI) for detection and localization of unobturated second mesial buccal (MB2) canals in cone-beam computed tomography (CBCT). Diagnostics. 2022;12(12):3214. https://doi.org/10.3390/diagnostics12123214.
22. Costa SM, Ribeiro BC, Bertelli Trivellato PF, Sverzut CE, Trivellato AE. Tridimensional analysis of the normal upper airways in non-dentofacial deformity patients. Morphologie. 2025;110(368):101078. https://doi.org/10.1016/j.morpho.2025.101078.
23. Dorris S, Anamali S, Castro JP, Dabdoub SM, Allareddy T. Comparisons of the reliability of airway measurements on cone beam computed tomography scans among human raters and a convolutional neural network. Oral Surg Oral Med Oral Pathol Oral Radiol. 2025; https://doi.org/10.1016/j.oooo.2025.10.001.
24. Kurt Bayrakdar S, Orhan K, Bayrakdar IS, Bilgir E, Ezhov M, Gusarev M, Shumilov E. A deep learning approach for dental implant planning in cone-beam computed tomography images. BMC Med Imaging. 2021;21(1):86. https://doi.org/10.1186/s12880-021-00618-z.

2 Automated Detection of Caries and Tooth Wear

Ana Paula Ayres, Adam Bartolo, Laura Godoy Ruíz, Guillermo Pradies, and Arthur Rodriguez Gonzalez Cortes

Dental caries remains a significant global and dental public health issue. Its early accurate detection is critical for enabling minimally invasive and cost-effective treatments. In this context, a previous systematic review found that experts were not able to detect a large amount of initial caries in dental radiographs [1]. Artificial intelligence (AI) tools have presented potential to meet this need, enhancing the diagnostic capabilities of clinicians and supporting the implementation of preventive care [2, 3]. Considering that AI technology is developing very fast in dentistry, the literature review of this chapter will focus on the most recent and high-impact studies, as well as on novel AI algorithms and software programs.

The choice of imaging method plays an important role in caries diagnosis. Bitewing radiographs are still considered the primary and most reliable method for routine diagnosis of interproximal caries, followed by periapical radiographs, as these offer an adequate balance of image quality, low radiation dose, and diagnostic accuracy. On the other hand, digital panoramic radiographs with modern devices are considered a suitable alternative for specific patient management challenges or when a panoramic survey is indicated for other clinical reasons. The use of modern extraoral bitewing modes is recommended to maximize diagnostic yield. Finally, 3D CBCT is not usually indicated for primary caries detection due to radiation dose

A. P. Ayres
University of São Paulo, São Paulo, Brazil

A. Bartolo · A. R. G. Cortes (✉)
Faculty of Dental Surgery, University of Malta, Msida, Malta
e-mail: adam.bartolo@um.edu.mt; arthur.nogueira@um.edu.mt

L. Godoy Ruíz · G. Pradies
Complutense University of Madrid, Madrid, Spain
e-mail: Gjpradie@ucm.es

A. R. G. Cortes (ed.), *Dental Clinical Procedures using Artificial Intelligence*,
https://doi.org/10.1007/978-3-032-24895-4_2

and cost considerations. However, the multiplanar reconstructions available on CBCT scans present a significant advantage in assessing surface cavitation without superimpositions, when a scan is available from an examination performed for other clinical indications. For these reasons, the AI-driven caries analyses of this chapter are basically illustrated by cases using routine 2D dental radiographs.

The role of digital workflows in preventive dentistry has been described in the literature, with the development of several tools such as the caries detection software tools of intraoral scanners and the respective fluorescence analysis [2]. Furthermore, numerous studies highlight the potential of AI in analyzing dental images to identify carious lesions, particularly non-cavitated and interproximal lesions that can be challenging for clinicians to diagnose in their early stages [3, 4]. This enhanced accuracy not only supports dentists in making precise diagnoses but also facilitates timely and noninvasive treatments.

These radiographic assessments can be performed by dentists using commercial dental AI-driven software programs that can be integrated with the radiographic imaging systems of the dental clinic. The Diagnocat (iCAT Solutions Ltd.) is a representative example of AI software program capable of performing caries assessments in both 2D and 3D dental radiographic modalities (Fig. 2.1). The steps to perform an adequate radiographic assessment using the tools of this software are explained below and further discussed in Chap. 6.

After selecting the imaging report category and uploading the respective original imaging files (e.g., JPG files for 2D radiographs and DICOM files for 3D CBCT scans), a detailed automated diagnostic report is made by the software (Fig. 2.2).

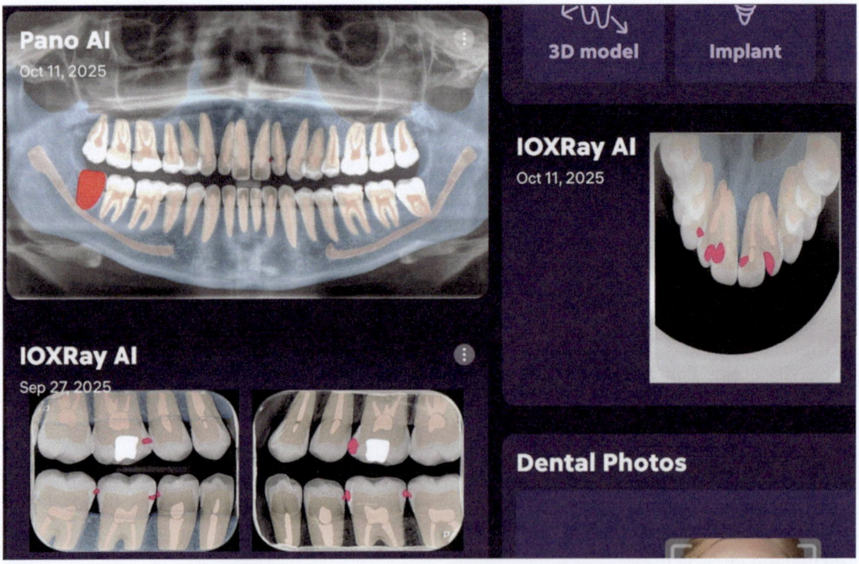

Fig. 2.1 Imaging reports of different categories created for the same patient with the Diagnocat software. Clicking on each image will open the respective detailed AI-driven diagnostic report

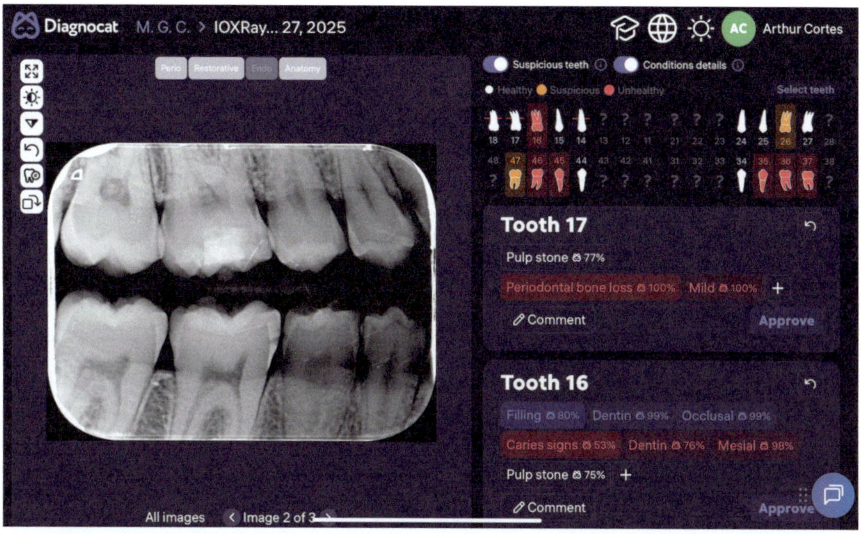

Fig. 2.2 Detailed imaging report of a bitewing radiography of a patient of Fig. 2.1. The diagnosis of each tooth can receive comments and be approved by the dental professional before finalizing the radiographic report document. Note that caries signs were detected for tooth 16, with an AI confidence percentage of 53%

Each present and missing tooth can then be selected by clicking on its number on the tooth chart. Any alterations of the selected teeth will show on the list of teeth analyzed, available in the report. Each tooth is classified into healthy (gray), suspicious (yellow), or unhealthy (red) category. Filters showing the alterations detected on the image, as well as tools to expand (Fig. 2.3), invert, edit tooth numbers, and control sharpness, brightness, and contrast, are available in the software interface.

2.1 Current Scientific Status of AI to Detect Caries

A meta-analysis in 2025 provided important quantitative performance metrics for AI in caries detection [3]. The analysis reported a mean sensitivity of 76% and a mean specificity of 91%. The area under the curve (AUC), a measure of overall diagnostic accuracy, was an impressive 92%. However, these figures are accompanied by a critical caveat: the same review found significant variability in performance across different studies and AI platforms, with reported accuracy ranging from as low as 41.5% to as high as 98.6%.

In this context, it is important to understand the performance of AI systems in comparison with human clinicians regarding specific and challenging tasks. A recent study performed in 1400 bitewing radiographs used a CNN algorithm (ResNet-152) to classify caries in primary dentition [4]. The accuracy results of this algorithm were comparable to the ones from leading human participants.

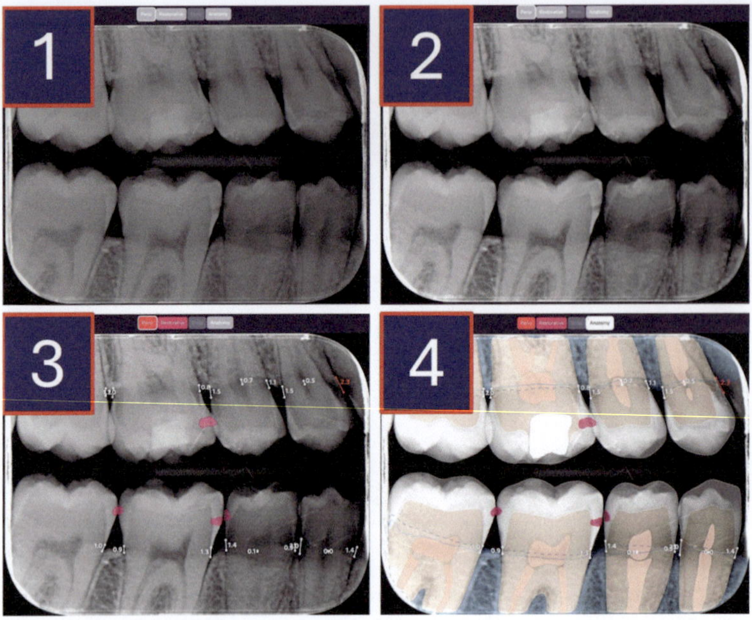

Fig. 2.3 Expanded images with different filters used in order as different steps of the assessment. (1) Original expanded bitewing radiography. (2) The same image after brightness and contrast optimization. (3) Filters of periodontal and restorative alterations activated. Areas with interproximal caries are marked in pink color. (4) Filter of anatomical segmentation activated on top of the others

Such finding suggests that CNN could serve as an alternative in caries classification, which could lead to improved restorative treatment planning.

On the other hand, a previous study compared the performance of an AI application with that of dental interns in assessing interproximal surfaces on bitewing and panoramic radiographs [5]. They found that for detecting secondary caries on bitewing radiographs, the AI performed significantly worse than the interns ($p < 0.05$). In contrast, the AI's accuracy was comparable to that of the interns for determining caries depth. The study also confirmed the statistically superior diagnostic value of bitewings as compared with panoramic radiographs for specific tasks such as caries detection ($p < 0.001$).

Furthermore, previous research findings indicate that AI sensitivity in caries detection may be lower for interproximal and buccal caries as compared to other types [6, 7]. One of the aforementioned studies also found that AI diagnostic results may also be affected by the tooth position [6]. This underscores the need for continuous algorithm refinement, the removal of dataset biases, and the implementation of techniques to prevent overfitting, where a model performs well on training data but fails to generalize to new, unseen cases.

2.2 Influence of Imaging Modalities

An analysis of the 45 reviewed studies reveals a primary reliance on two distinct imaging modalities for training and testing AI models [3]. Dental radiographs were the predominant data source, used in 33 of the 45 studies, obtaining a general mean accuracy of 78.2%. The main radiographic modalities used are bitewing, periapical and panoramic radiographs, as well as CBCT images. Clinical images, in turn, were utilized in the remaining 12 studies, obtaining a general mean accuracy of 81.5%. The datasets were composed of photographs compiled from various sources, including digital single lens reflex (DSLR) cameras, mobile phones, and intraoral cameras.

The choice of imaging modality appears to influence diagnostic performance of AI systems in caries diagnosis [3]. A subgroup analysis conducted by the aforementioned study found that AI demonstrates superior sensitivity and equal specificity when detecting caries from clinical images compared to traditional bitewing radiography. This finding highlights the versatility of AI in leveraging diverse imaging techniques to enhance diagnostic precision.

This performance variability ranging from 41.5% to 98.6% is a direct consequence of the systemic data and methodological challenges that are common in the field of AI in dentistry. For this reason, a deeper examination of the limitations that currently affect the consistency and reliability of these methods in real-world clinical settings is still needed.

A different study using clinical intraoral photographs achieved accuracy values higher than 90% for the general detection of caries lesion in single teeth photographs available as JPG files [8]. On the other hand, a second assessment specifically performed among the different caries classifications found worsen results for cavitated lesions, as compared with non-cavitated lesions and caries-free surfaces. It is also suggested that the diagnostic performance of this method could be affected by the quality and resolution of the photography. In this context, the radiographic images taken with optimized parameters could lead to superior diagnostic performance of commercial dental AI-driven software programs (Fig. 2.4).

It is important that the AI software is able to describe the surfaces involved in order to differentiate between occlusal caries leading to class I restorations, or those involving interproximal surfaces, leading to class II (Fig. 2.5), III, and IV restorations. Indication of pulp chamber exposure (Fig. 2.6) and root caries (Fig. 2.7) as well as classification of recurrent caries and cervical lesions are equally essential to be highlighted by the software for an appropriate AI-driven imaging diagnosis, which will be used as part of a comprehensive radiographic interpretation and as a tool for the definition of the restorative treatment plan by the dental professional.

The opinion of the AI software on the quality of the existing restorations (Fig. 2.8) can also be checked using the software, as alterations such as interproximal overhangs (Fig. 2.9) and voids in the restored area can be detected and highlighted in different colors on the AI-driven radiographic report.

With the advent of these features participating in the decision-making process of the professional treatment plan, the dental professional should upload to the system any future radiographic and dental images taken after the restorative treatment is

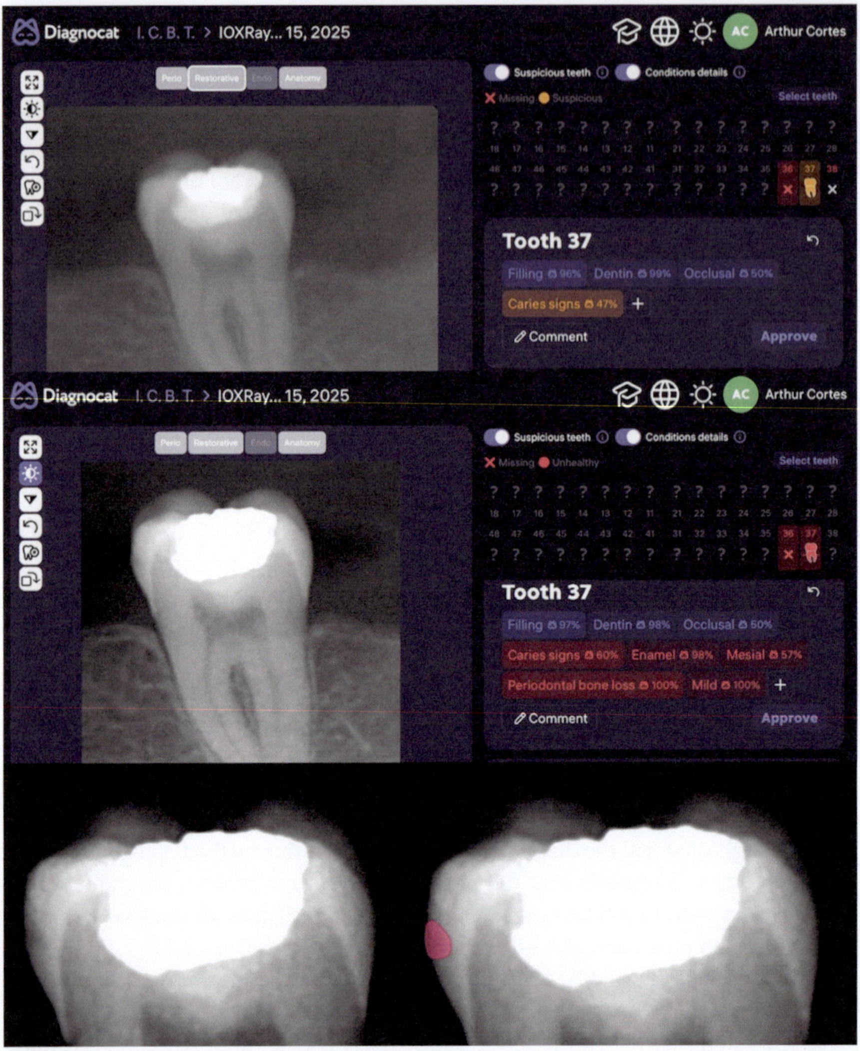

Fig. 2.4 Automated reports of two different radiographic images of the same tooth. The first image has inferior quality and resolution (top), resulting in misdiagnosis of an initial interproximal caries, classifying the tooth as suspicious. After retaking the radiography (middle), the tooth was considered unhealthy. The area with caries on enamel was depicted by the software with satisfactory precision (bottom)

performed. This enables an adequate and organized AI-driven imaging follow-up of the dental treatment (Fig. 2.10), in which the opinions of the AI software from different time points in the treatment can be now compared to orient further professional decisions.

The literature also highlights several successful applications of other methods. Optical coherence tomography (OCT) is a diagnostic imaging method that uses

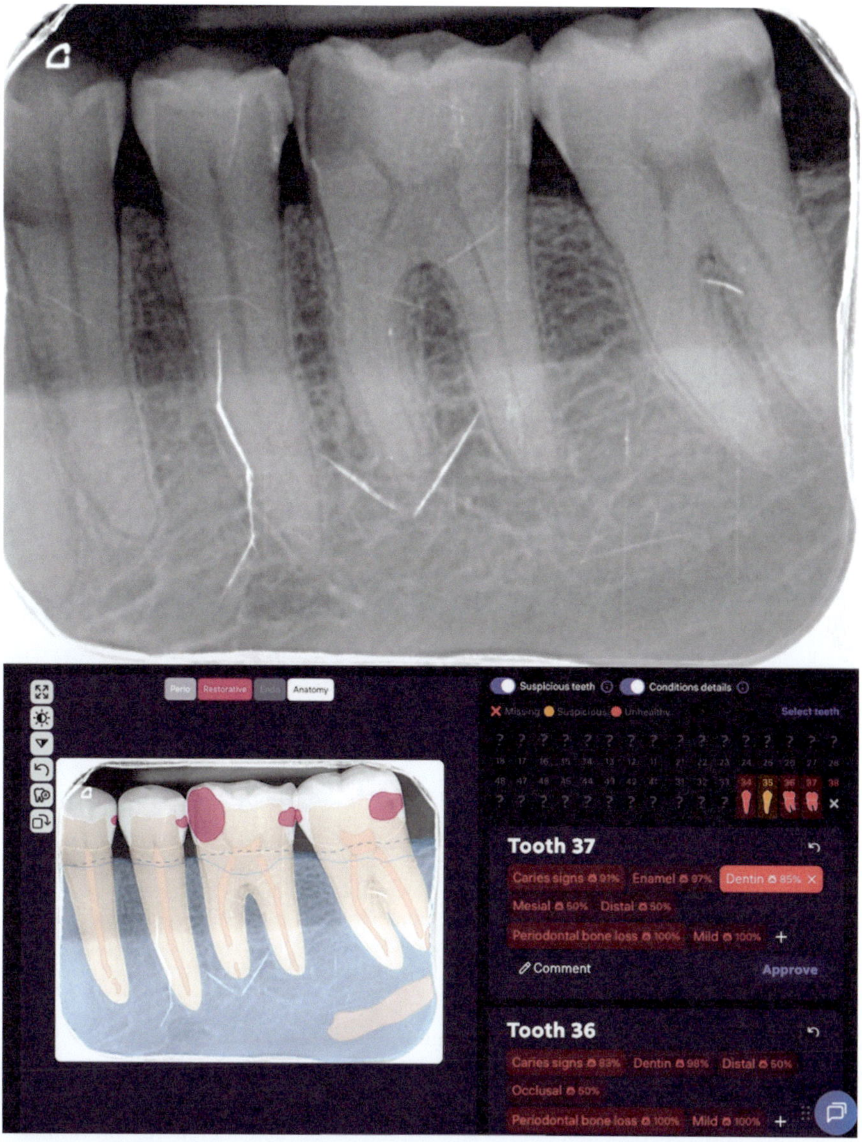

Fig. 2.5 Automated detection of interproximal caries with the Diagnocat software

infrared light waves to obtain cross-sectional images of the teeth structure. In a previous study, OCT was used with a CNN-based model that achieved 95.21% accuracy in detecting caries from OCT images [9], underscoring the potential of this noninvasive modality when paired with advanced AI. Furthermore, as previously mentioned, digital dental radiographic images, including bitewing [10, 11] and panoramic radiographs [12], have consistently served as effective inputs for AI, with

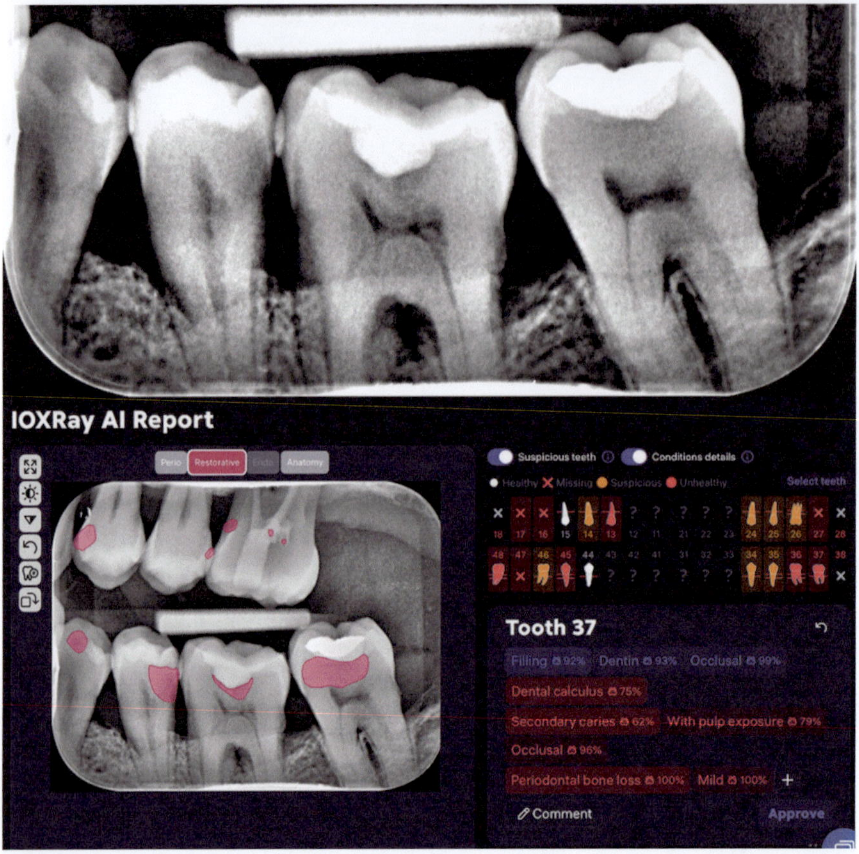

Fig. 2.6 Automated detection of recurrent (secondary) caries with the Diagnocat software. Note that the software reports tooth 37 with pulp exposure by caries with 79% of AI confidence. The dental professional should use these findings carefully as part of a comprehensive radiographic interpretation and always correlate with clinical data and patient's symptoms

models frequently achieving accuracy higher than 90% in detecting carious lesions. Finally, smartphone photographs were also used to detect occlusal caries [13], achieving a notable accuracy of up to 92.37%. This demonstrates the potential for accessible and low-cost imaging technologies to be considered for preliminary screening and teledentistry.

Finally, automated caries detection can also be performed with the AI tools of some of the modern intraoral scanners, such as the TRIOS 6 (3Shape A/S), which uses a combination of advanced hyperspectral imaging and AI algorithms within its accompanying software (TRIOS Dx Plus) to detect loss of mineralization in enamel and dentin. For this purpose, this intraoral scanner captures data using three different light sources simultaneously during a single scan. These include white light for capturing the true geometry and natural color of the teeth. Fluorescence detection is also performed using a blue/UV light source to help identify areas of

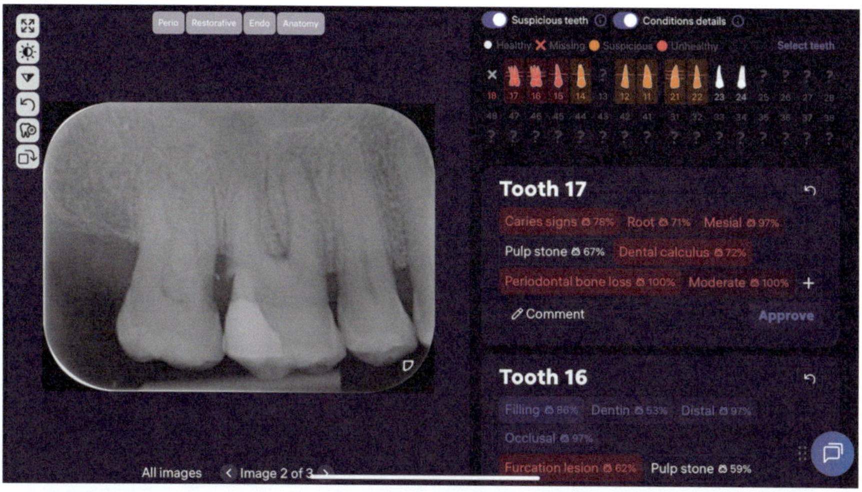

Fig. 2.7 Automated detection of root caries on the mesial surface of tooth 17, with the Diagnocat software. Note that the software also detected the presence of pulp stone with an AI confidence of 67%

demineralization, as carious tissue exhibits different fluorescence properties than healthy tissue. Near-infrared imaging is also used for enhanced visualization, particularly of interproximal surfaces. Nevertheless, this AI tool is to be used as an assistive diagnostic aid for caries (Fig. 2.11) and tooth wear (Fig. 2.12) but does not replace the professional judgment of the clinician responsible for the treatment and the traditional diagnostic methods such as the clinical examination following the ICDAS classification (still considered a gold standard method for occlusal caries) and bitewing radiographs (still considered a gold standard method for interproximal caries).

A final report with the diagnostic outcome for caries and tooth wear can be exported to be recorded and presented to the patient and assessed by the dental team involved in the respective treatment (Fig. 2.13).

2.3 Influence of Training Dataset Size and Quality

A clear trend identified across multiple studies is the positive correlation between the size of the training dataset and the resulting accuracy of the AI model. For instance, the study by Kühnisch and collaborators utilized a substantial dataset of 2417 images to train a CNN, achieving a high accuracy of 92.50% [8]. Larger datasets allow deep learning models to learn a more comprehensive range of features and variations, leading to more robust and generalizable performance. However, this dependency on extensive and diverse datasets presents a significant challenge in the dental context. The acquisition of such data is often hampered by critical barriers, including the need to ensure data privacy and security, as well as the need for

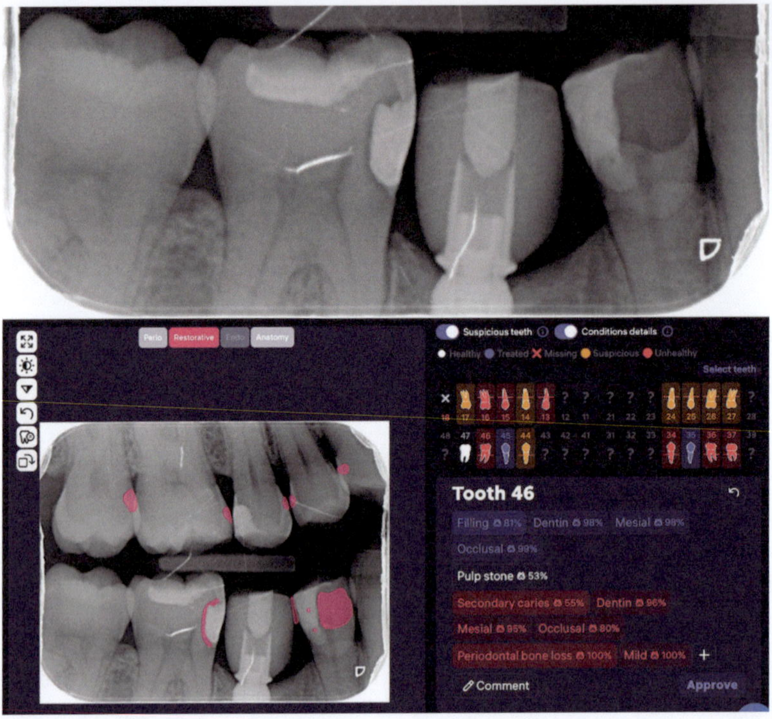

Fig. 2.8 The software detected the presence of secondary caries on the mesial surface of tooth 46 with an AI confidence of 55% with the Diagnocat software. However, a regular radiolucent contour underneath a restoration could be due to the bond or lining material thickness. Note also that the AI software detected a lack of interproximal contact between teeth 44 and 45. For this reason, bitewing radiographs should be taken with the horizontal angle as parallel as possible to the interproximal surfaces of the teeth

ethical transparency and interpretability in AI decision-making processes [14]. To compensate for limited dataset sizes, the majority of the diagnostic studies on AI to detect caries employed preprocessing augmentation. This is a method to artificially increase the size of the training dataset by creating modified copies of existing images, a common practice that does not replace the need for diverse, real-world data. The use of poorly annotated, nondiverse, or biased datasets can lead to suboptimal model performance, potentially introducing inaccuracies when applied in real-world clinical scenarios.

One of the studies with the largest sample size was conducted on 1349 panoramic radiographs, to analyze the AI system CariesNet in a total of 3217 caries lesions, distributed among shallow, medium, and deep categories [15]. The authors found an accuracy value of 0.94 for caries detection considering a control group composed of four experienced dentists. The authors have also confirmed the role of CariesNet in the segmentation of caries regardless of their classification.

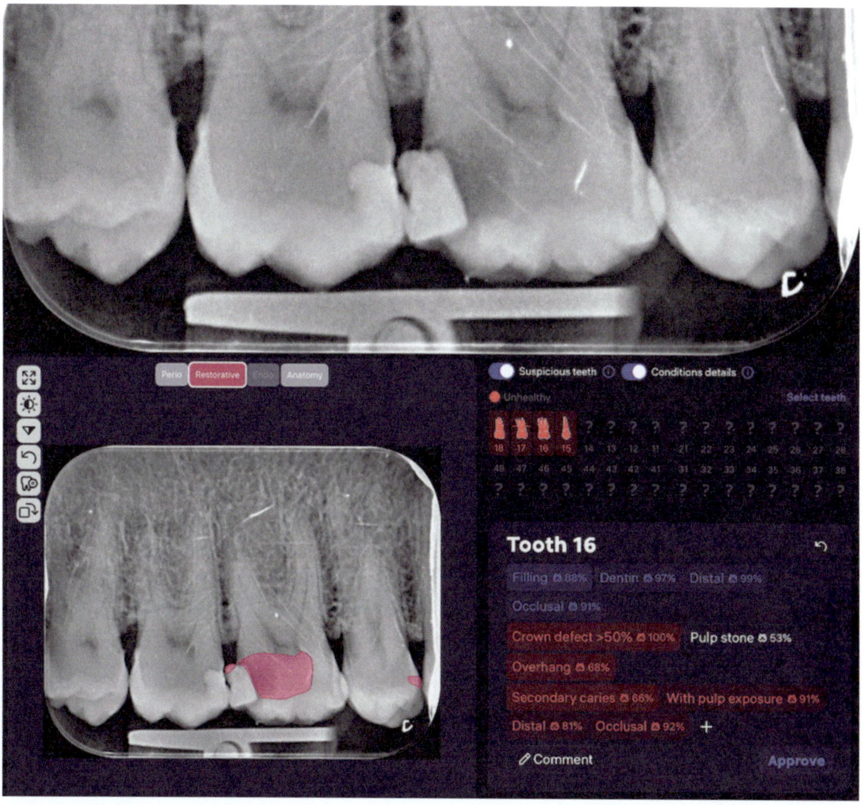

Fig. 2.9 Automated detection of a distal restoration overhang on tooth 16. Note that the software also detected the presence of pulp exposure by the caries with an AI confidence of 91%

Similar results in panoramic radiographs were shown by a different study that also described a multistage approach to detect caries using a deep learning system [16].

Another important issue is the lack of standardization in how dental caries is identified and classified. Studies used varying scales (from two-point to seven-point systems) to define and label carious lesions, making it impossible to meaningfully compare the performance of different AI platforms. This problem is compounded by extreme cases, such as one study that used image editing software to artificially create dental caries on images of sound teeth. Such practices, while perhaps useful for initial model training, create AI platforms that fundamentally restrict their ability to be replicated, compared against other models, and generalized to external, real-world clinical datasets.

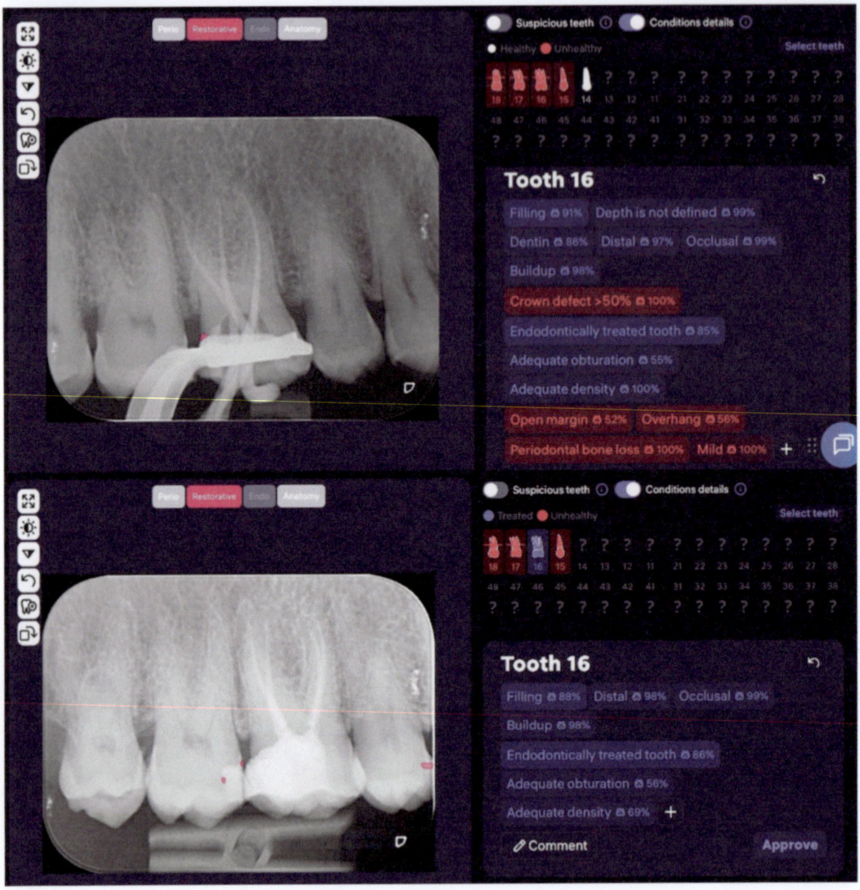

Fig. 2.10 AI-driven imaging follow-up of the clinical case of Fig. 2.9. Tooth 16 underwent root canal treatment (top). Note that this tooth is depicted in blue color since it is no longer considered "unhealthy" after the endodontic treatment (bottom)

2.4 Clinical Case Studies

2.4.1 Diagnostic Support for Deep Restorations (Case by Dr. Ana Paula Ayres)

The treatment of deep subgingival caries presents a significant clinical challenge for dental practitioners. Historically, such cases often led to invasive procedures or even tooth loss. This case report describes a modern, conservative solution that prioritizes the preservation of natural tooth structure.

Conventional treatment options for teeth with deep subgingival caries lesions are often aggressive and present significant biological and financial drawbacks. These alternatives include clinical crown lengthening and orthodontic extrusion or

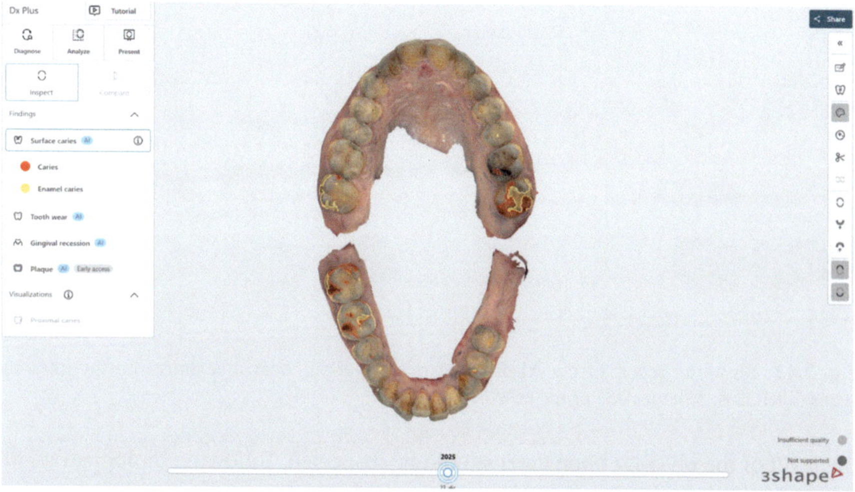

Fig. 2.11 AI-driven caries detection on the enamel (yellow) and dentin (red) using the Trios 6 intraoral scanner (3Shape A/S)

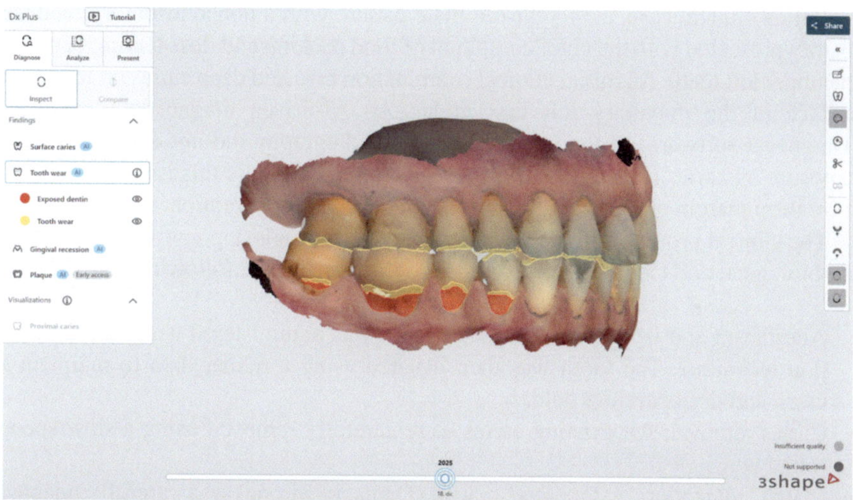

Fig. 2.12 AI-driven detection of tooth wear involving only the enamel (yellow) and areas with dentin exposed (red), using the Trios 6 intraoral scanner (3Shape A/S)

extraction followed by implant placement [17]. Each of these traditional methods presents challenges related to biological cost, treatment duration, and invasiveness.

Deep margin elevation is a procedure designed to manage deep, localized subgingival margins by bonding a dental resin composite base to the tooth structure, effectively elevating the restorative margin to a supragingival position [18]. Ideally, a minimum distance of at least 3 mm from the cervical margin of the restoration to

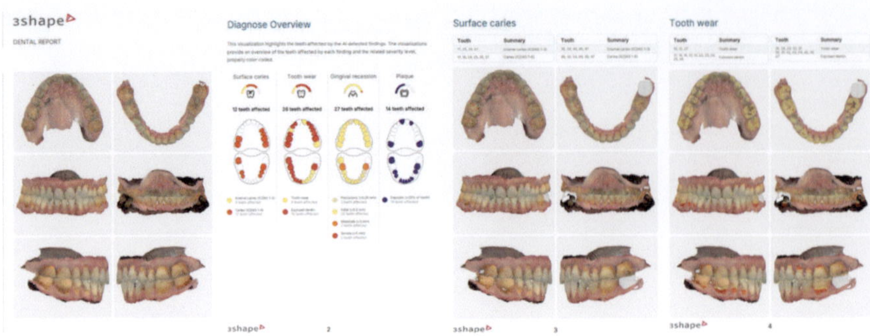

Fig. 2.13 Resulting report of the AI-driven caries and tooth wear assessment on the intraoral scans (TRIOS 6, 3Shape A/S) of the case of Fig. 2.12

the level of the alveolar bone crest should be respected, following biological width principles [19]. In this procedure, a complex restorative scenario becomes manageable by using proper rubber dam isolation, which in turn simplifies subsequent endodontic and prosthodontic procedures while preserving tooth structure and respecting periodontal integrity.

In this clinical case, a 54-year-old male patient with a noncontributory medical history presented with the chief complaint of food packing and floss tearing between the upper left teeth. An initial clinical examination revealed deep caries on the distal surface of the maxillary left first molar. An AI-driven diagnostic assessment (Diagnocat software) of the initial periapical radiography did not detect any pulp exposure by caries (Fig. 2.14). The treatment plan to address this issue was to perform deep margin elevation with subsequent composite restoration.

The clinical procedures below were planned for a single appointment, to manage the biological and technical complexities of this case, in the following order:

- Anesthesia and isolation: Local anesthesia was administered using the infiltration technique. The tooth was then isolated using a rubber dam to maintain a clean and dry operating field.
- Caries removal: All existing caries were carefully removed using a slow-speed round bur.
- Matrix adaptation: A Palodent matrix (Dentsply-Sirona) was carefully adapted around the tooth and secured with wooden wedges and Teflon tape to create a tight seal at the deep margin. A bitewing radiograph was taken to confirm that the matrix band was positioned correctly below the apical extent of the preparation.
- Adhesion protocol: The tooth surface was etched with 37% phosphoric acid, thoroughly rinsed, and thin dried. A universal adhesive system (Scotchbond Universal, 3M) was applied and light-cured according to the manufacturer's instructions.
- Composite layering and direct restoration: Carefully performed with composite resin (Filtek Z350 XT Universal, 3M) to optimize adaptation and marginal integrity (Fig. 2.15).
- Polishing: Performed with a composite polish system (Sof-Lex, 3M).

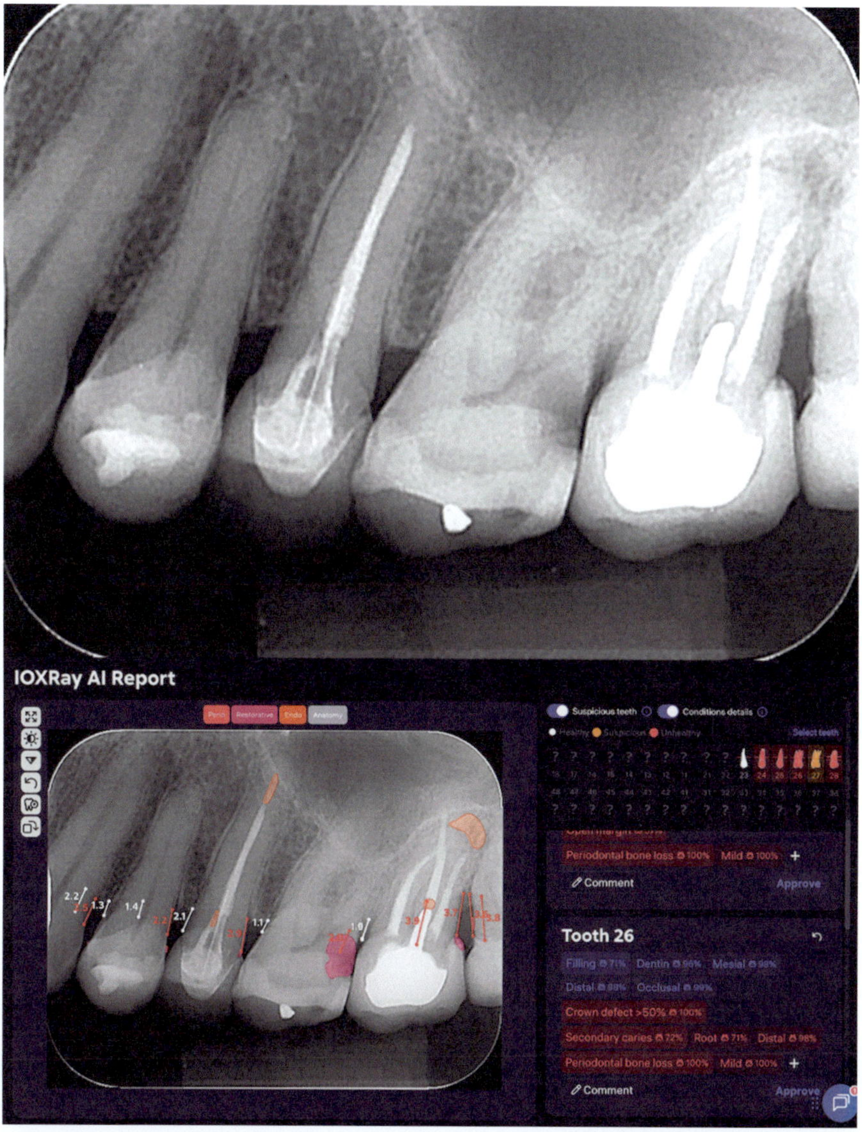

Fig. 2.14 Initial situation of tooth 26 and corresponding AI-driven report (Diagnocat)

The patient attended a follow-up visit at 6 months, which included clinical and radiological examinations and reinforcement of oral hygiene practices. At both appointments, the clinical outcome was deemed highly successful. The patient remained asymptomatic. No discomfort or other complications were reported. At the clinical follow-up examination, the restoration and surrounding periodontal tissues were healthy, with no evidence of gingival inflammation or recurrent dental

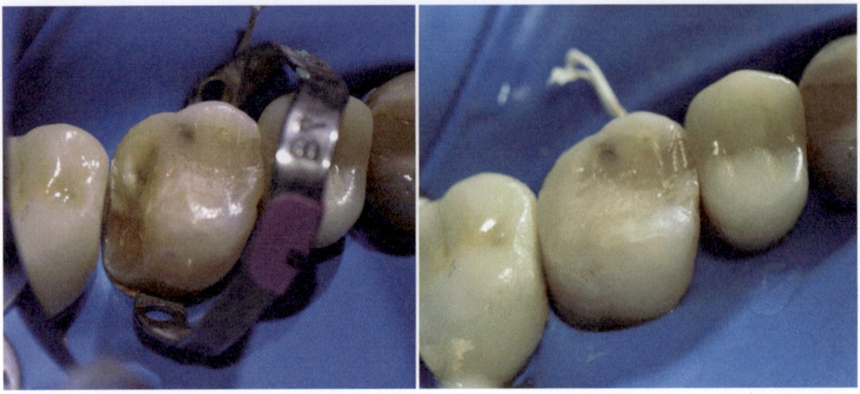

Fig. 2.15 Clinical restorative procedure of deep margin elevation and subsequent direct composite restoration of tooth 26

caries, as further confirmed by a follow-up periapical radiography, which was analyzed by the dental professional and with the AI software program (Fig. 2.16), confirming the treatment success.

2.4.2 Failing Single Crown Replacement and Adjacent Interproximal Restoration (Case by Dr. Ana Paula Ayres)

A 47-year-old male patient in good general health presented with the chief complaint of bad smell and floss tearing on the region of upper left posterior teeth. An initial AI-driven radiographic examination revealed the presence of a failing prosthetic crown with a post on the endodontically treated tooth 26 and presence of distal caries on tooth 27 (Fig. 2.17). Both teeth were firm with no signs of mobility, and with probing depths within a normal range of 2–3 mm, although bleeding on probing was noted.

The endodontic treatment of tooth 26 was considered satisfactory to enable the placement of a new single crown. Treatment options were discussed with the patient, and the final treatment sequence was established as placement of a new full-coverage indirect restoration on tooth 26 (Fig. 2.18), as well as a direct composite restoration on the mesial surface of tooth 27.

A three-appointment approach was selected for this case:

- First appointment: Initial clinical and radiographic examination, failing crown removal, review of the conditions of the preparation of tooth 26, and new temporary crown
- Second appointment: Distal composite restoration on tooth 27 and intraoral scans (Itero Element 5D, Align Technology) of the tooth 26 preparation, antagonist arch and bite registration of the patient

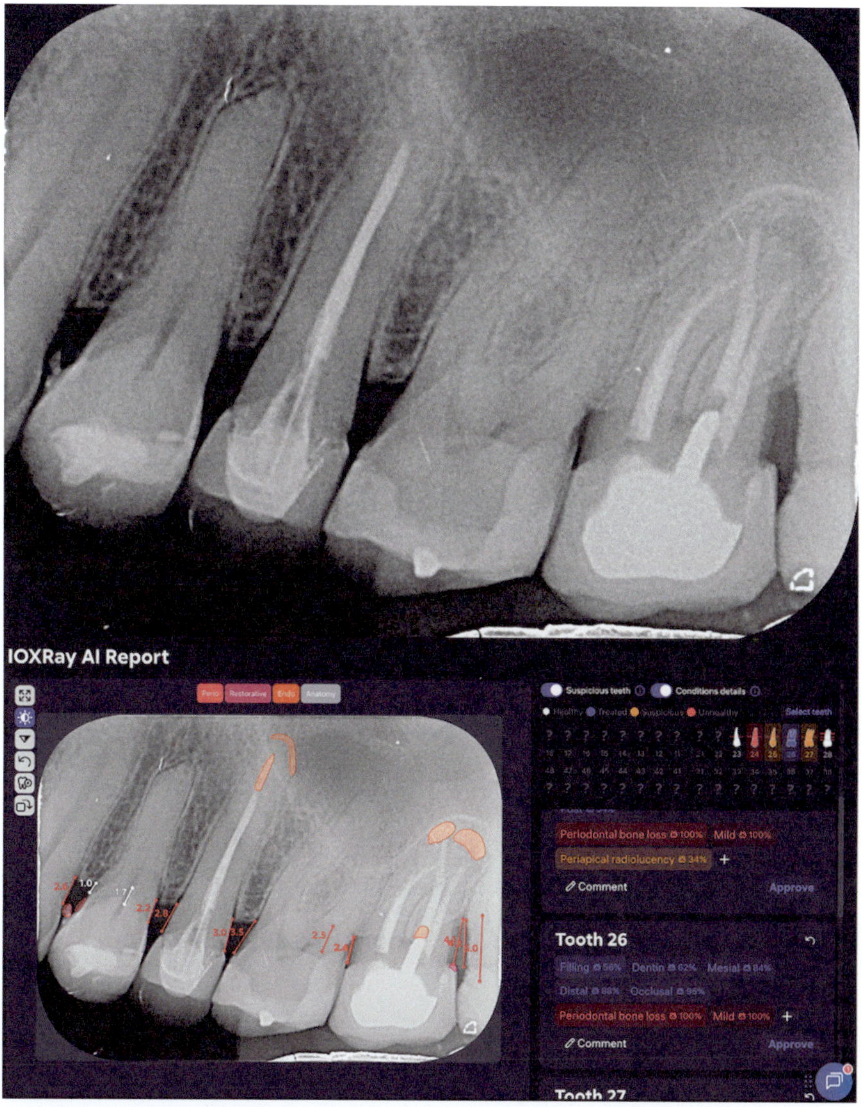

Fig. 2.16 Follow-up periapical radiography of tooth 26 and corresponding AI-driven report (Diagnocat). Note that the restoration is reasonably distant from the alveolar crest

- Third appointment: Cementation of the final lithium disilicate crown (emax, Ivoclar) with Panavia V5 (Kuraray Noritake), followed by chairside occlusal check with articulating paper

Follow-up clinical and radiographic examinations were conducted after 3 months, revealing satisfactory conditions of both restorations (Fig. 2.19).

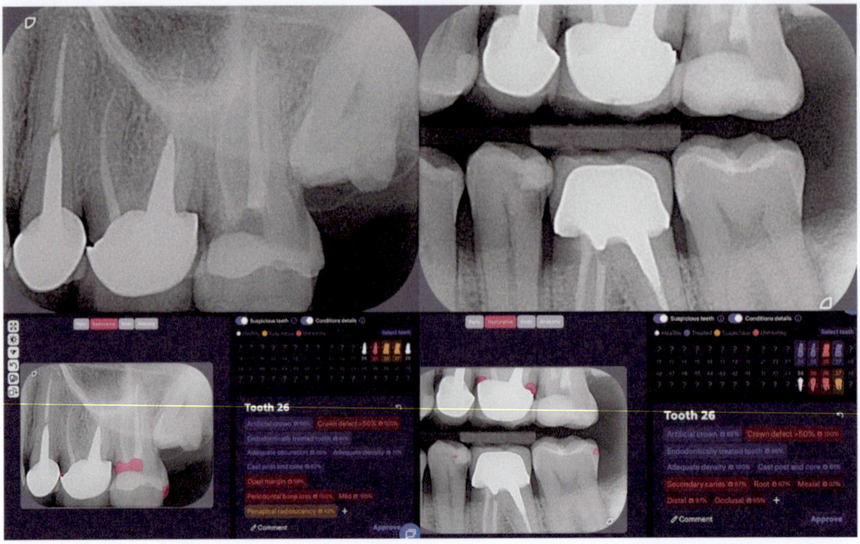

Fig. 2.17 AI-driven report (Diagnocat) of the initial periapical (left) and bitewing (right) radiographs. Note the lack of adaptation of the prosthetic crown on tooth 26

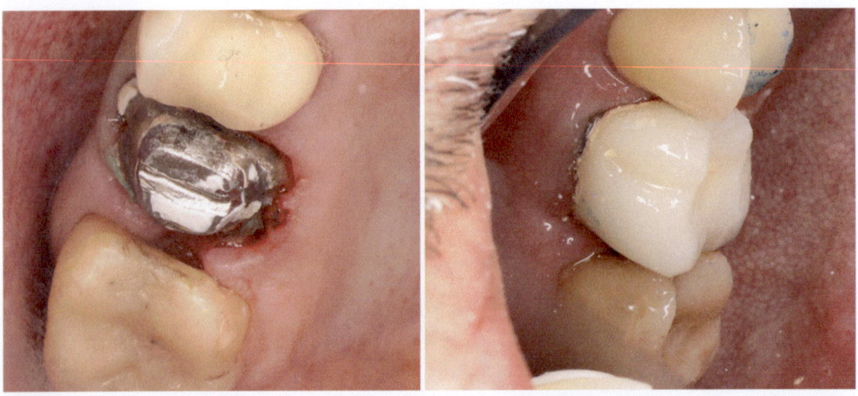

Fig. 2.18 Intraoral photographs of the clinical situation after the failing crown removal (left) and after mesial restoration of tooth 27 and a new temporary crown on tooth 26

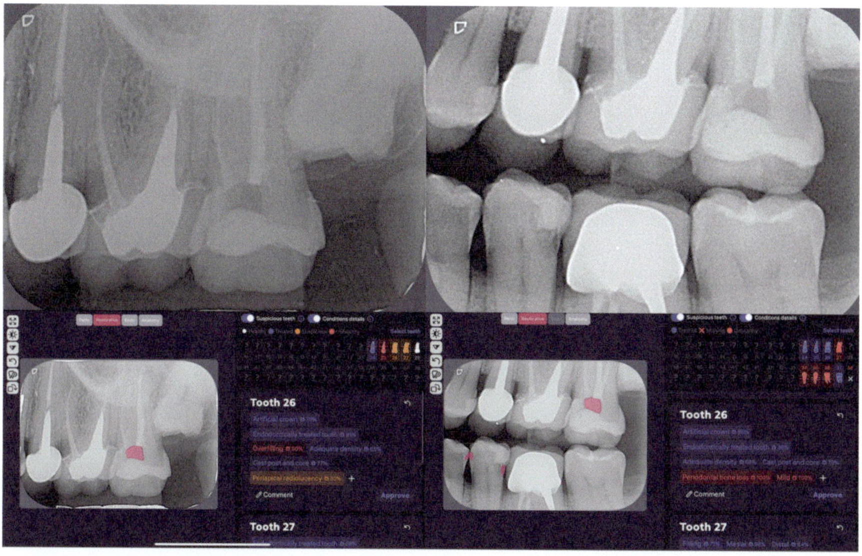

Fig. 2.19 AI-driven report (Diagnocat) of the final periapical (left) and bitewing (right) radiographs, confirming treatment success

2.4.3 Images of the Assessment of Tooth Wear and Caries Using an Intraoral Scanner (Courtesy of Dr. Jan Paulics and 3Shape A/S)

One of the most important aspects of the detection of tooth wear and caries is the classification of the severity of each case. The following images of clinical cases are shown as examples of AI-driven automated detection of mild (Fig. 2.20) and severe tooth wear (Fig. 2.21). Furthermore, it is always important to check the level of confidence reported by the AI system being utilized to detect alterations. For this reason, two different images of AI-driven detection of caries are available to show examples of different AI confidence levels to detect initial and severe caries (Fig. 2.22).

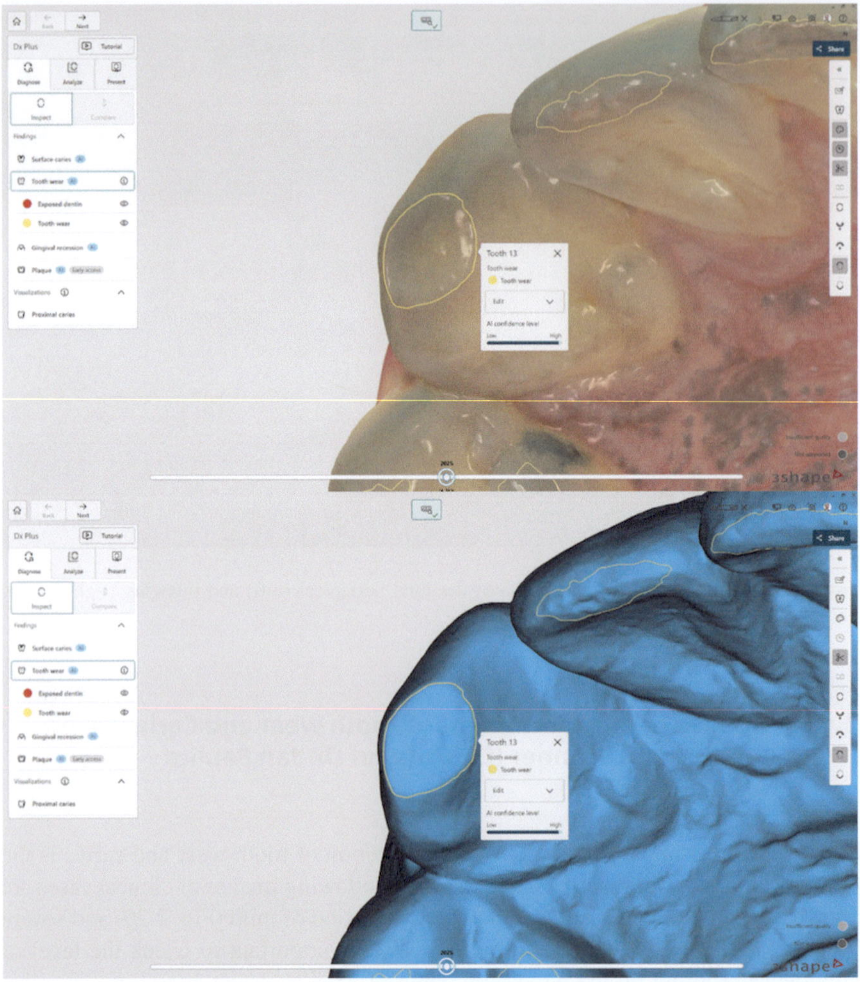

Fig. 2.20 AI-driven detection of mild tooth wear on an intraoral scan (TRIOS 6)

2.5 Conclusion

Given the significant variability in performance reported in the literature, with accuracy rates spanning from 41.5% to 98.6%, AI tools should not be considered reliable enough to replace traditional diagnostic methods for dental caries. Current systems lack the consistency required for independent clinical decision-making. Therefore, at present, AI should be considered a useful supplementary aid that requires careful human oversight. It can assist clinicians by highlighting potential areas of concern or providing a second opinion, but the final diagnostic responsibility must remain with the dental professional.

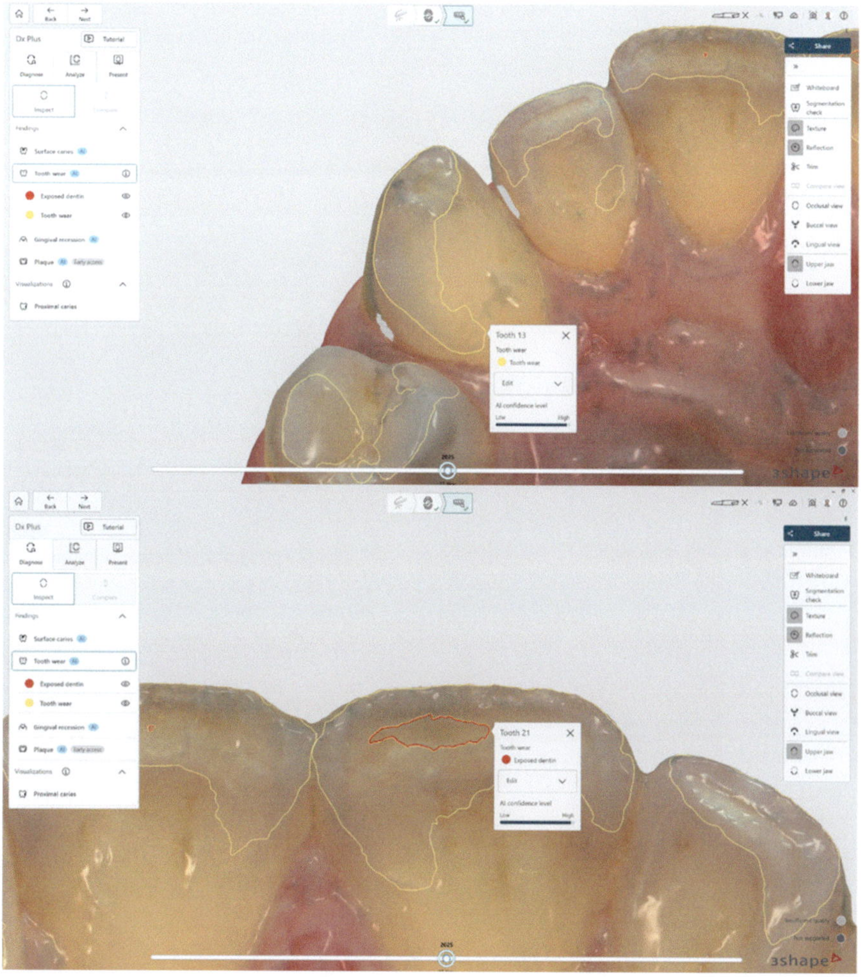

Fig. 2.21 AI-driven detection of severe tooth wear on an intraoral scan (TRIOS 6)

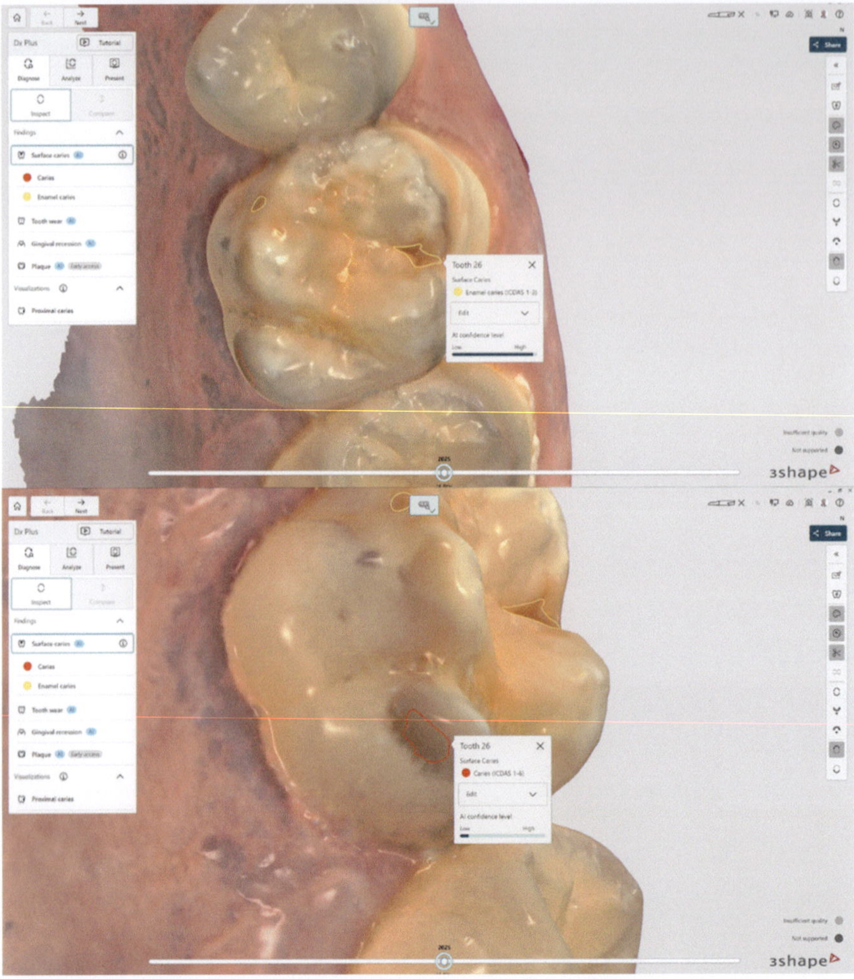

Fig. 2.22 AI-driven detection of initial caries showing high AI confidence (top) and of severe caries with very low AI confidence (bottom) on an intraoral scan (3shape Dx software, TRIOS 6, 3Shape A/S)

References

1. Schwendicke F, Tzschoppe M, Paris S. Radiographic caries detection: a systematic review and meta-analysis. J Dent. 2015;43(8):924–33. https://doi.org/10.1016/j.jdent.2015.02.009. Epub 2015 Feb 24. Erratum in: J Dent. 2021;114:103783.
2. Agius A, Attard NJ, Gatt G, Cortes ARG. Digital workflow in dental publichealth, preventive dentistry, and dental education. In: Cortes ARG, editor. Digital dentistry: a step-by-step guide and case atlas. Wiley-Blackwell Publishing Ltd.; 2022. p. 287–92. https://doi.org/10.1002/9781119852025.ch10.
3. Abbott LP, Saikia A, Anthonappa RP. Artificial intelligence platforms in dental caries detection: a systematic review and meta-analysis. J Evid Based Dent Pract. 2025;25(1):102077. https://doi.org/10.1016/j.jebdp.2024.102077.

4. Nampim N, Panyarak W, Suttapak W, Wantanajittikul K, Nirunsittirat A, Wattanarat O. Deep learning-based caries lesion classification of primary teeth using bitewing radiographs and its comparison with dental professionals. Eur Arch Paediatr Dent. 2025; https://doi.org/10.1007/s40368-025-01129-z.
5. Köse E, Hoşgör S. Assessment of posterior interproximal surfaces on bitewing and panoramic radiographs by dental interns and an artificial intelligence application. Oral Radiol. 2025; https://doi.org/10.1007/s11282-025-00872-9.
6. Zhang JW, Fan J, Zhao FB, Ma B, Shen XQ, Geng YM. Diagnostic accuracy of artificial intelligence-assisted caries detection: a clinical evaluation. BMC Oral Health. 2024;24(1):1095. https://doi.org/10.1186/s12903-024-04847-w.
7. Ourang SA, Sohrabniya F, Mohammad-Rahimi H, Dianat O, Aminoshariae A, Nagendrababu V, Dummer PMH, Duncan HF, Nosrat A. Artificial intelligence in endodontics: fundamental principles, workflow, and tasks. Int Endod J. 2024;57(11):1546–65.
8. Kühnisch J, Meyer O, Hesenius M, Hickel R, Gruhn V. Caries detection on intra-oral images using artificial intelligence. J Dent Res. 2022;101(2):158–65. https://doi.org/10.1177/00220345211032524.
9. Huang Y, Lee S. Deep learning for caries detection using optical coherence tomography. 2021. https://www.semanticscholar.org/paper/Deep-Learning-for-Caries-Detection-using-Optical-Huang-Lee/99c4e6c0b3cb7c4555397424682d7241ebe4c5f2.
10. Bayraktar Y, Ayan E. Diagnosis of interproximal caries lesions with deep convolutional neural network in digital bitewing radiographs. Clin Oral Investig. 2022;26(1):623–32. https://doi.org/10.1007/s00784-021-04040-1.
11. Piipari L, Anttonen V, Lussi A, Laitala ML, Tanner T, Karki S. Reliability of an artificial intelligence software in the detection of approximal caries lesions using bitewing radiographs. Caries Res. 2025:1–8. https://doi.org/10.1159/000547245.
12. Lian L, Zhu T, Zhu F, Zhu H. Deep learning for caries detection and classification. Diagnostics (Basel). 2021;11(9):1672. https://doi.org/10.3390/diagnostics11091672.
13. Duong DL, Kabir MH, Kuo RF. Automated caries detection with smartphone color photography using machine learning. Health Informatics J. 2021;27(2):14604582211007530. https://doi.org/10.1177/14604582211007530.
14. Carrillo-Perez F, Pecho OE, Morales JC, Paravina RD, Della Bona A, Ghinea R, Pulgar R, Pérez MDM, Herrera LJ. Applications of artificial intelligence in dentistry: a comprehensive review. J Esthet Restor Dent. 2022;34(1):259–80.
15. Zhu H, Cao Z, Lian L, Ye G, Gao H, Wu J. CariesNet: a deep learning approach for segmentation of multi-stage caries lesion from oral panoramic X-ray image. Neural Comput Appl. 2022:1–9. https://doi.org/10.1007/s00521-021-06684-2.
16. Pornprasertsuk-Damrongsri S, Vachmanus S, Papasratorn D, Kitisubkanchana J, Chaikantha S, Arayasantiparb R, Mongkolwat P. Clinical application of deep learning for enhanced multistage caries detection in panoramic radiographs. Sci Rep. 2025;15(1):33491. https://doi.org/10.1038/s41598-025-16591-4.
17. Iqbal MK, Kim S. A review of factors influencing treatment planning decisions of single-tooth implants versus preserving natural teeth with nonsurgical endodontic therapy. J Endod. 2008;34(5):519–29. https://doi.org/10.1016/j.joen.2008.01.002.
18. Blatz MB, Eggmann F. Deep margin elevation: next-level adhesive dentistry to avoid surgical crown lengthening. Compend Contin Educ Dent. 2023;44(9):530–1.
19. Padbury A Jr, Eber R, Wang HL. Interactions between the gingiva and the margin of restorations. J Clin Periodontol. 2003;30(5):379–85.

Automated Detection of Oral Lesions

3

Adam Bartolo, Ji Yong Han, Min Suk Heo, Nicholas Busuttil Dougall, Faleh Tamimi, and Arthur Rodriguez Gonzalez Cortes

Clinical and radiographic diagnosis of oral lesions are among the most important tasks of the routine of a dental professional. Traditional diagnostic methods have been considered foundational, but with important drawbacks. The process of interpreting radiographic images is inherently subjective, leading to interobserver variability and the potential for human error. This challenge is particularly significant given the prevalence of the condition; apical periodontitis, for instance, accounts for approximately 75% of periapical radiolucent lesions. Dental clinicians attempt to identify subtle changes in bone density and structure, which is a task that can be complicated by imaging artifacts, anatomical superimpositions, imaging noise, and the usual underestimation of bone loss that is inherent of most radiographic methods. This reliance on subjective interpretation can lead to diagnostic inconsistencies and potentially delay necessary treatment, highlighting the need for more objective and reliable tools.

A. Bartolo · N. Busuttil Dougall · A. R. G. Cortes (✉)
Faculty of Dental Surgery, University of Malta, Msida, Malta
e-mail: adam.bartolo@um.edu.mt; nicholas.busuttil-dougall@um.edu.mt; arthur.nogueira@um.edu.mt

J. Y. Han · M. S. Heo
Seoul National University, Seoul, South Korea
e-mail: jiyong@snu.ac.kr; hmslsh@snu.ac.kr

F. Tamimi
McGill University, Montreal, Canada
e-mail: Faleh.tamimimarino@mcgill.ca

A. R. G. Cortes (ed.), *Dental Clinical Procedures using Artificial Intelligence*,
https://doi.org/10.1007/978-3-032-24895-4_3

3.1 Radiographic Methods to Detect Oral Lesions

Intraoral periapical radiographs and orthopantomographs (panoramic radiographs) are the most frequently used 2D diagnostic techniques in routine clinical practice. They are valued for their accessibility and low radiation dose. However, their primary limitation is the inherent inaccuracy that results from compressing complex three-dimensional anatomy into a flat and two-dimensional image. The resulting superposition of anatomical structures can obscure subtle pathological changes, making the early detection of periapical lesions challenging.

To overcome the limitations of 2D imaging, CBCT was developed. This modality provides accurate 3D views of the maxillofacial region, allowing clinicians to accurately detect periapical lesions and assess their 3D location and extent without anatomical superpositions. The diagnostic superiority of CBCT for this task has been quantified in meta-analyses, which report significantly higher accuracy compared to 2D methods [1], as further explained in this chapter. It is important to remember, however, that the quality and resolution of the radiographic images may affect the accuracy and reliability of the automated detection of lesions, as it also affects conventional diagnostic assessments by dental professionals and oral and maxillofacial radiologists [2]. One previous study in dry rabbit mandibles, for instance, found that the AI system tested for automated segmentation and volume calculation of intraosseous lesions achieved a significantly higher volumetric accuracy in high-resolution CBCT scans of 0.1 mm voxel size, as compared with other scans of 0.2 mm [3]. Other factors affecting image quality and assessments of CBCT scans are the field-of-view, kilovoltage peak, and slice thickness, among others [2]. These findings indicate that dental clinicians should have knowledge on imaging parameters and software tools to ensure an adequate use of these images with AI systems.

3.1.1 Automated Diagnosis of Periapical Radiolucencies

Several studies have focused on the primary task of automatically identifying periapical lesions from radiographs [4–9]. One of these studies developed a deep learning algorithm that could identify periapical radiolucencies on radiographic images as effectively as a group of 24 experienced oral and maxillofacial surgeons [8]. Another quantitative study assessed an AI system that correctly identified 142 out of 153 periapical lesions, achieving a detection accuracy rate of 92.8% [9]. These findings demonstrate the potential of AI models to diagnose lesions with a high degree of reliability.

Commercial AI-driven dental diagnostic software programs can also be used by dental clinicians to perform automated diagnostic reports (Fig. 3.1). For this purpose, dental clinicians should be well-trained and updated regarding imaging diagnosis of oral lesions (Fig. 3.2). The accurate differentiation of odontogenic lesions

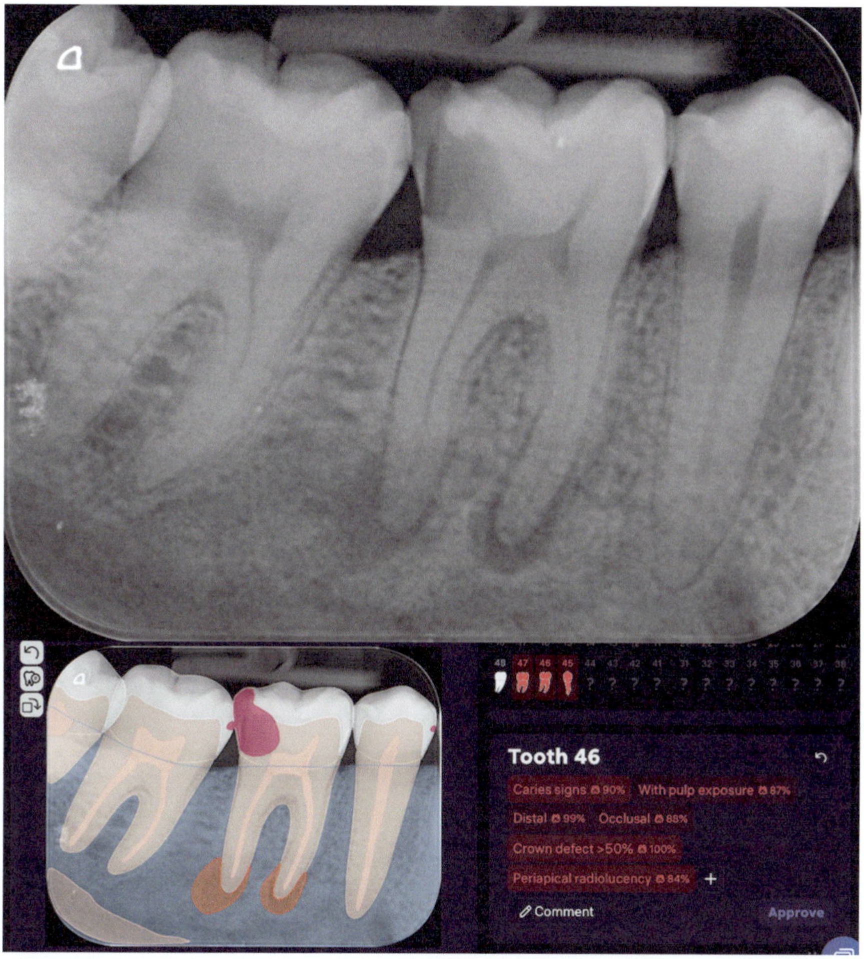

Fig. 3.1 AI-driven diagnostic report (Diagnocat) detecting two radiolucent lesions suggestive of periapical granuloma versus radicular cyst, associated with pulp chamber exposure by caries

represents a fundamental challenge in clinical practice, directly informing therapeutic strategy and patient prognosis. These lesions, originating from the tooth-forming apparatus, are broadly categorized based on their underlying cause as either inflammatory or developmental. Inflammatory lesions arise as a host response to microbial or traumatic insults, while developmental lesions form from entrapped epithelial remnants of odontogenesis. Both types of lesions should be well understood by the dental professional operating an AI-driven diagnostic system.

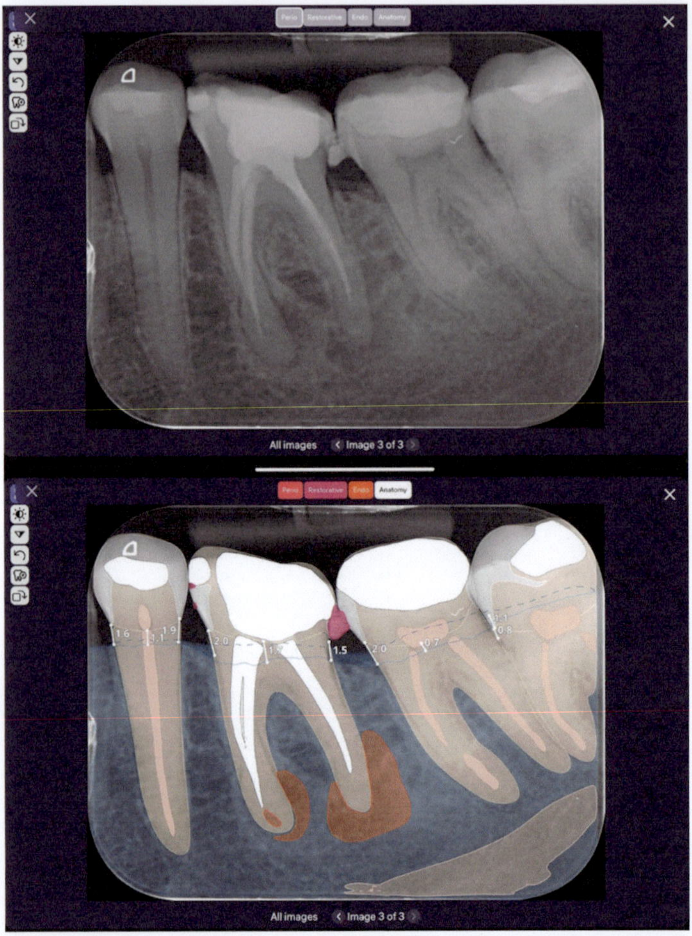

Fig. 3.2 Maximized images of the AI-driven report (Diagnocat) of case with periapical lesions on tooth 36. Note the relatively large trabecular spaces of the posterior mandible, which could be a challenge for the diagnosis due to undesired superimpositions

3.1.2 Automated Detection of Periapical Lesions in 3D Images

As previously mentioned, CBCT has emerged as the 3D imaging gold standard, providing high-resolution volumetric data that allows for a precise evaluation of the size, location, and morphology of periapical lesions. However, the interpretation of CBCT scans can still be affected by significant interobserver variability and the potential for fatigue-related diagnostic errors. In this context, AI represents a transformative technology capable of automating and augmenting CBCT analysis. By using deep learning algorithms, AI systems can enhance diagnostic accuracy, thus improving interpretation consistency and clinical efficiency [10].

Across the reviewed studies, convolutional neural network (CNN)-based architectures, particularly U-Net variants, were the most frequently applied. These deep learning models are consistently effective due to their inherent strength in spatial pattern recognition and image segmentation, making them exceptionally well-suited for analyzing volumetric CBCT data. One of the foundational works on this topic utilized a U-Net model to achieve strong segmentation performance (AUC: 93%; Dice Similarity Coefficient: 0.67), demonstrating the viability of deep learning in this domain [11]. Similar findings were described by another study that employed the GoogLeNet Inception-v3 model to directly demonstrate the superior diagnostic performance of AI models trained on 3D CBCT data, as compared to models trained on 2D panoramic images [12].

Besides CBCT, recent scientific research has also tested CNN and other AI systems such as vision transformers (ViTs) on medical CT images to perform paranasal sinuses segmentation in the presence of sinusitis [13]. This study assessed medical CT of 200 patients. Diagnostic performance in cases with sinusitis were compared with scans of normal paranasal sinuses, which include the maxillary sinuses. According to the findings, a hybrid network outperformed all other AI systems included, with a reduced number of false positives.

It is noteworthy that not all commercial dental AI-driven diagnostic software programs work with CBCT or 3D images. With the Diagnocat software, a CBCT AI report can be generated by uploading original DICOM (Digital Imaging and Communications in Medicine) files (which have the extension ".dcm"). While the scan output of several CBCT devices is an entire folder of .dcm files (usually one per axial slice), other modern devices allow for clustering or compressing the entire scan into a single .dcm file.

Once the CBCT AI report is generated, a coronal panoramic view of the scan will show with the filters of alterations discussed in the previous chapters. Clicking on a tooth of the chart will open the specific report of that tooth (Fig. 3.3), from which it

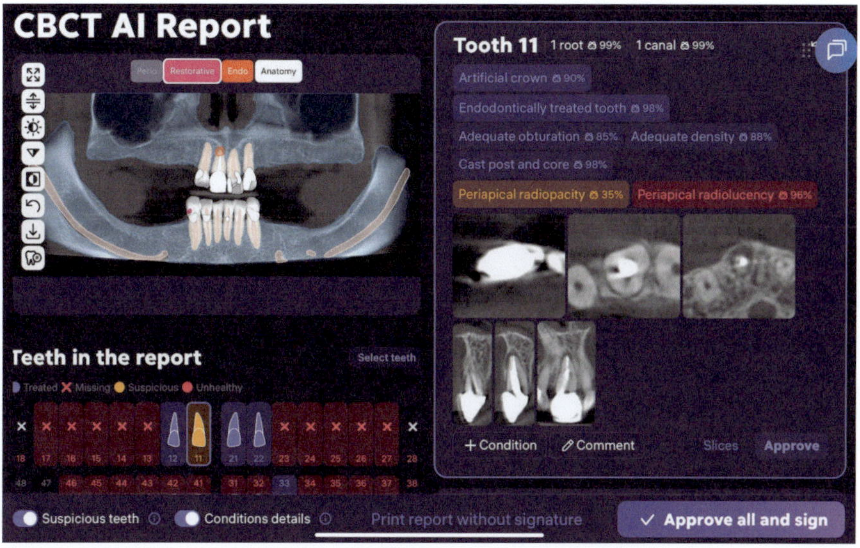

Fig. 3.3 AI-driven CBCT report (Diagnocat) showing a periapical radiolucency associated with tooth 11. The professional should click on "slices" to assess the multiplanar reconstruction to navigate through the three orthogonal planes: sagittal, coronal, and axial

is possible to access multiplanar reconstructed images (Fig. 3.4) and automated volume calculations (Fig. 3.5).

While the tool "CBCT AI report" lists and describes all alterations detected, a 3D-reconstructed model can also be rendered from the original DICOM files using the tool "3D model AI" to depict all CBCT segmentations and respective alterations (Fig. 3.6). The usefulness of this tool will be further discussed on Chap. 6.

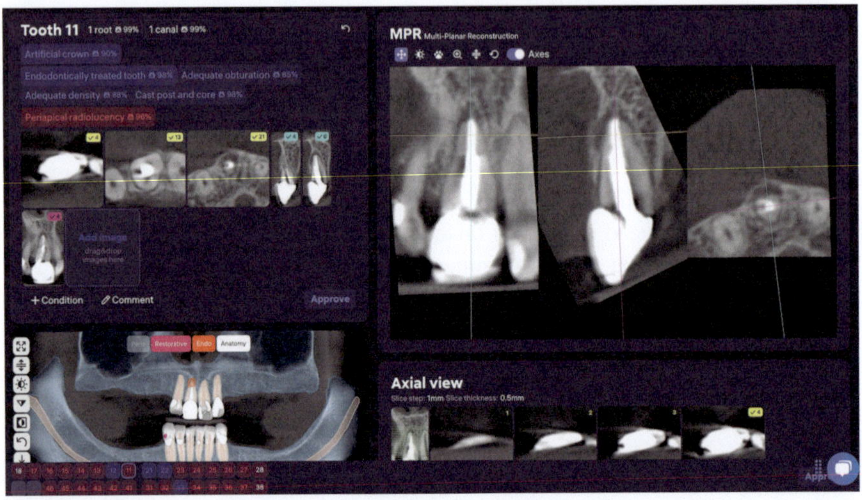

Fig. 3.4 CBCT multiplanar reconstruction of the case of Fig. 3.3, showing, from left to right, coronal, sagittal, and axial windows with navigation axes

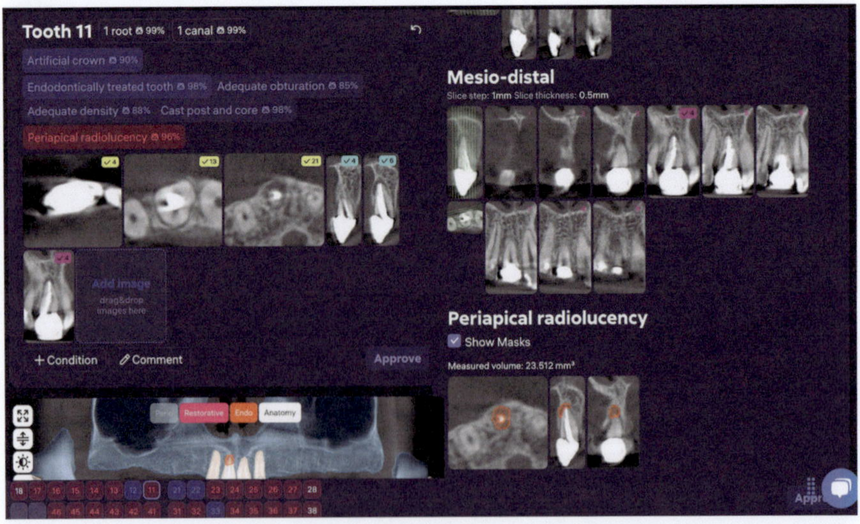

Fig. 3.5 CBCT cross-sectional slices and automated volume calculation of the lesion shown in Figs. 3.3 and 3.4

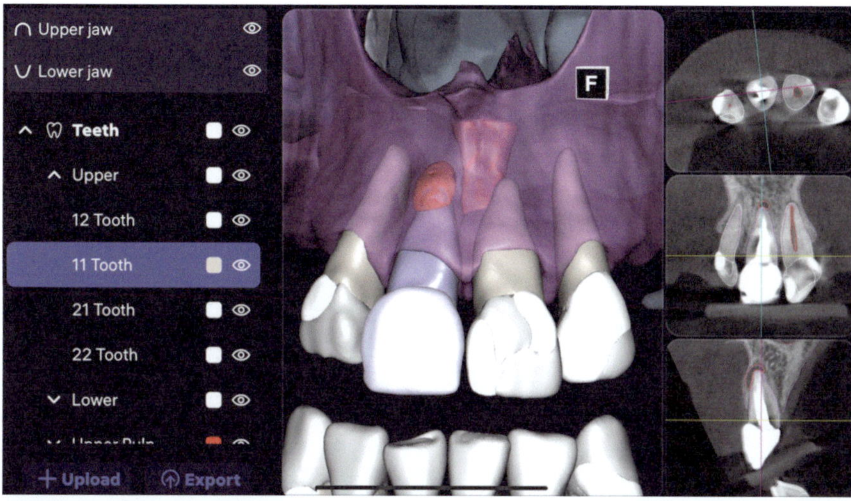

Fig. 3.6 CBCT AI reconstructed model showing a 3D view of the alterations listed on the CBCT AI report

3.1.3 Review of the Most Common Periapical Radiolucencies

Inflammatory odontogenic lesions are the direct result of the host's defense mechanisms responding to stimuli, most commonly microbial invasion from a necrotic dental pulp or physical trauma. This category includes a spectrum of conditions that often represent different stages of the same disease process, such as acute and chronic apical periodontitis, the periapical granuloma, as well as the periapical or radicular cyst. The differentiation between these stages and other conditions requires a careful analysis of the existing 2D (Fig. 3.7) and/or 3D (Fig. 3.8) radiographic images of the case. This confirmation needs to be performed by the dental professional, as AI software programs will generally just indicate the presence of a periapical radiolucency, regardless of its actual diagnosis.

The process begins with acute apical periodontitis, the initial inflammatory response in the tissues surrounding the root apex following the egress of microbial invaders from an infected root canal system. This acute phase is dominated by the infiltration of polymorphonuclear leukocytes, which attack the offending microorganisms and release inflammatory mediators such as prostaglandins and leukotrienes, intensifying the host response. Patients with acute apical periodontitis typically report symptoms of pain, tenderness on pressure or chewing, and a sensation that the tooth feels elevated in its socket. The involved tooth is characteristically tender to percussion. The dental pulp may be vital in cases of trauma and in the early stages of infection or necrotic in severe cases. Radiographic changes are often minimal, such as slight widening of the periodontal ligament space, or absent.

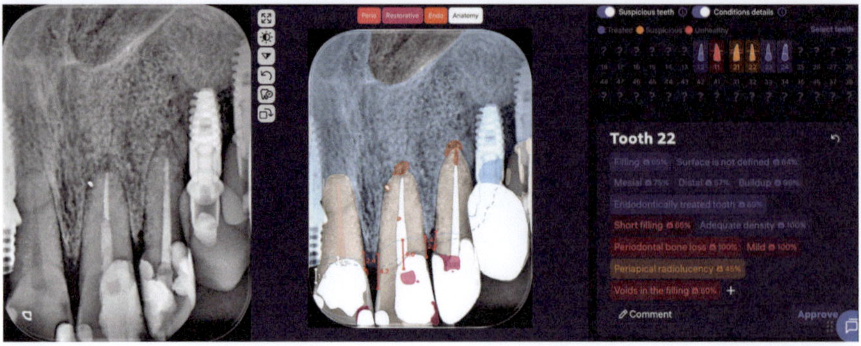

Fig. 3.7 AI-driven report (Diagnocat) of a periapical radiograph detecting a periapical radiolucency on tooth 22 with AI confidence of 45%

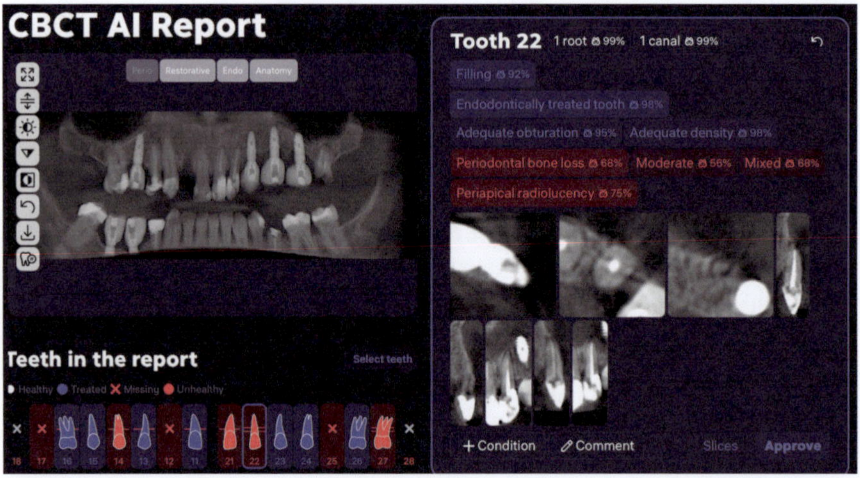

Fig. 3.8 AI-driven report (Diagnocat) of the CBCT of the case of Fig. 3.7, detecting a periapical radiolucency on tooth 22 with AI confidence of 75%

When the acute inflammatory response fails to eliminate the microbial stimulus, a chronic lesion develops. Chronic apical periodontitis represents this progression, in which the lesion becomes encapsulated in connective tissue. These lesions are often asymptomatic and are frequently discovered as incidental findings on routine radiographs. The pulp of the associated tooth is usually necrotic, and the tooth will not respond to thermal or electric sensibility tests. The most common radiographic pattern is a small well-limited radiolucent space, representing moderate or severe periodontal ligament space widening (Fig. 3.9).

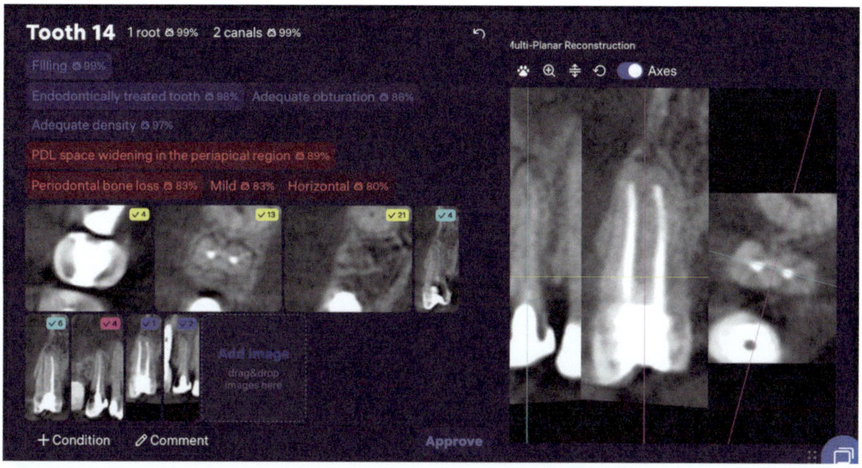

Fig. 3.9 AI-driven CBCT report (Diagnocat) detecting periodontal ligament space widening on tooth 14

A periapical granuloma consists of inflamed granulation tissue that forms at the apex of a non-vital tooth. While initial acute radiographic alterations have ill-defined limits (Fig. 3.10), periapical granulomas are chronic well-defined radiolucent lesions (Fig. 3.11). Histologically, it is distinguished by the absence of an epithelial lining and is considered a precursor to an inflammatory radicular cyst (also known as periapical cyst). The radicular cyst forms when the chronic inflammation within a granuloma stimulates the proliferation of the epithelial cell rests of Malassez (ERM), which are residual cells from root formation [1, 2]. This proliferation leads to the formation of a true epithelial-lined cavity, the defining feature of a cyst. Clinically, the associated tooth is non-vital, typically due to a history of extensive dental caries or trauma. Similar to chronic apical periodontitis, these lesions are often asymptomatic and identified during radiographic examination. Periapical granulomas are usually seen in routine dental radiographs as a small well-defined homogeneous radiolucent lesion at the apex of the non-vital tooth. Radicular cysts have similar radiographic aspects, but usually slightly more aggressive, often with corticated borders, round and symmetrical shapes. In several cases, CBCT images of these lesions are taken to plan a surgical removal approach, such as enucleation and apicoectomy (Fig. 3.12).

The association between a vertical bone defect and a periapical lesion may be suggestive of an endo-perio lesion (Fig. 3.13). The marginal bone of every tooth, especially those with alterations listed by the AI reports, should be carefully checked by the dental professional to correctly diagnose this and related conditions.

Developmental odontogenic lesions arise spontaneously from the proliferation of epithelial remnants of tooth development that become entrapped within the jawbones or gingiva. Unlike their inflammatory counterparts, their formation is not initiated by infection or trauma. The two most prominent examples discussed here are the dentigerous cyst and the odontogenic keratocyst (OKC).

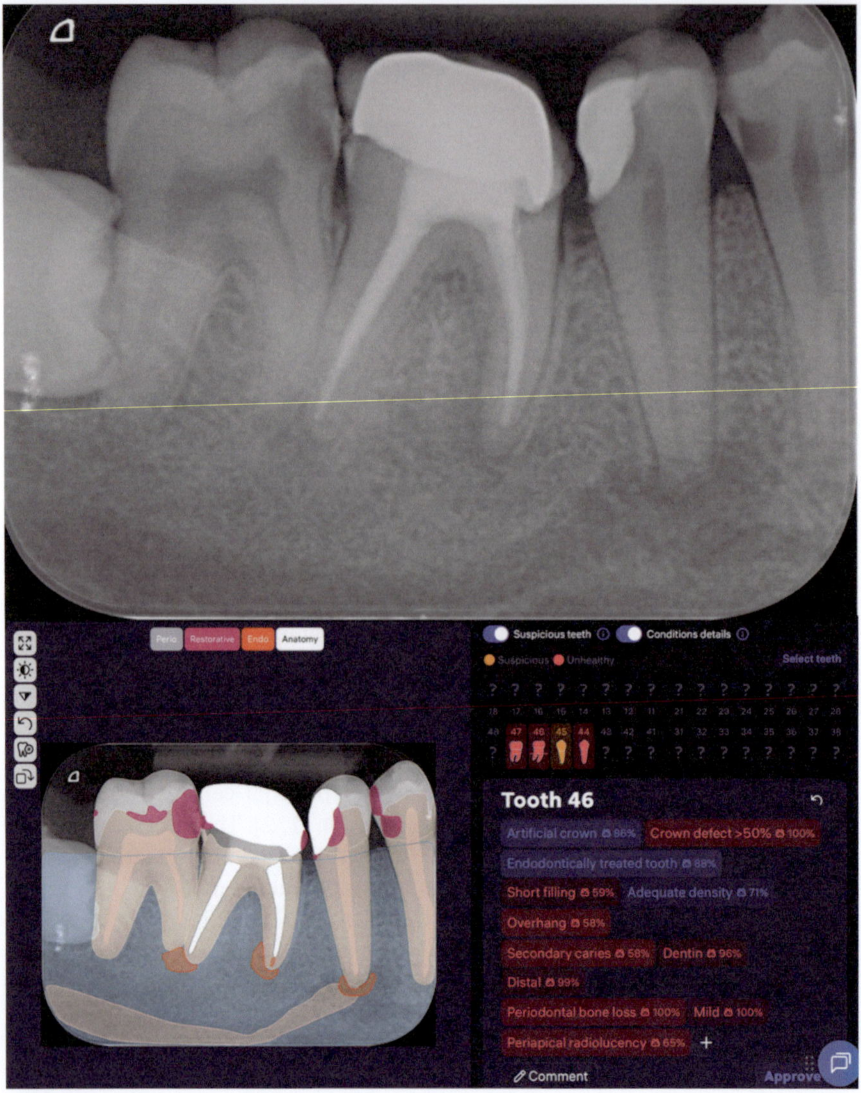

Fig. 3.10 AI-driven CBCT report (Diagnocat) detecting periapical radiolucent alterations with ill-defined limits on right mandibular first and second molars

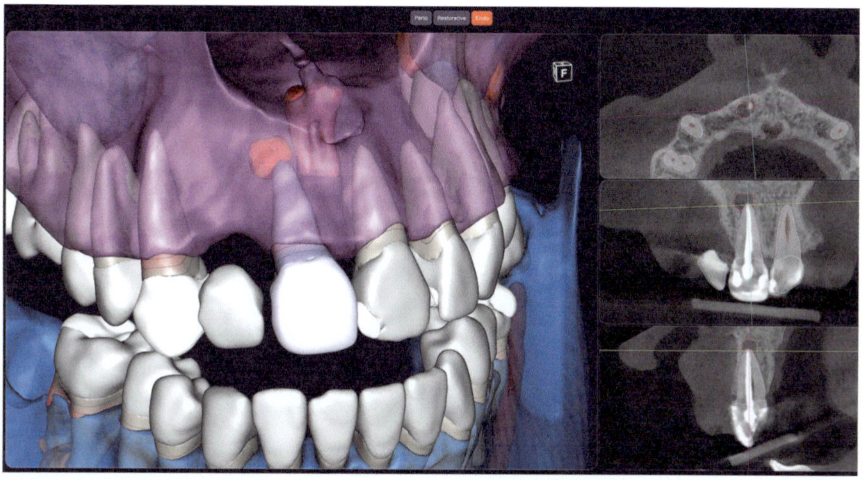

Fig. 3.11 3D model AI showing a periapical granuloma on tooth 11

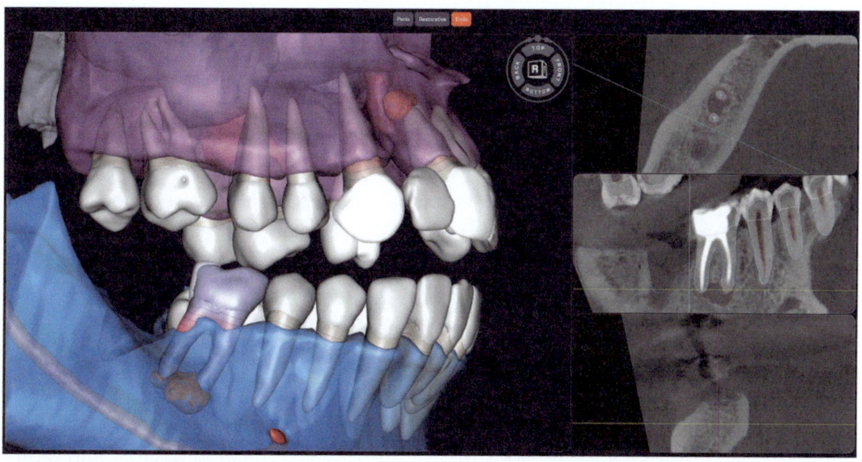

Fig. 3.12 Lateral view of the 3D model AI of Fig. 3.11 showing a radicular cyst on tooth 46

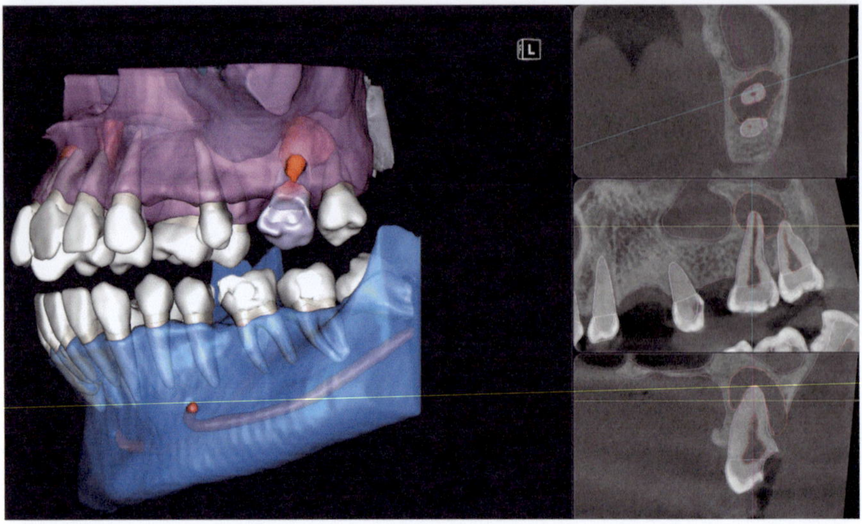

Fig. 3.13 Lateral view of the 3D model AI of Figs. 3.11 and 3.12, showing an endo-perio lesion associated with a radicular cyst on tooth 27. Note the proximity of the lesion with the maxillary sinus floor

A dentigerous cyst develops when fluid accumulates between the crown of an unerupted or impacted tooth and the reduced enamel epithelium. This accumulation dilates the dental follicle, forming a cystic cavity that surrounds the crown and prevents its eruption. Dentigerous cysts are characteristically associated with an impacted or unerupted tooth, most commonly the third molars and maxillary canines. It is usually asymptomatic unless it becomes secondarily inflamed. Radiographically, dentigerous cysts are well-limited unilocular radiolucencies usually attached to the cementoenamel junction of the crown of an impacted tooth, although lesions can be more aggressive, resembling the radiographic aspects of OKCs (Figs. 3.14, 3.15, and 3.16).

OKCs originate from remnants of the dental lamina, known as the rests of Serres. These distinct etiologies are responsible for the varied clinical behaviors and radiographic appearances of odontogenic lesions, which are essential for forming a differential diagnosis. OKCs are often asymptomatic because they tend to expand in an anterior-posterior direction within the bone without causing significant buccolingual expansion (Fig. 3.17). However, larger lesions can present with pain, edema, trismus, infection, or neurosensory deficits. The presence of multiple OKCs should prompt an evaluation for nevoid basal cell carcinoma syndrome or Gorlin-Goltz syndrome (Fig. 3.18).

Radiographically, OKCs can show several patterns, from a relatively small unilocular radiolucency (Figs. 3.19, 3.20, 3.21, and 3.22) to a large lesion with scalloped borders, or a multilocular lesion resembling an ameloblastoma. OKCs are often associated with an impacted tooth, but unlike dentigerous cysts, not necessarily attached to the CEJ of the tooth.

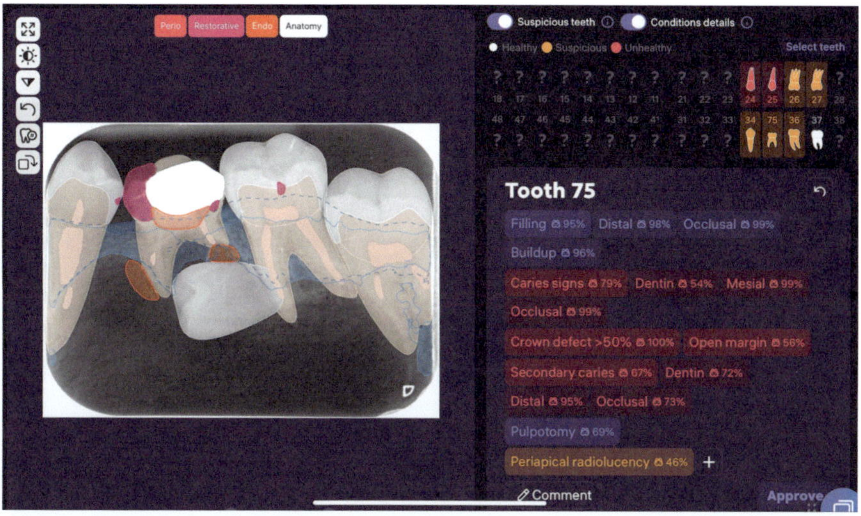

Fig. 3.14 AI-driven CBCT report (Diagnocat) showing an incorrect segmentation of a large radiolucent lesion contiguous with the apices of tooth 75 and the crown of impacted tooth 35. A 3D CBCT was then requested to further investigate the region

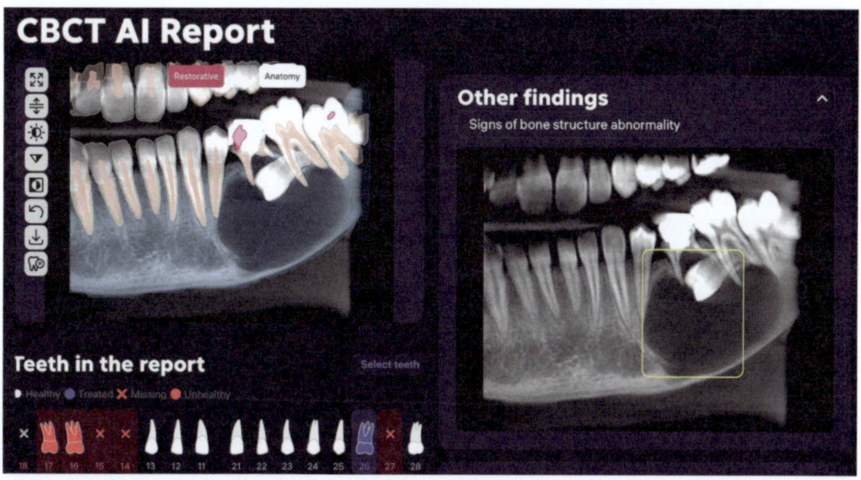

Fig. 3.15 AI-driven CBCT report (Diagnocat) of the case of Fig. 3.14, classifying the existing radiolucent lesion as "bone abnormality," rather then being associated to a specific tooth

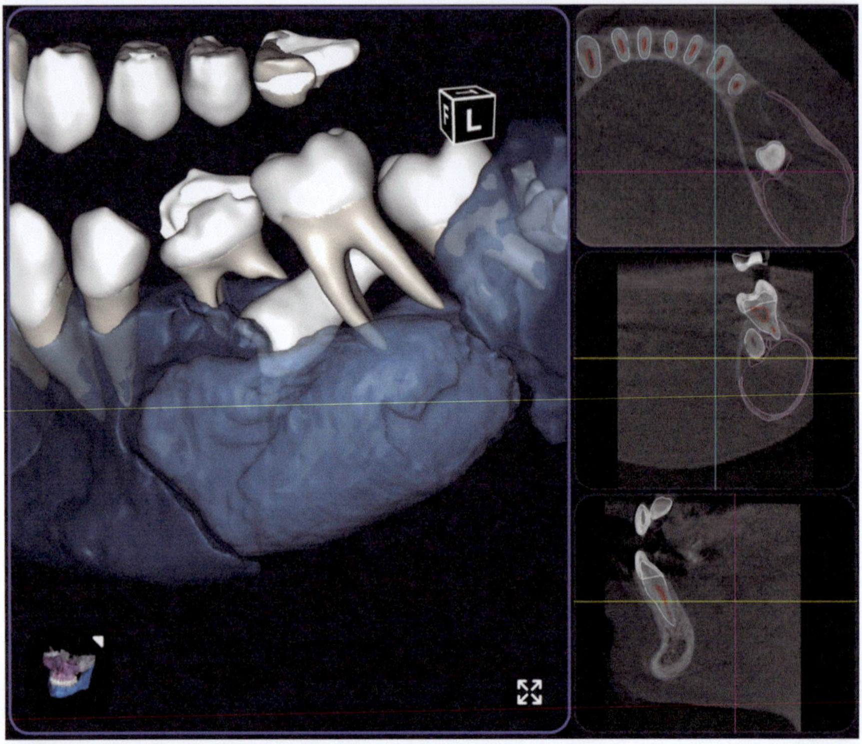

Fig. 3.16 3D model AI of the case of Figs. 3.14 and 3.15. The lesion was confirmed by histological analysis to be an OKC associated with tooth 75

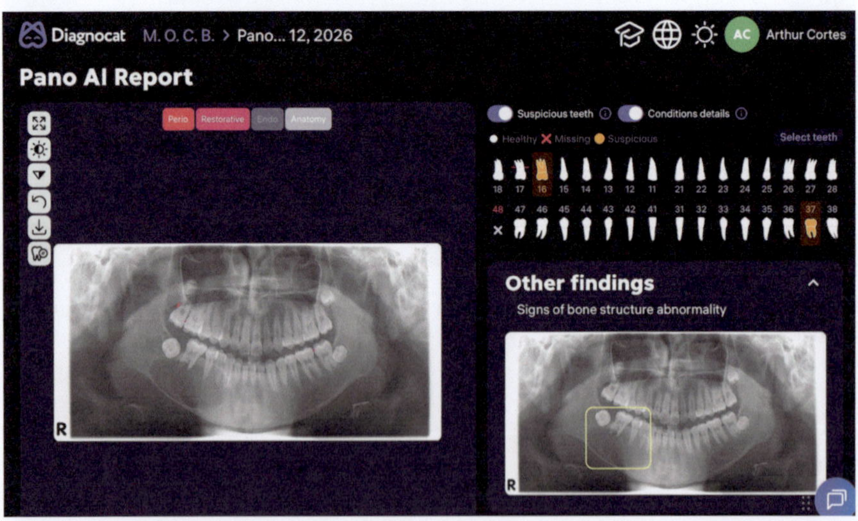

Fig. 3.17 Pano AI report (Diagnocat) of a case of OKC. The cyst on right posterior mandible was classified as "bone abnormality," rather than being associated to a specific tooth. However, the lesion on the right posterior maxilla superimposed to the maxillary sinus to the zygomatic bone was not detected by the AI tool

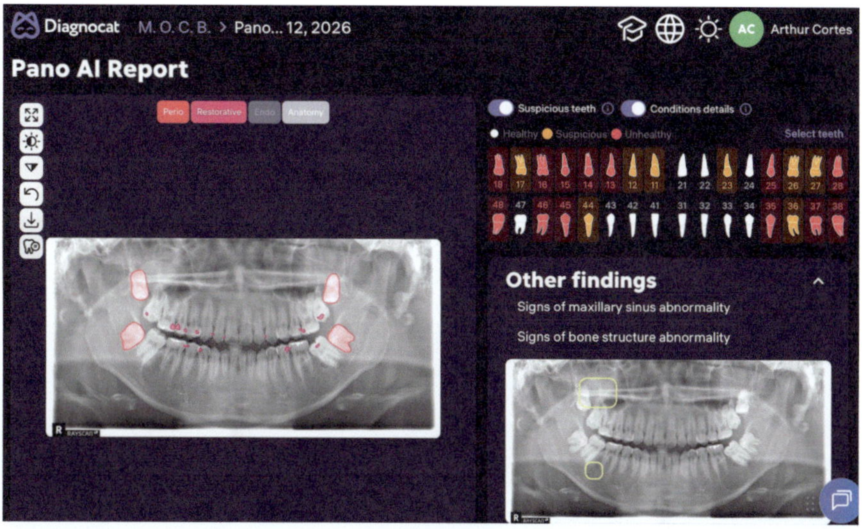

Fig. 3.18 Pano AI report (Diagnocat) of a case of multiple OKCs. The cyst on the right posterior mandible was classified as "bone abnormality," rather than being associated to a specific tooth. However, the lesion on the left posterior mandibular body was not detected by the AI tool. Note that an antral pseudocyst was also detected as a "sinus abnormality," on the right maxillary sinus

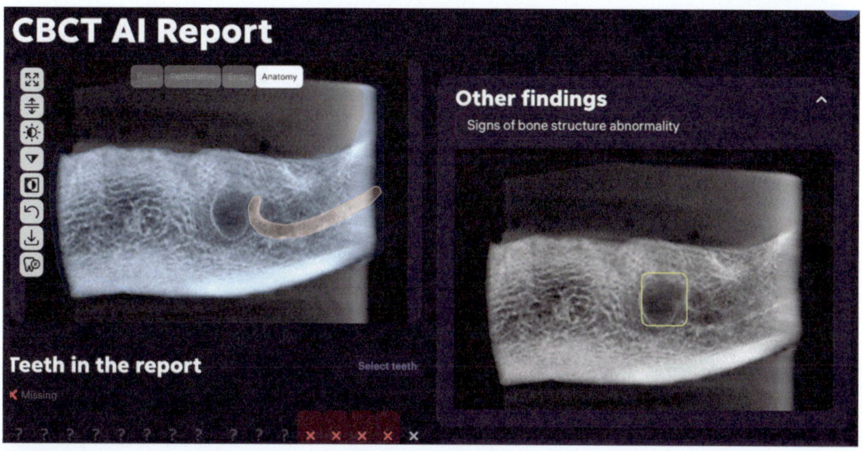

Fig. 3.19 AI-driven CBCT report (Diagnocat) of an edentulous patient, classifying an existing radiolucent lesion as "bone abnormality," rather than being associated to a specific tooth. The lesion was confirmed by histological analysis to be an OKC

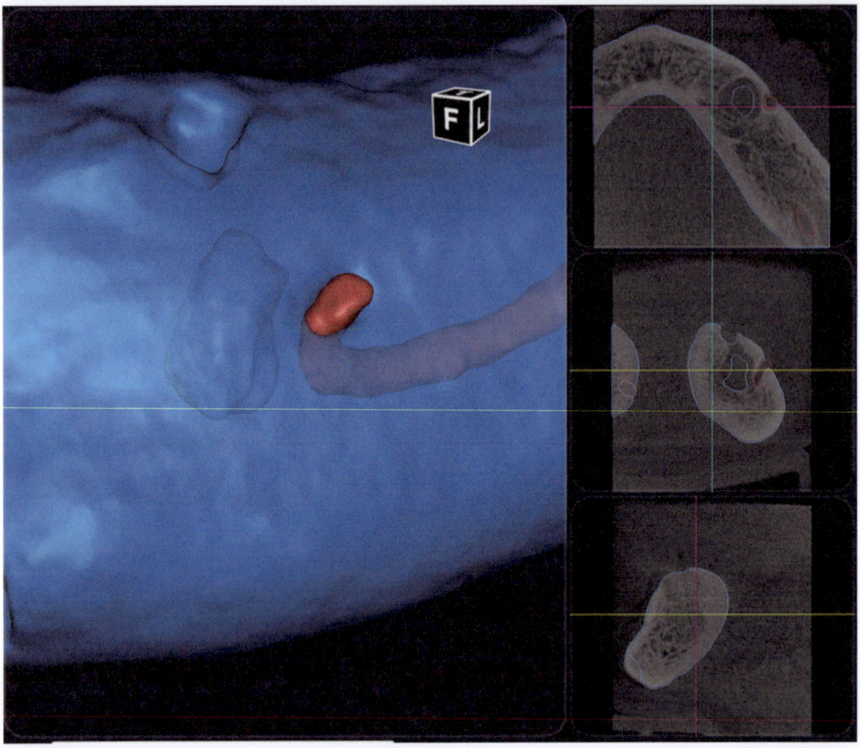

Fig. 3.20 3D model AI of the case of Fig. 3.19. The lesion was confirmed by histological analysis to be an orthokeratinized odontogenic cyst, which has characteristics similar to OKCs. Note the proximity of the lesion to the mental foramen and to a bone defect on the alveolar crest

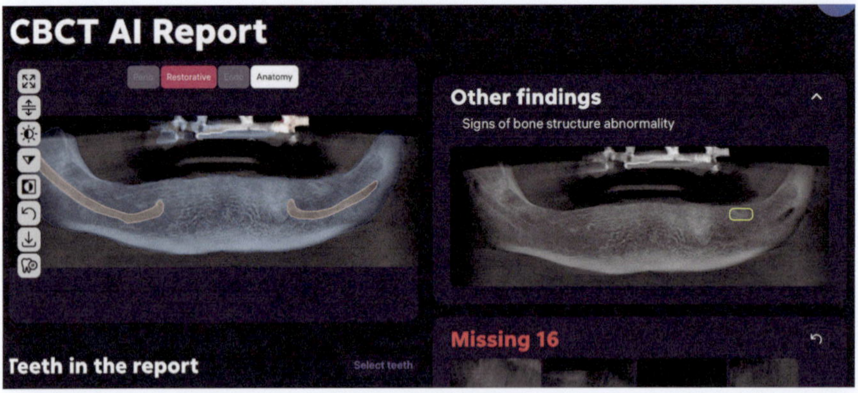

Fig. 3.21 AI-driven report (Diagnocat) of a second CBCT scan taken after surgical removal of the lesion of Figs. 3.19 and 3.20 (surgery by Dr. Adam Bartolo). For this scan, the AI algorithm only classified an existing area of bone sclerosis as a new "bone structure abnormality." Note the healing of the lesion site

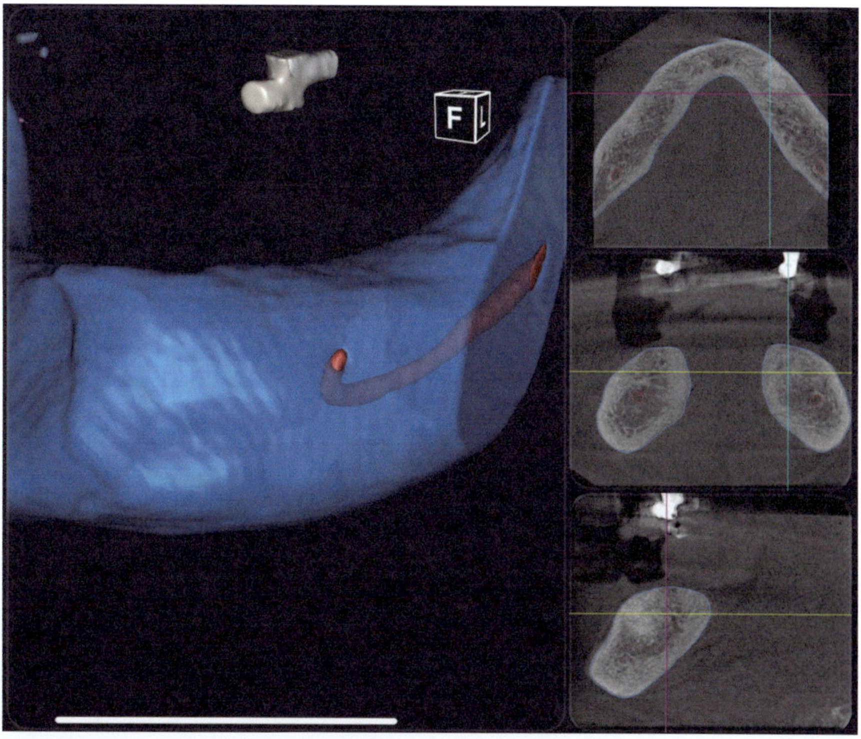

Fig. 3.22 3D model AI of the second CBCT of the case of Figs. 3.19, 3.20, and 3.21. Note the healing of the alveolar bone at the lesion site

Although most of the radiolucent lesions from currently available research have an odontogenic origin, several AI deep convolutional neural networks (DCNNs) have also proven useful to detect nasopalatine duct cysts and periapical cysts on panoramic radiographs [14]. The aforementioned study included a total of 1209 panoramic radiographs, for which the DCNN systems (Fig. 3.23) tested presented satisfactory diagnostic performance in comparison with two general dental practitioners. Of note, one of the DCNN systems (EfficientDet-D3) presented accuracy, sensitivity, and specificity higher than 90%, as explained in detail below (Fig. 3.24) [14].

Radiographically, a nasopalatine duct cyst is typically a well-defined, heart-shaped, oval, or round radiolucency between the roots of the central maxillary incisors. It is usually found in the anterior maxilla, is generally painless, and can be an incidental finding on dental radiographs. Differential diagnoses include a wide incisive foramen or inflammatory periapical lesions, reason why pulp vitality tests are essential to rule out a dental origin. The superimposition of the anterior nasal spine and the narrow focal through area on panoramic radiographs can represent challenges in the diagnosis of this lesion. To address these diagnostic challenges, the AI networks mentioned in the previous paragraph were used, following two main important processes:

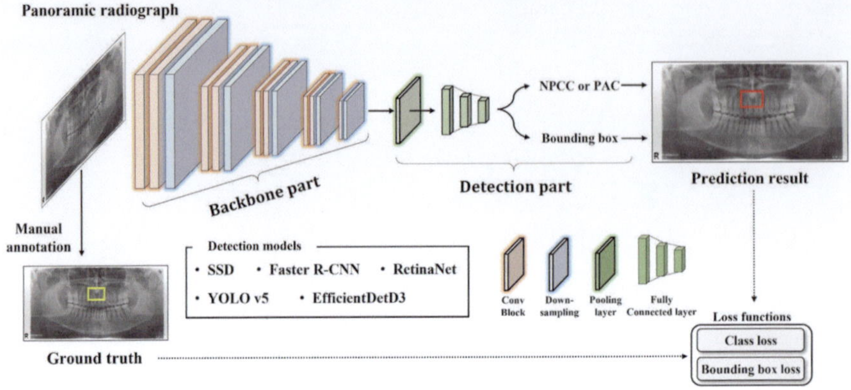

Fig. 3.23 Flowchart of the AI deep learning approaches developed for detection of nasopalatine duct cyst and periapical cyst on panoramic radiographs. NPCC, nasopalatine canal cyst; PAC, periapical cyst

Fig. 3.24 Detection of nasopalatine duct cyst (top) and periapical cyst (bottom) using the deep convolutional neural network system EfficientDet-D3 on panoramic radiographs. Note the comparison between the actual diagnosis (ground tooth, marked in yellow) and predicted result by the algorithm (marked in red). NPCC, nasopalatine canal cyst; PAC, periapical cyst

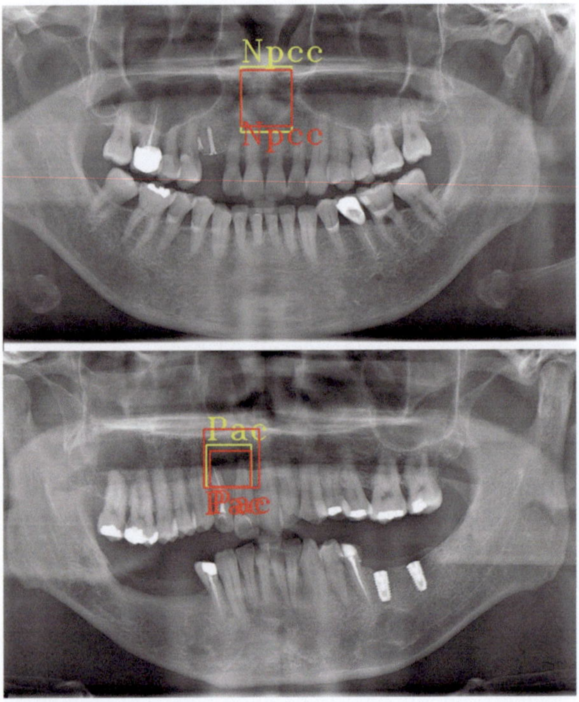

1. Data Collection and Preparation: Building the Training Ground for AI

   To teach an AI to recognize dental cysts, researchers first needed a large and reliable dataset of annotated images. The process involved collecting radiographs and meticulously preparing them for the models. The Radiograph Dataset was composed of a total of 1209 panoramic radiographs. The dataset groups were balanced, containing 606 images of NPDC and 603 images of PAC. All radiographs were sourced from the Seoul National University Dental Hospital. Every diagnosis was verified and validated against histopathologic reports from biopsy results, ensuring the "ground truth" for the AI was accurate.
2. Image Preparation Process
   (a) Image annotation: An oral and maxillofacial radiologist labeled each cyst by drawing a tight bounding box around it using the VGG Image Annotator software.
   (b) Image formatting: The original images, in DICOM format, were resized to a standard resolution of 800 × 1344 pixels for consistent training.
   (c) Data splitting: The 1209 images were divided into training (967 images), validation (121 images), and test (121 images) sets using an 8:1:1 ratio.
   (d) Data augmentation: To make the models more robust, data augmentation techniques—such as rotation, width/height shifting, and zooming—were applied to the training images. This simulates variations and helps the AI generalize better.

   With the data prepared, the next step was to select and train the AI architectures for the detection task.

The study mentioned herein did not rely on a single AI model but instead conducted a comparative evaluation of five different deep convolutional neural network (DCNN) architectures to identify the most effective one. These models fall into two main categories:

- Single-stage detectors: These models treat object detection as a simple regression problem, performing it in a single step to predict both the bounding box location and the class (NPDC or PAC) simultaneously. The models tested were EfficientDet-D3, YOLO v5, RetinaNet, and SSD.
- Two-Stage Detectors: These models first use a "region proposal network" to generate regions of interest where a lesion might be and then classify the object within that region. The model tested was Faster R-CNN.

Based on the results, EfficientDet-D3 was identified as the model that achieved the highest performance, with approximately 94% diagnostic accuracy. This top-performing model was then advanced to a head-to-head comparison with human clinicians. This comparison analyzed diagnostic errors and revealed a fundamental and clinically significant difference between AI and human practitioners. The most common AI error was generating false positives (detecting additional lesions where none existed), often by misidentifying normal anatomic structures like the lateral fossa or radiolucent airspaces. In contrast, the most common and critical error made by the GPs was generating false negatives (missing an existing NPDC lesion and marking the image as "no lesion"). This distinction is a very important insight of the study. In a clinical screening setting, a false negative could lead to more dangerous situations than a false positive. A false positive prompts further review, which would quickly reveal the finding as a normal structure, causing no patient harm. A false negative, however, leads to a missed diagnosis, delayed treatment, and potentially worse patient outcomes.

3.1.4 Differentiating Types of Lesions with AI

A clinically significant application of AI is in differential diagnosis, particularly distinguishing between pathologies that may appear similar on radiographs but require different treatment approaches. A previous study demonstrated a method using CBCT images to distinguish between periapical cysts and granulomas [15]. This capability carries immense clinical value, as it can help clinicians identify periapical granulomas that are likely to heal following nonsurgical root canal treatment. This differentiation allows for the avoidance of unnecessary surgical intervention, aligning with a more conservative and patient-centric approach to care.

Another type of alteration with different pathological causes and imaging manifestations is the opacification of the maxillary sinus. Although the Diagnocat software is usually able to detect these alterations, they are usually classified as "signs of maxillary sinus abnormalities" by the software AI report (Fig. 3.25). As usual, the professional should be the one investigating possible tooth-related causes and the radiographic diagnosis of the alteration.

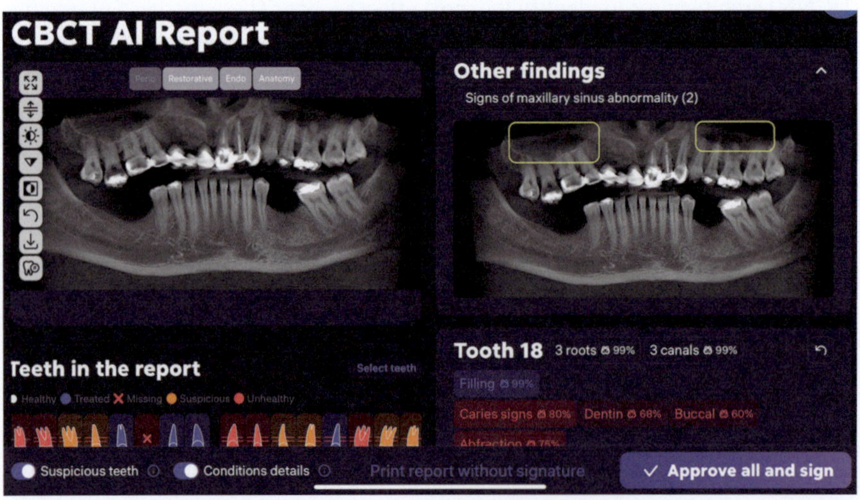

Fig. 3.25 CBCT AI report (Diagnocat) detecting areas of maxillary sinus opacification, suggestive of sinus membrane thickening

3.2 Automated Diagnosis of Lesions on the Oral Mucosa

The diagnosis of oral mucosal lesions presents a critical and persistent challenge for clinicians, complicated by the diverse manifestations of these conditions and the potential for malignant transformation. This challenge is particularly acute in the context of oral cancer, which accounts for over 377,000 newly diagnosed cases and 177,000 deaths annually worldwide. Diagnostic delays can have severe consequences for patient outcomes. Studies indicate that patients may consult up to four different specialists over an average of 16.8 months before receiving a definitive clinical diagnosis. Such delays are especially detrimental for oral cancer, where early diagnosis can elevate 5-year survival rates from approximately 60% to over 80%.

To address the complexity of such diagnosis, clinical algorithms have been developed as tools to support practitioners. In a healthcare context, a clinical algorithm is a structured flowchart that represents a sequence of decisions designed to guide the diagnostic and management processes by clinician. By providing a concise, systematic approach, these algorithms aim to save time, improve efficiency, and enhance the consistency of clinical decision-making. Despite their potential, the quality, applicability, and overall state of development of these tools for oral lesions have not been comprehensively synthesized.

A relatively recent scoping review revealed that the field of diagnostic algorithms for oral lesions is highly specialized [16]. Rather than universal diagnostic tools, researchers have developed a series of distinct algorithms tailored to specific categories of lesions. This specialization reflects the clinical reality that different lesion types present with unique characteristics and requires targeted diagnostic pathways.

3.2.1 Existing AI Tools to Detect Oral Mucosal Lesions

The aforementioned scoping review included a total of 17 algorithms, covering ten distinct categories of oral mucosal alterations [16]: exophytic lesions (two algorithms), oral immune-mediated disorders (one algorithm), oral pigmented lesions (three algorithms), white lesions (three algorithms), gingival growth or swelling (one algorithm), oral lichen planus (one algorithm), oral lesions of viral, bacterial, and fungal origin (one algorithm), ulcerative lesions and recurrent oral ulcers (two algorithms), desquamative gingivitis and associated mucocutaneous diseases (two algorithms), and general oral mucosal lesions (one algorithm).

The single most significant knowledge gap identified in the review is that none of the 17 identified algorithms had been validated in a clinical setting. Algorithm development is only the first step; validation is the essential process of testing whether the tool performs accurately, reliably, and safely in the real world with actual patients. Without validation through rigorous clinical trials and consensus-building among multiple experts, the diagnostic accuracy and safety profile of these tools remain empirically unverified.

Beyond formal validation, none of the studies had assessed the clinical utility of their algorithms—that is, whether they actually improve diagnostic outcomes, save time, or are practical for clinicians to use in a busy practice. One of the related studies that intended to test the reproducibility and reliability of their pediatric decision tree stands as a rare and notable exception, highlighting an awareness of this crucial but unfulfilled next step [17]. Nonetheless, the general lack of validation and utility assessment indicates that these tools, while academically analyzed, are not yet ready for clinical implementation.

Another recent study aimed to develop and evaluate DCNN models for the automated classification of glossitis and oral squamous cell carcinoma (OSCC) from clinical tongue photographs [18]. The four DCNN architectures tested were fine-tuned utilizing a dataset of 652 images by means of transfer learning. The results demonstrated strong performance for glossitis classification, with accuracy values ranging around 90%. For OSCC detection, the models achieved near-perfect performance, with two of the DCNN models tested reaching 100% of accuracy. The findings of this study indicate that DCNN models, augmented with Grad-CAM for interpretability, provide a robust and accurate tool for AI-driven tongue diagnosis. The study highlights the significant potential of this technology for enhancing early detection of oral pathologies and expanding access to healthcare by means of remote and telemedicine-based applications.

3.2.2 Future Directions and Implications

To advance the field of AI in oral diagnosis from theoretical algorithm design to the creation of practical and validated clinical tools, the research community must address the identified gaps with a clear and concerted strategy. The following steps are essential for building a foundation of evidence-based diagnostic support.

3.2.2.1 Clinical Validation

The most urgent priority is to conduct research that investigates the clinical validity, utility, and usability of existing algorithms. This requires designing studies where these tools are tested in real-world clinical settings to measure their diagnostic accuracy, impact on decision-making, and practicality from the perspective of the clinical end user.

3.2.2.2 Pedagogical Applications

Once validated, these algorithms hold significant potential as teaching tools. They can be used to assist dental students and residents in learning the complex process of differential diagnosis. By providing a structured framework, these tools can help trainees develop and refine their clinical reasoning skills in a systematic way.

3.2.2.3 Standardization and Integration

To overcome the existing barriers for clinical adoption, the development of a centralized repository of standardized and validated clinical decision-making algorithms is recommended. Such a resource would ensure that clinicians have access to trustworthy tools, being able to provide a valuable, knowledge-based foundation for informing the development of next-generation, AI-based diagnostic aids. By pursuing these directions, the field would be able to move toward producing diagnostic aids that are not only well-designed but also rigorously tested and clinically effective.

3.3 Clinical Case Studies

3.3.1 Aggressive Dentigerous Cyst with Perforation of the Base of the Mandible (Case by Dr. Adam Bartolo; Scientific Review by Dr. Nicholas Busuttil Dougall)

As previously mentioned in this chapter, dentigerous cysts (DCs) occur in association with unerupted teeth, mostly mandibular third molars (75% of findings) and second premolars, as well as maxillary third molars and canines. Rarely, DCs are associated with supernumerary teeth and odontomas and are most commonly seen in 10- to 30-year-old patients with a slight male predilection. The lesions are usually asymptomatic and often detected as incidental findings. However, they can sometimes grow considerably in size and present with bony expansion, which is usually painless until the occurrence of secondary infection. Pathological fracture of the jaws due to DCs is rare [19].

In the present case, a 13-year-old male patient with no relevant medical conditions presented with a panoramic radiograph showing a large, well-defined, unilocular, radiolucent lesion in the left posterior body of the mandible with a clear demarcated sclerotic border around the crown of an impacted and ectopic mandibular second molar (Fig. 3.26). Considering the position and presentation of the cyst, a CBCT was indicated for surgical planning and to help establishing a differential diagnosis list. CBCT was taken with a Orthophos SL (Sirona) using an imaging protocol composed of s 85 kVp, 10 mA, and 5 s, while the low dose (LD) exposure protocol 85 kVp, 10 mA, 5 s of exposure, field-of-view of 5 × 5.5 cm^2 and a voxel size of 0.16 × 0.16 × 0.16 mm^3. The resulting multiplanar reconstruction (MPR) was analyzed with a commercial AI software (Diagnocat), showing bone plate expansion, perforation of the lingual aspect of the base of the mandible by the tooth apices, as well as mandibular canal displacement (Fig. 3.27). These are characteristics of a large slow growing cyst. A 3D-reconstructed AI model was also rendered to orient the treatment planning for accessing and surgically removing the lesion (Fig. 3.28).

Treatment options for DC in adults usually consist of enucleation and extraction of affected tooth. If the lesion is very large or very close to an important structure such as the inferior alveolar nerve, coronectomy with cystectomy or cyst decompression and marsupialization can be performed in the order of preference. While this approach ensures a safe removal of the cyst, it could also substantially delay treatment completion.

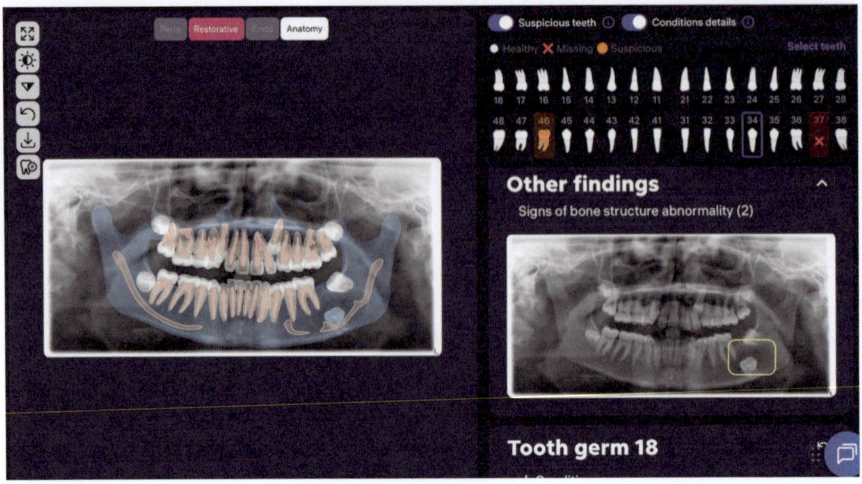

Fig. 3.26 AI report (Diagnocat) of the initial panoramic radiograph detecting classifying the cystic lesion associated with the impacted second molar as "bone structure abnormality"

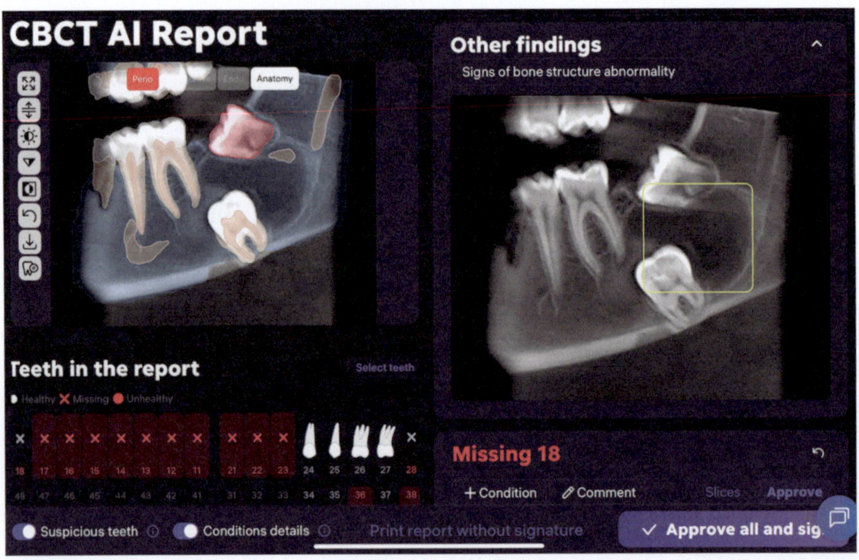

Fig. 3.27 AI report (Diagnocat) of the preoperative CBCT detecting classifying the cystic lesion as "bone structure abnormality." Note the disrupted segmentation of the mandibular canal

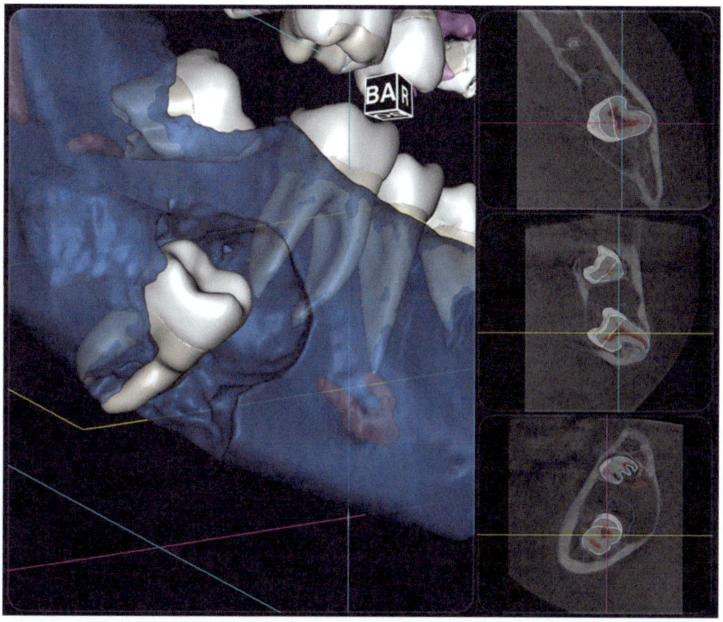

Fig. 3.28 Lingual view of the 3D AI model of the CBCT. Note the lingual plate expansion and thinning

In children and preadolescents, treatment should focus around allowing the affected tooth to erupt spontaneously or through orthodontic means. Several articles in the literature support decompression and marsupialization of the cyst. Apart from leading the lesion to decrease in size and reducing damage risk to adjacent structures, this approach also encourages spontaneous eruption of the teeth involved [20]. However, apart from the disadvantages already mentioned for adults, child patients may present the added difficulty of noncompliance leading to possible cyst cavity infection and other complications. An even more serious disadvantage is leaving the cyst lining behind, which may be different from the lining examined histopathologically. Recent studies have also shown approaches where the complete removal of dentigerous cysts is carried out while preserving the associated teeth in situ [19]. This allows for fast treatment with minimal morbidity while preserving the tooth for spontaneous/orthodontic eruption.

As differential diagnosis, odontogenic keratocyst (OKC) and ameloblastoma are usually considered for dentigerous cysts. In the present case, however, OKC was more likely as a hypothesis because of the patient's age, considerable resorption of the bone in the mesial-distal direction, and location in the posterior body of the mandible. The lesion was also associated with expansion of buccal and lingual plates and severe inferior displacement of the mandibular canal and the associated tooth. The origin of the lesion appeared to be slightly below the CEJ.

Histopathological analysis of the lesion should always be carried out to determine if further management is needed. For this purpose, a container with 10%

neutral buffered formalin should be available at the time of the surgery, ensuring that the volume of formalin is at least ten times the volume of the tissue specimen. After opening a flap, the cyst was located and could be carefully enucleated, together with the associated tooth 37, which was deemed to have poor potential for proper eruption. Primary closure of tissues was obtained with monofilament sutures, and the wound healed uneventfully (Fig. 3.29). The definitive diagnosis of a DC was confirmed by histological analysis from the biopsy, so no further treatment was needed. A postoperative panoramic radiograph taken 6 months after the enucleation showed satisfactory bone healing and maturation (Fig. 3.30).

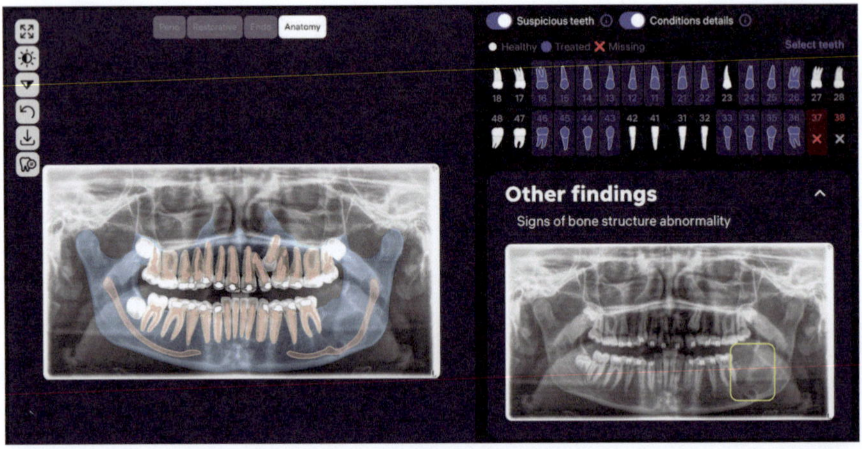

Fig. 3.29 AI report (Diagnocat) of the immediate postoperative panoramic radiograph indicating the site of the removed lesion as a "bone structure abnormality"

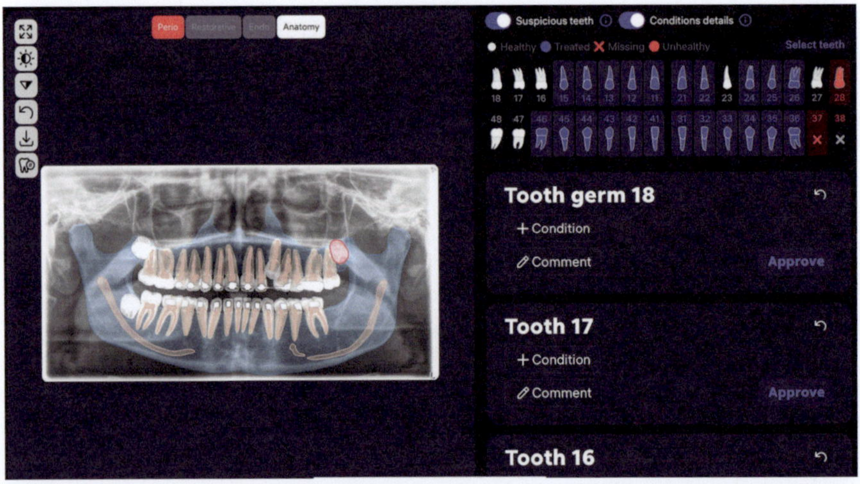

Fig. 3.30 AI report (Diagnocat) of the 6-month follow-up panoramic radiograph, confirming satisfactory alveolar bone healing at the treated site

3.3.2 Apicoectomy of a Large Radicular Cyst Contiguous to the Nasopalatine Canal (Case by Prof. Arthur Cortes)

Radicular cysts represent the most common cystic lesions affecting the tooth root, presenting a frequent challenge in endodontic practice. Understanding the escalating hierarchy of treatment, from conservative nonsurgical approaches to definitive surgical intervention, is a cornerstone of effective clinical management. The decision to progress to surgery is critical, and evaluating the necessity of each surgical step is essential for optimizing patient outcomes and clinical efficiency.

The conventional treatment pathway for persistent periapical lesions is methodical and conservative. The first line of defense is conventional root canal therapy (RCT), followed by nonsurgical retreatment if the initial therapy fails. Endodontic surgery is reserved for cases where these conservative measures are unsuccessful, in cases of cystic lesions that keep growing, or when retreatment is complicated by factors such as a large intracanal post.

Standard endodontic surgery for these conditions involves a dual procedure: apical resection (apicoectomy) and retrograde filling. An apicoectomy consists of the surgical removal of the 2–3 mm of the contaminated apex of tooth, an area often containing lateral and accessory canals that can harbor bacteria. Following this resection, a retrograde filling can be placed to seal the root canal system apically. The primary purpose of this seal is to prevent any remaining bacteria from leaking out of the root canal into the surrounding periapical tissues, thereby promoting healing [21]. Reported survival rates for these conventional procedures range from 69% to 76% [22], underscoring the critical nature of optimizing every aspect of treatment. However, the necessity of this retrograde filling, particularly in cases where high-quality orthograde endodontic treatment has already been performed, has become a subject of clinical debate.

Reevaluating the necessity of retrograde filling is a strategic clinical question aimed at simplifying surgical protocols, reducing resource utilization, and avoiding potential complications associated with filling materials without compromising treatment success. This approach challenges a long-held component of endodontic surgery by questioning its universal applicability, especially in the context of radicular cyst enucleation.

The main hypothesis is that the prognosis for teeth affected by cysts can be highly favorable after apicoectomy alone, provided that a high-quality and definitive endodontic treatment has been completed beforehand. This premise suggests that if the coronal and middle portions of the root canal system are effectively disinfected and sealed, the primary source of periapical inflammation is already controlled, potentially rendering an additional apical seal redundant.

This reevaluation is further supported by the clinical challenges and potential drawbacks associated with the retrograde filling procedure itself. In a clinical setting, achieving a perfect apical seal can be difficult due to factors such as persistent bleeding and limited visibility at the surgical site. These conditions can hinder the precise manipulation of retrograde filling materials like mineral trioxide aggregate (MTA), potentially leading to voids or an incomplete filling that compromises the seal [23].

In the present case, a 63-year-old female patient with no relevant medical conditions presented with tenderness to percussion on the endodontically treated tooth 12. The single most important preoperative requirement is that the current endodontic treatment of the tooth undergoing the procedure must have high-quality and adequate conditions. This was confirmed via CBCT multiplanar reconstruction and supported by the respective AI-driven report (Diagnocat), which confirmed the presence of a dense and well-compacted root canal obturation extending to the desired length (Figs. 3.31 and 3.32). This enables the possibility of a treatment plan based on apicoectomy without retrograde filling [23].

The surgical procedure was then performed by accessing the root apex, followed by apicoectomy performed with a spherical bur under irrigation with saline solution (Fig. 3.33). This step was performed simultaneously with the complete enucleation (removal of lesion along with the surrounding epithelial wall) of the radicular cyst with no subsequent retrograde filling, following a previously described methodology that led to satisfactory clinical outcomes [24]. In this case, this surgical approach could be successfully performed despite the proximity of the lesion to the nasopalatine canal. By removing the entire cystic lesion along with the problematic root apex, the pathological stimulus is eliminated. The resulting cavity was then grafted with a particulate synthetic bone substitute basically composed of biphasic calcium phosphate (Boneceramic, Straumann), which is an adequate material to graft bone defects even immediately after the removal of a lesion [25]. The diagnosis of radicular cyst was confirmed histologically. A postoperative panoramic radiograph taken after 3 months showed satisfactory healing conditions of the lesion site (Fig. 3.34). No complications were noted in a total follow-up period of 3 years.

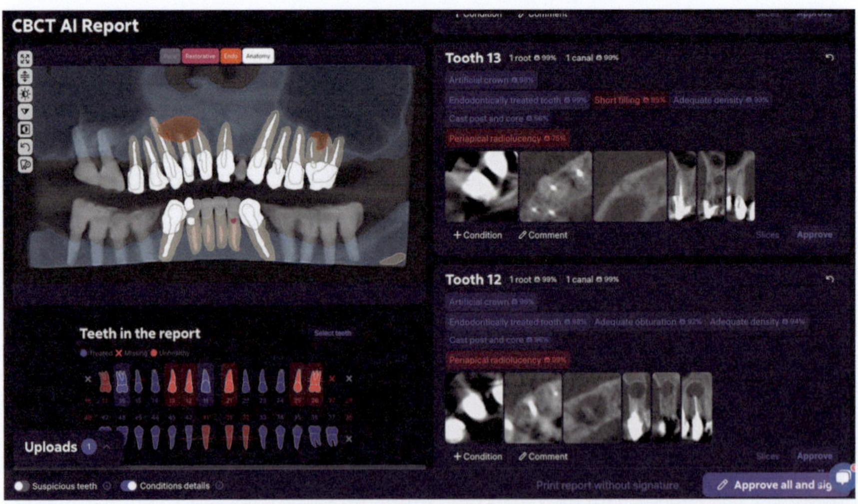

Fig. 3.31 CBCT AI report (Diagnocat) showing a well-limited, homogeneous, round, periapical hypodense (radiolucent) lesion with corticated borders associated with tooth 12, which presented satisfactory condition of the existing endodontic treatment

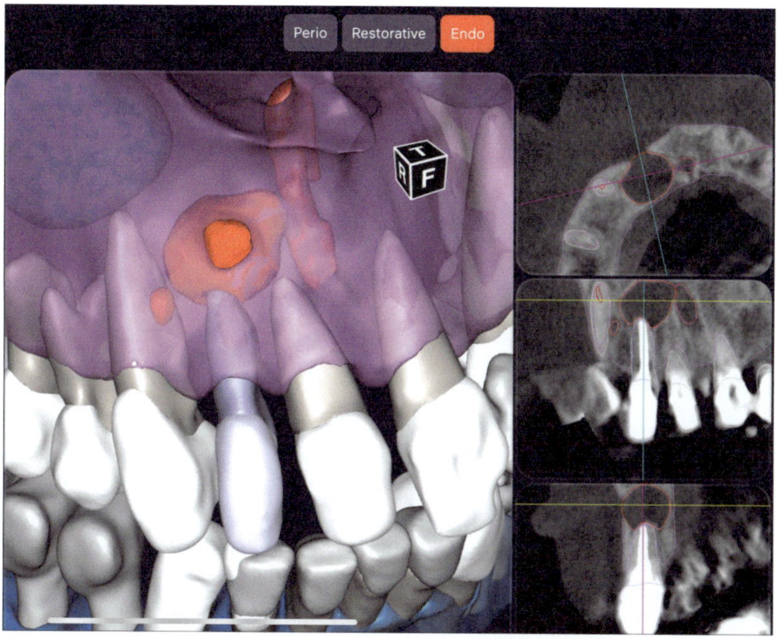

Fig. 3.32 3D-reconstructed model of the case with automated segmentations showing that the lesion was contiguous with the nasopalatine canal wall and associated with buccal plate resorption, suggestive of radicular cyst. Note that the lesion was not affecting the lamina duras of the adjacent teeth 13 and 11

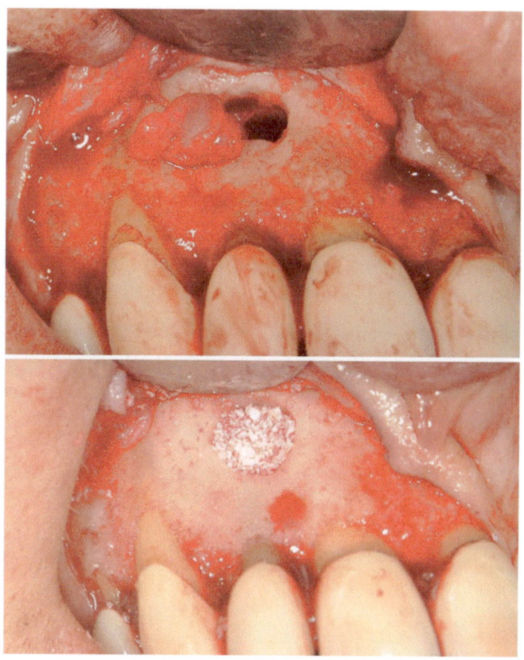

Fig. 3.33 Apicoectomy approach performed along with lesion enucleation (top), with subsequent bone grafting of the resulting cavity (bottom)

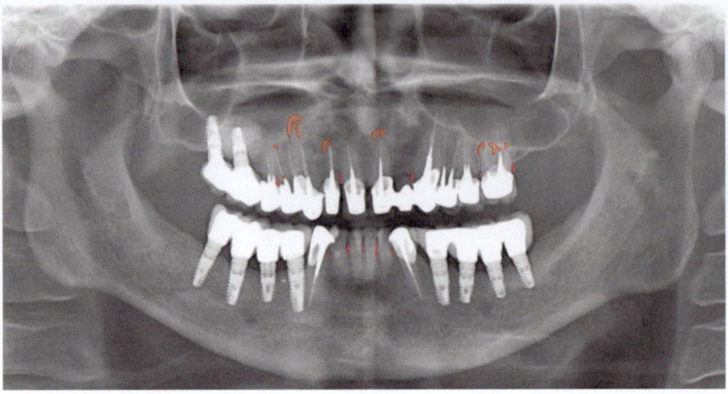

Fig. 3.34 AI report (Diagnocat) of the 3-month follow-up panoramic radiograph, confirming satisfactory process of alveolar bone healing at the treated site

3.3.3 CBCT Volumetric Follow-Up of Multiple Conditions (Technique Report by Prof. Arthur Cortes)

In the present case, two CBCT scans of the same patient taken in different time point (2 years apart) to diagnose and plan different treatments were retrospectively analyzed (Fig. 3.35). The CBCT DICOM image files from the CBCT scans were obtained using the same device (ProMax, Planmeca) with the same imaging protocol (90 KvP, 8 mA, 0.2-mm slice thickness and 0.02-mm^3 voxel size). Both scans could be compared regarding several remaining conditions with the aid of an AI-driven software program (Diagnocat), including maxillary sinus opacification (Fig. 3.36) and the volume of a periapical hypodense or radiolucent area on tooth 24, which was not treated during the period between the scans.

The volume of this radiolucent area was automatically measured in cubic millimeters by the AI software on both scans, showing that the area increased in size over time (Figs. 3.37 and 3.38). All volumetric measurements were also performed by an oral radiologist with a semiautomatic segmentation procedure using a robust DICOM viewer (OsiriX MD, Pixmeo; Fig. 3.39) following a previous methodology [26], which involved the definition of an outlined volumetric region of interest containing the radiolucent area (Fig. 3.40). It was noted that the lesion volume was slightly overestimated by the AI software. Future prospective research studies are recommended to assess the impact of different imaging protocols and volumetric measurement methods on the diagnosis and follow-up of periapical lesions.

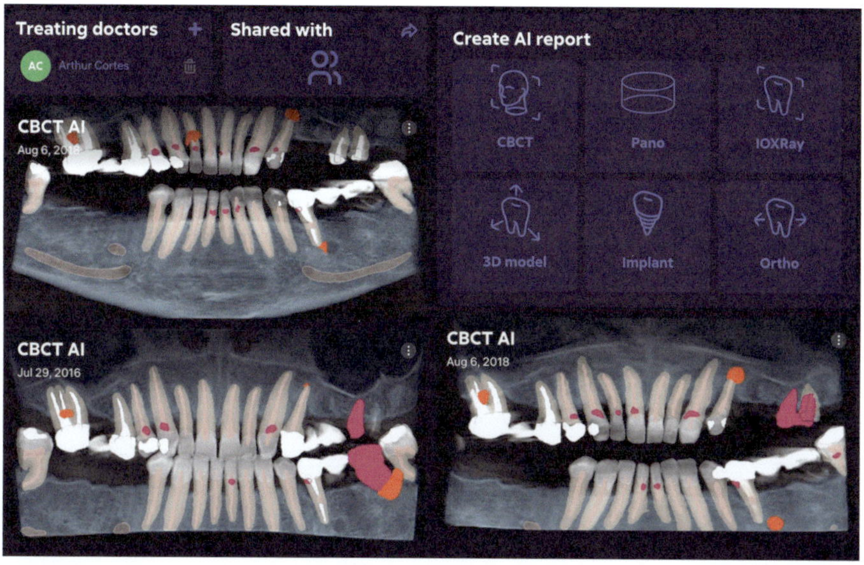

Fig. 3.35 AI reports (Diagnocat) of CBCT scans taken in 2016 (maxilla) and 2018 (maxilla and mandible)

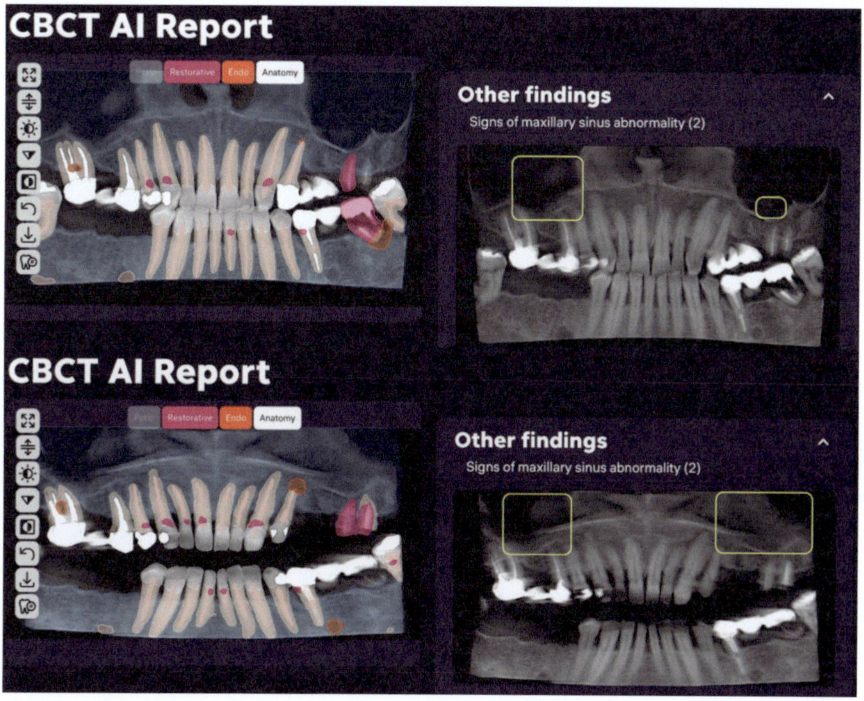

Fig. 3.36 Comparison of the CBCT AI reports (Diagnocat). Note that the left maxillary sinus hyperdense (radiopaque) area and the periapical lesion of tooth 24 increased in size Also note that other conditions were depicted differently between the scans

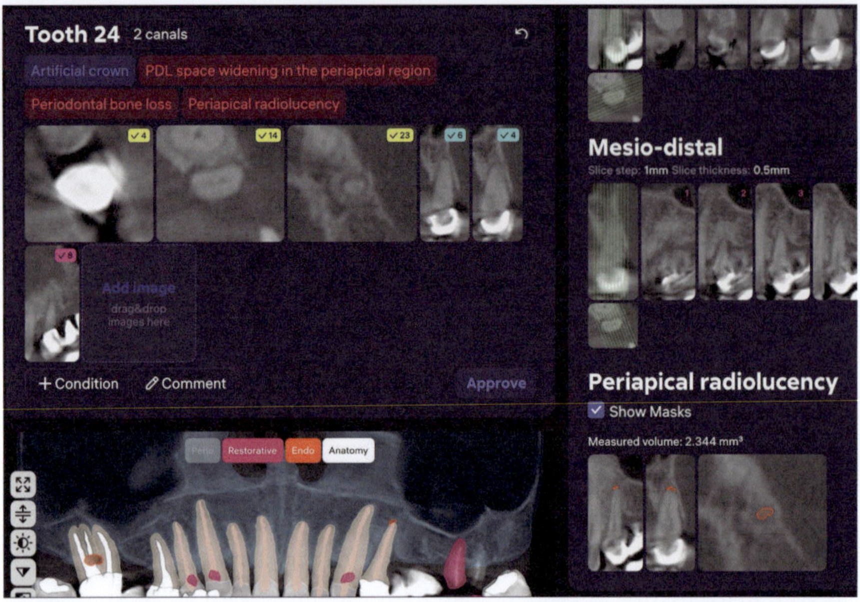

Fig. 3.37 AI automated volumetric measurements of the periapical radiolucent area shown in the first CBCT scan

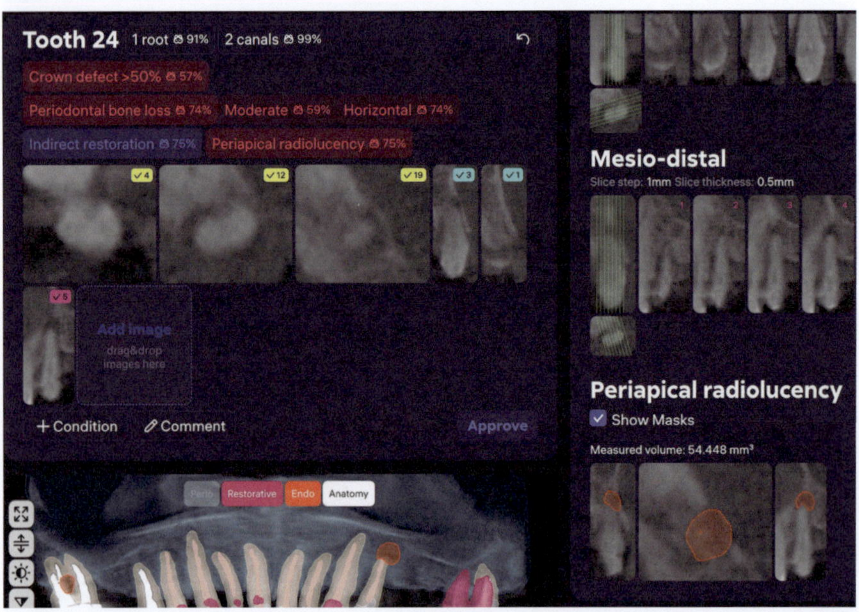

Fig. 3.38 AI automated volumetric measurements of the periapical radiolucent area shown in the second CBCT scan. Note the difference in volume between the scans

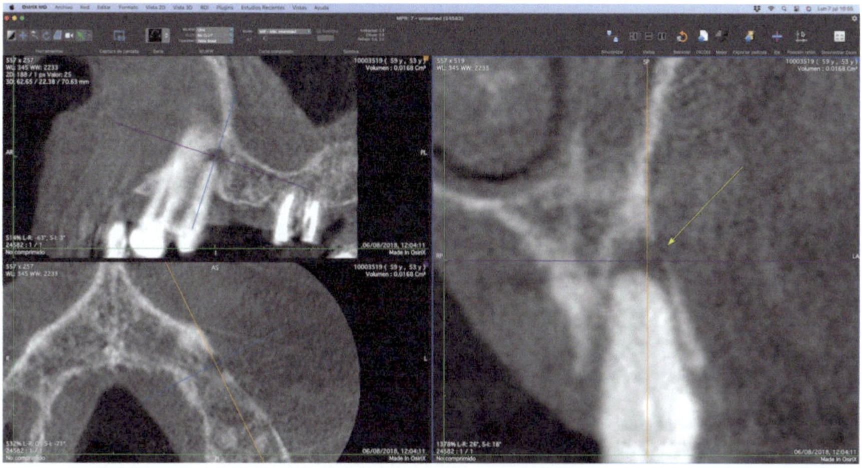

Fig. 3.39 Screenshot of the OsiriX MD software, used by the oral radiologist to assess the second CBCT scan of the lesion, which caused buccal plate resorption (yellow arrow)

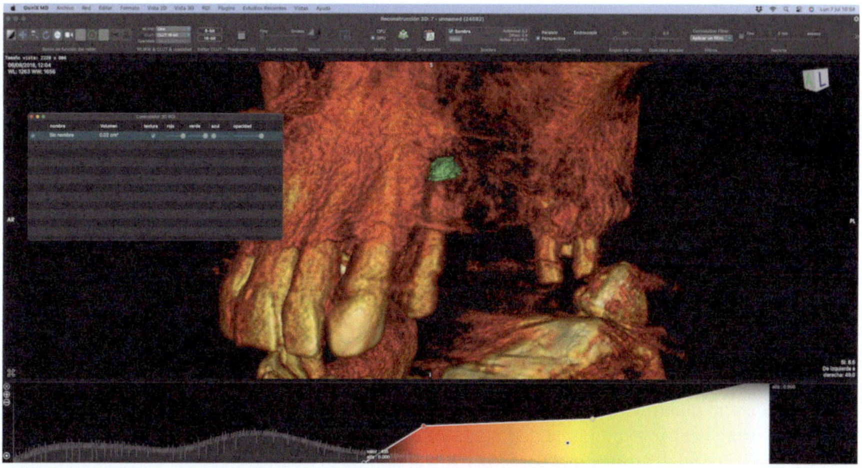

Fig. 3.40 Screenshot of the OsiriX MD software showing the volumetric measurement output of the lesion superimposed to a 3D reconstruction of the second CBCT scan

References

1. Dennis D, Suebnukarn S, Heo MS, Abidin T, Nurliza C, Yanti N, Farahanny W, Prasetia W, Batubara FY. Artificial intelligence application in endodontics: a narrative review. Imaging Sci Dent. 2024;54(4):305–12. https://doi.org/10.5624/isd.20240321.
2. Cortes ARG. Digital dentistry: a step-by-step guide and case atlas. Hoboken, NJ: Wiley; 2022. https://doi.org/10.1002/9781119852025.

3. Shalalvand M, Haghanifar S, Moudi E, Bijani A. Deep learning-assisted CBCT segmentation provides reliable volumetric assessment of mandibular defects compared with micro-CT for 3D printing and surgical planning. Sci Rep. 2025;15(1):37561. https://doi.org/10.1038/s41598-025-24748-4.
4. Ba-Hattab R, Barhom N, Osman SAA, Naceur I, Odeh A, Asad A, Al-Najdi SARN, Ameri E, Daer A, Silva RLBD, et al. Detection of periapical lesions on panoramic radiographs using deep learning. Appl Sci. 2023;13(3):1516. https://doi.org/10.3390/app13031516.
5. Kaygısız ÖF, Uranbey Ö, Gürsoytrak B, Gür ZB, Çiçek A, Canbal MA. A deep learning approach based on YOLO v11 for automatic detection of jaw cysts. BMC Oral Health. 2025;25(1):1518. https://doi.org/10.1186/s12903-025-06767-9.
6. Saber S, Abou El Nasr H, Torky AA, Saif N. Automated assessment of periapical health based on the radiographic periapical index using YOLOv8, YOLOv11, and YOLOv12 one-stage object detection algorithms. Sci Rep. 2025;15(1):36487. https://doi.org/10.1038/s41598-025-21761-5.
7. Pauwels R, Brasil DM, Yamasaki MC, Jacobs R, Bosmans H, Freitas DQ, Haiter-Neto F. Artificial intelligence for detection of periapical lesions on intraoral radiographs: comparison between convolutional neural networks and human observers. Oral Surg Oral Med Oral Pathol Oral Radiol. 2021;131(5):610–6. https://doi.org/10.1016/j.oooo.2021.01.018.
8. Endres MG, Hillen F, Salloumis M, Sedaghat AR, Niehues SM, Quatela O, et al. Development of a deep learning algorithm for periapical disease detection in dental radiographs. Diagnostics (Basel). 2020;10:430. https://doi.org/10.3390/diagnostics10060430.
9. Orhan K, Bayrakdar IS, Ezhov M, Kravtsov A, Özyürek T. Evaluation of artificial intelligence for detecting periapical pathosis on cone-beam computed tomography scans. Int Endod J. 2020;53:680–9. https://doi.org/10.1111/iej.13265.
10. Karobari MI, Adil AH, Mathur A, Snigdha NT. Applications and clinical translation of artificial intelligence in CBCT-based detection of endodontic lesions: a scoping review. Oral Radiol. 2025. https://doi.org/10.1007/s11282-025-00876-5.
11. Setzer FC, Shi KJ, Zhang Z, Yan H, Yoon H, Mupparapu M, Li J. Artificial intelligence for the computer-aided detection of periapical lesions in cone-beam computed tomographic images. J Endodont. 2020;46(7):987–93. https://doi.org/10.1016/j.joen.2020.03.025.
12. Lee JH, Kim DH, Jeong SN. Diagnosis of cystic lesions using panoramic and cone beam computed tomographic images based on deep learning neural network. Oral Dis. 2020;26(1):152–8. https://doi.org/10.1111/odi.13223.
13. Song D, Yang S, Han JY, Kim KG, Kim ST, Yi WJ. Comparison of segmentation performance of cnns, vision transformers, and hybrid networks for paranasal sinuses with sinusitis on CT images. Sci Rep. 2025;15(1):32087. https://doi.org/10.1038/s41598-025-17266-w.
14. Lee HS, Yang S, Han JY, Kang JH, Kim JE, Huh KH, Yi WJ, Heo MS, Lee SS. Automatic detection and classification of nasopalatine duct cyst and periapical cyst on panoramic radiographs using deep convolutional neural networks. Oral Surg Oral Med Oral Pathol Oral Radiol. 2024;138(1):184–95. https://doi.org/10.1016/j.oooo.2023.09.012.
15. Okada K, Rysavy S, Flores A, Linguraru MG. Noninvasive differential diagnosis of dental periapical lesions in cone-beam CT scans. Med Phys. 2015;42:1653–65. https://doi.org/10.1118/1.4914418.
16. Al-Shehri M, Dillibabu T, Nicolau B, Magalhaes M, Makhoul N, Tamimi F, Chauvin P, Madathil S. The current state of clinical diagnostic algorithms for mucosal oral lesions: a scoping review. Oral Dis. 2025. https://doi.org/10.1111/odi.15388.
17. Guillouet C, Riou MC, Duong LT, de La Dure-Molla M, Fournier BPJ. Oral lesions of viral, bacterial, and fungal diseases in children: a decision tree. Front Pediatr. 2022;10:937808. https://doi.org/10.3389/fped.2022.937808.
18. Lee YH, Jeon S, Jung J, Auh QS, Lee JS, Chaurasia A, Noh YK. DCNN models with post-hoc interpretability for the automated detection of glossitis and OSCC on the tongue. Sci Rep. 2025;15(1):31940. https://doi.org/10.1038/s41598-025-16760-5.

19. Hauer L, Seidlová P, Merglová V, Hrusak D, Böhmová H, Posta P, Gencur J, Netolicky J. Complete removal of dentigerous cysts with preservation of associated teeth as an alternative to marsupialization in children and preadolescents. J Craniomaxillofac Surg. 2020;48(8):808–14. https://doi.org/10.1016/j.jcms.2020.05.014.
20. Allon DM, Allon I, Anavi Y, Kaplan I, Chaushu G. Decompression as a treatment of odontogenic cystic lesions in children. J Oral Maxillofac Surg. 2015;73(4):649–54. https://doi.org/10.1016/j.joms.2014.10.024.
21. Lieblich SE. Current concepts of periapical surgery: 2020 update. Oral Maxillofac Surg Clin North Am. 2020;32:571–82.
22. Ng YL, Gulabivala K. Factors that influence the outcomes of surgical endodontic treatment. Int Endod J. 2023;56(Suppl 2):116–39.
23. Villa-Machado PA, Botero-Ramírez X, Tobón-Arroyave SI. Retrospective follow-up assessment of prognostic variables associated with the outcome of periradicular surgery. Int Endod J. 2013;46:1063–76.
24. Ku JK, Jeon WY, Ko SO, Yoon JY. Assessing the efficacy of apicoectomy without retrograde filling in treating periapical inflammatory cysts. J Korean Assoc Oral Maxillofac Surg. 2024;50(3):140–5. https://doi.org/10.5125/jkaoms.2024.50.3.140.
25. Cortes AR, Cortes DN, Arita ES. Correction of buccal dehiscence at the time of implant placement without barrier membranes: a retrospective cone beam computed tomographic study. Int J Oral Maxillofac Implants. 2013;28(6):1564–9. https://doi.org/10.11607/jomi.3093.
26. Aoki EM, Abdala-Júnior R, de Oliveira JX, Arita ES, Cortes AR. Reliability and reproducibility of manual and automated volumetric measurements of periapical lesions. J Endodont. 2015;41(9):1555–9. https://doi.org/10.1016/j.joen.2015.06.015.

Artificial Intelligence in Periodontal Diagnosis

4

Pierre Lahoud, Reinhilde Jacobs,
Alexandre Domingues Teixeira-Neto,
Claudio Mendes Pannuti, Giuseppe Alexandre Romito,
Arthur Rodriguez Gonzalez Cortes, and Ana Paula Ayres

Periodontal diseases comprise a group of inflammatory conditions that affect the periodontium, including both the protective tissues (gingiva) and the supporting structures of the teeth (periodontal ligament, cementum, and alveolar bone). There are two main forms of periodontal disease: gingivitis and periodontitis. Gingivitis is a reversible inflammatory condition confined to the gingival tissues, induced by

P. Lahoud
Division of Periodontology and Oral Microbiology, Department of Oral Health Sciences, Faculty of Medicine, KU Leuven, Leuven, Belgium

OMFS-IMPATH Research Group, Department of Imaging and Pathology, Faculty of Medicine, KU Leuven, Leuven, Belgium

Department of Conservative Dentistry, Periodontology and Digital Dentistry, LMU University Hospital, LMU Munich, Munich, Germany
e-mail: pierre.lahoud@uzleuven.be

R. Jacobs
OMFS-IMPATH Research Group, Department of Imaging and Pathology, Faculty of Medicine, KU Leuven, Leuven, Belgium

Department of Oral and Maxillofacial Surgery, University Hospitals Leuven, Leuven, Belgium

Department of Dental Medicine, Karolinska Institute, Stockholm, Sweden
e-mail: reinhilde.jacobs@kuleuven.be

A. D. Teixeira-Neto
GoBeyond Dental Institute, Curitiba, Brazil
e-mail: alexandre@batelsoho.com

C. M. Pannuti · G. A. Romito · A. P. Ayres
University of São Paulo, São Paulo, Brazil
e-mail: Pannuti@usp.br; ana.ayres.lima@gmail.com

A. R. G. Cortes (✉)
Faculty of Dental Surgery, University of Malta, Msida, Malta
e-mail: arthur.nogueira@um.edu.mt

A. R. G. Cortes (ed.), *Dental Clinical Procedures using Artificial Intelligence*,
https://doi.org/10.1007/978-3-032-24895-4_4

dental biofilm. Its diagnosis is based primarily on clinical features, particularly the presence of gingival inflammation and bleeding on probing, in the absence of clinical attachment loss or radiographic bone loss. In contrast, periodontitis is a chronic, multifactorial, host-mediated inflammatory disease associated with dysbiotic biofilms and characterized by progressive destruction of the tooth-supporting tissues, with diagnosis requiring evidence of clinical attachment loss and radiographically assessed alveolar bone loss. Periodontitis stands as a primary cause of tooth loss in the adult population. Furthermore, periodontal diseases remain among the most prevalent chronic inflammatory conditions worldwide, representing a major cause of tooth loss and contributing significantly to systemic health burdens [1, 2]. The effective management of these diseases depends on early and accurate diagnosis, a process that has traditionally faced significant challenges.

According to the 2017 AAP/EFP classification, periodontitis is characterized using a multidimensional framework based on staging and grading. Staging is primarily determined by disease severity and complexity using clinical parameters together with radiographically assessed alveolar bone loss and tooth loss attributable to periodontitis [3]. Grading reflects the rate of disease progression, preferentially estimated from longitudinal radiographic evidence of bone loss over time or, when unavailable, from indirect measures such as the ratio of radiographic bone loss to patient age, underscoring the central role of radiographic imaging in both staging and grading of periodontitis [4].

4.1 Biological and Clinical Foundations of Periodontal Diagnosis

Periodontal diagnosis is anchored in the biological mechanisms governing host-microbe interactions and the clinically observable consequences of periodontal tissue breakdown [3, 5]. In this context, tissue breakdown in periodontitis is neither linear nor uniform and is influenced by many factors, including genetic susceptibility, systemic modifiers, environmental exposures, and behavioral factors [5]. This complex biology underlies the inherent diagnostic challenges in accurately identifying disease activity, severity, and future risk.

4.1.1 Biological Determinants of Periodontal Tissue Breakdown

At the biological level, periodontal destruction is driven by sustained activation of innate and adaptive immune pathways, leading to connective tissue degradation and osteoclastic bone resorption. Important mediators include pro-inflammatory cytokines, chemokines, and proteolytic enzymes, which collectively disrupt periodontal homeostasis [6].

It is noteworthy that clinical signs of inflammation and tissue destruction often lag behind molecular and cellular changes, limiting the sensitivity of conventional diagnostics for detecting early or subclinical disease. The episodic nature of periodontal breakdown further complicates interpretation of cross-sectional clinical data, particularly when attempting to distinguish historical tissue loss from current disease activity [7, 8].

4.1.2 Clinical Metrics as Surrogates of Disease Expression

Clinical periodontal parameters should be regarded as surrogate markers rather than direct measures of disease activity. Measures such as probing-derived attachment loss and pocket depth primarily quantify the cumulative consequences of inflammatory destruction, while bleeding indices reflect the inflammatory status of the periodontal tissues at the time of examination. Although these metrics are indispensable for disease classification and treatment planning, they remain indirect and context dependent [5]. Their diagnostic value is influenced by tissue phenotype, examiner calibration, probing methodology, and the inherent limitations of manual measurement resolution. Moreover, other clinical findings such as furcation involvement, pathological tooth mobility, and occlusal trauma-related changes signal biomechanical compromise and disease complexity rather than an active inflammatory burden alone [5]. As such, they contribute to assessing functional prognosis and therapeutic complexity but provide limited insight into short-term disease dynamics.

4.2 The Importance of Imaging Diagnosis in Periodontal Therapy

As discussed above, according to the current AAP/EFP classification, the primary clinical indicator of periodontitis is clinical attachment loss (CAL), which is determined by the combined assessment of gingival recession and probing depth [9]. These measurements, however, show considerable inter- and intra-examiner variability, which directly affects the reliability of diagnostic data. These fluctuations can distort important clinical findings, such as the detection of periodontal pockets and the quantification of probing pocket depth and attachment loss. As a result, such variabilities may lead to the overestimation or underestimation of disease severity and limit overall diagnostic precision.

To minimize the inherent limitations of clinical measurements, radiographic assessment emerges as an important component of periodontal evaluation. Radiographs provide an objective and more standardized visualization of hard tissues, including alveolar bone levels, defect morphology, and the degree of furcation involvement. This complementary information reduces the influence of examiner-dependent variability and supports a more consistent interpretation of periodontal status. Moreover, radiographic imaging is essential for accurate staging by defining the extent of bone loss and for grading by enabling the estimation of past and ongoing disease progression (Fig. 4.1). However, conventional imaging must be interpreted within the biological and physical constraints inherent to radiographic technique [5].

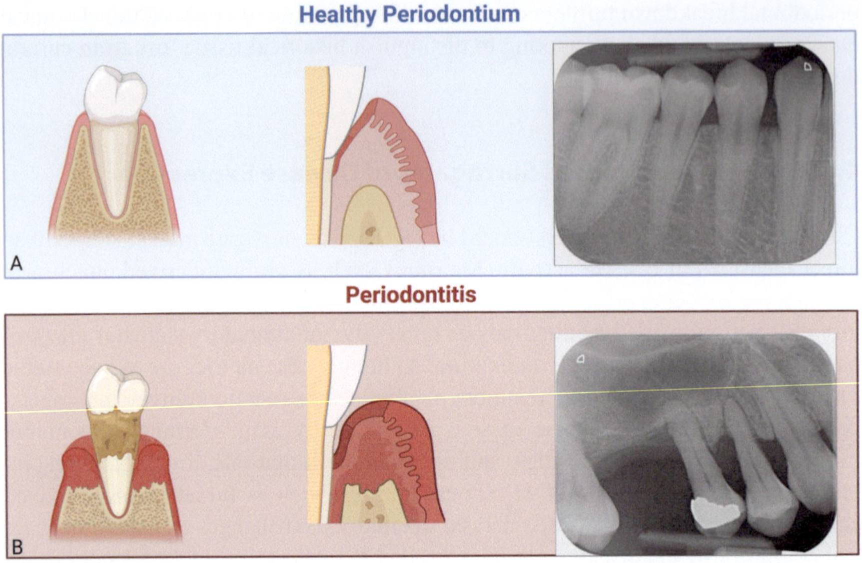

Fig. 4.1 Comparison of (**a**) healthy periodontium versus (**b**) periodontitis. Image created using a premium license of the BioRender software. (Clinical cases are courtesy of Dr. Reinhilde Jacobs and Dr. Pierre Lahoud)

4.2.1 Clinical Guidelines for the Use of Imaging Methods in Periodontology

Among ionizing imaging modalities, intraoral radiographs remain the primary tools for assessing teeth, alveolar bone levels, periodontal ligament space, and lamina dura integrity. The selection of the radiographic technique depends on the clinical presentation of periodontal pockets. Horizontal bitewings provide sufficient visualization for patients with generalized probing depths below 5 mm, while deeper or irregular pockets require vertical bitewings combined with periapical radiographs to capture the full extent of the supporting bone. In cases of generalized periodontal involvement, a complete full-mouth intraoral radiographic survey is recommended to provide a comprehensive assessment of disease distribution and severity [10].

Digital image receptors, including phosphor storage plates and solid-state sensors, allow efficient radiographic capture with lower radiation exposure than films while maintaining diagnostic accuracy. Using minimal exposure settings and rectangular collimation further reduces unnecessary radiation, directing the X-ray beam only to the area of interest and supporting essential radioprotection principles.

A common method for interpreting these images involves measuring the vertical distance between the cementoenamel junction (CEJ) and the alveolar crest. When this measurement exceeds 1.9 mm, within a confidence interval ranging from 0.4 to 1.9 mm, it may indicate the presence of bone loss. It is essential to recognize, however, that this radiographic measurement appears smaller than the physical measurement of alveolar crestal bone height obtained during intraoperative procedures. In addition, these radiographs allow clinicians to identify local predisposing factors for periodontal disease, such as subgingival calculus deposits, root morphology anomalies, and overhanging dental restorations, which may exacerbate periodontal breakdown and require targeted management [11, 12].

The accuracy and reliability of intraoral radiographs depend critically on the standardization of the X-ray beam geometry. To achieve optimal results with minimal distortion, the X-ray beam should be directed perpendicularly to the long axis of the teeth and the image receptor plane. Consequently, the paralleling technique for periapical radiographs is strongly recommended over the bisecting-angle technique, due to the superior geometric configuration and more precise diagnostic information. The use of positioning holders is essential for ensuring adequate geometric relationship, offering consistency, and reducing the need for retakes [12].

4.2.2 The Rationale to Apply 3D Imaging in Periodontal Treatment Planning

Radiographs support periodontitis grading by helping estimate disease progression, either by means of comparison with previous images or by relating the amount of bone loss to the patient's age, allowing better distinction between stable and rapidly progressing disease. Despite their usefulness, conventional radiographic findings of marginal radiographic bone loss should not serve as the main determinant in diagnosing periodontal disease, due to two significant limitations. First, two-dimensional radiographs compress three-dimensional anatomical structures into a single plane, causing superimposition that may obscure critical details. As a result, measurements of alveolar bone loss and bone defects are limited to the parasagittal plane and fail to represent the full 3D morphology of the alveolar ridge. Furthermore, due to these spatial and structural constraints, clinical and intraoral radiographic measurements cannot fully depict the 3D configuration of infrabony defects or furcation involvement. Information on both these alterations is essential for planning effective and targeted periodontal therapy.

When 3D information is required for periodontal diagnosis, cone-beam computed tomography (CBCT) provides volumetric data and multiplanar reconstructions in the sagittal, axial, and coronal planes, providing adequate contrast resolution and eliminating structural overlap (Fig. 4.2). Image acquisition is extraoral, rapid, and technically simple, and the field of view can be collimated to the region of interest to minimize radiation exposure. Adjustable exposure parameters also allow optimization of image quality, ensuring reliable visualization of infrabony defects, bone dehiscences, furcation involvement, as well as alterations of alveolar crest height and the periodontal ligament space. A previous systematic review confirmed CBCT as the most accurate imaging modality for assessing these periodontal alterations [13].

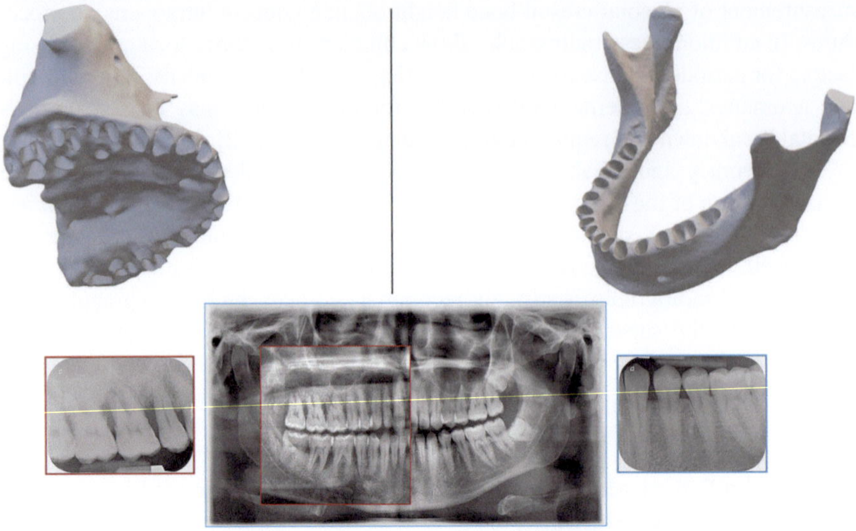

Fig. 4.2 Comparison of 2D and 3D visualization in a healthy (right) versus periodontally compromised patient (left)

4.3 AI-Powered Automated Periodontal Analyses

Artificial intelligence (AI) has recently emerged as a potential adjunct in periodontal diagnostics, addressing the interpretative variability and technical constraints inherent to 2D and 3D imaging. While conventional radiographic and tomographic modalities remain essential for detecting and characterizing periodontal conditions, their analysis is susceptible to inconsistency and limited in sensitivity, prompting growing interest in AI-based systems capable of enhancing diagnostic accuracy and efficiency [14–19]. In this context, machine and deep learning models have demonstrated the ability to analyze complex clinical and imaging datasets with high speed and consistency and create models of oral and maxillofacial structures that can be used for patient-specific modeling [20, 21]. The potential of these models includes the detection periodontal bone loss, classification of defect morphology, and support for disease staging with increasing reliability, as discussed below.

Building on these advances, the strategic use of AI in periodontology has aimed to enable objective, reproducible, and earlier identification of pathological changes. By processing complex datasets with a level of precision beyond human capability, AI can automate time-consuming tasks, highlight subtle alterations that might otherwise be overlooked, and provide clinicians with robust decision-support tools. The main current AI applications in periodontology described in the current literature are discussed below.

4.3.1 Detection of Plaque and Gingival Recession

Dental biofilm is recognized as the primary etiological factor in periodontal diseases, as its accumulation at or below the gingival margin triggers inflammatory responses that may progress to periodontal tissue destruction. Accordingly, identifying and quantifying supragingival biofilm remains essential for assessing disease risk, guiding preventive measures, and supporting effective periodontal therapy [14].

An early study explored the use of an AI-assisted approach for dental biofilm detection in animals using quantitative light-induced fluorescence images. The proposed system showed a high level of agreement with human evaluation, suggesting a satisfactory potential for objective and reproducible plaque assessment. An important advantage of this approach was the combination of automated analysis with simple clinician interaction, allowing rapid correction of misclassified areas and improving usability in a clinical setting. The method reduced subjectivity associated with conventional visual indices and enabled more detailed quantification of biofilm coverage over time. However, the approach depended on fluorescence-based imaging and still required limited expert supervision, indicating that full automation was not achieved. Despite these limitations, the study highlighted the potential of AI-assisted tools to support clinicians in monitoring biofilm and treatment outcomes more consistently than traditional visual scoring methods [15].

Two studies investigated the use of AI to detect supragingival dental plaque from intraoral photographs, aiming to provide a more objective and reproducible alternative to traditional visual plaque indices. Both approaches demonstrated clinically acceptable performance, with AI systems achieving plaque detection results comparable to experienced clinicians and showing particular strength in identifying more mature or extensive plaque deposits. An important advantage highlighted was the use of conventional intraoral or mobile cameras, suggesting a potential applicability in routine clinical practice and even in dental public health or home-based settings. However, relevant limitations were observed. The AI performance was influenced by image quality, lighting conditions, and camera angulation, and both studies relied on two-dimensional photographs, which restrict visualization of interproximal and lingual surfaces. In addition, detection of early or thin plaque remained more challenging, as subtle plaque deposits can visually blend with tooth or gingival tissues. Despite these limitations, the findings support the potential role of AI-assisted plaque detection as a supportive clinical tool to reduce examiner subjectivity, improve consistency in plaque assessment, and aid in patient education while emphasizing the need for more diverse datasets and integration with three-dimensional imaging technologies to enhance clinical reliability [16, 17].

Furthermore, intraoral scanners have recently introduced AI tools for automated plaque detection (Fig. 4.3). Although these tools show potential to improve diagnosis and help orienting periodontal treatment planning, future clinical studies are still needed to address the diagnostic accuracy and usefulness of these AI tools.

Overall, the studies discussed above indicate that the primary value of AI-based plaque detection lies in improving objectivity and consistency rather than replacing clinical judgment. While current systems show performance comparable to

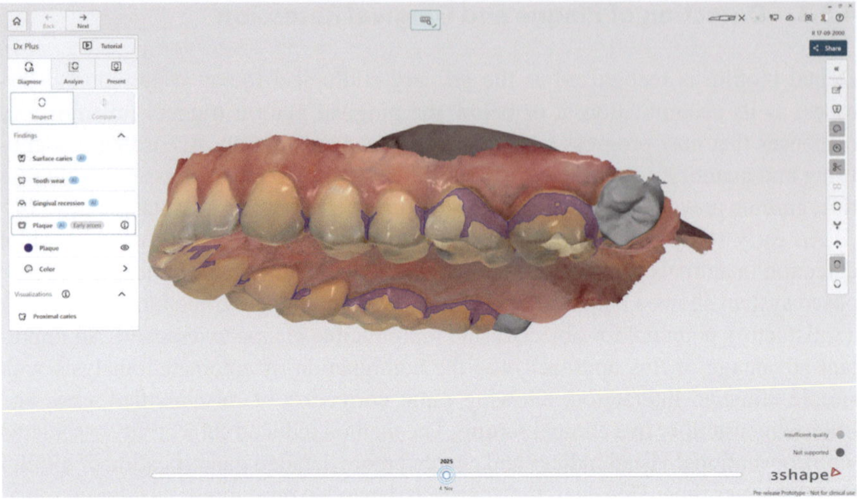

Fig. 4.3 Screenshot of the 3Shape Dx software showing AI-powered automated plaque detection on an intraoral scan (Trios 6, 3Shape A/S). (Courtesy of Dr. Jan Paulics)

experienced clinicians, their effectiveness is influenced by imaging limitations and reduced sensitivity for early plaque deposits. Thus, AI tools should be viewed as complementary aids that can help standardize assessments, support longitudinal monitoring, and enhance patient education, with further advances relying on more diverse datasets and integration with three-dimensional digital workflows.

A similar potential of AI tools is also suggested by techniques for diagnosing gingival recession with intraoral scanners (Fig. 4.4). Such diagnosis can provide understanding of the underlying causes, severity, and progression of periodontal tissue loss. In this context, gingival recession is multifactorial arising from factors such as periodontitis, traumatic toothbrushing, thin gingival phenotype, and orthodontic movement. Accurate diagnosis allows clinicians to identify etiologic factors and proceed with adequate treatment or prevention. Establishing precise measurements from the cementoenamel junction and documenting baseline conditions enable effective monitoring over time, which is critical because recession often progresses slowly and may remain unnoticed by patients. The early diagnosis of gingival recession could allow for prevention, enhanced plaque control, and management of related conditions such as dentin hypersensitivity, root caries susceptibility, and aesthetic concerns, all of which influence patient comfort and quality of life.

4.3.2 Diagnosis of Gingivitis

Gingivitis represents a reversible inflammatory response of the marginal gingiva triggered primarily by biofilm accumulation. Cross-sectional and prospective epidemiological studies consistently show that gingival inflammation is almost always

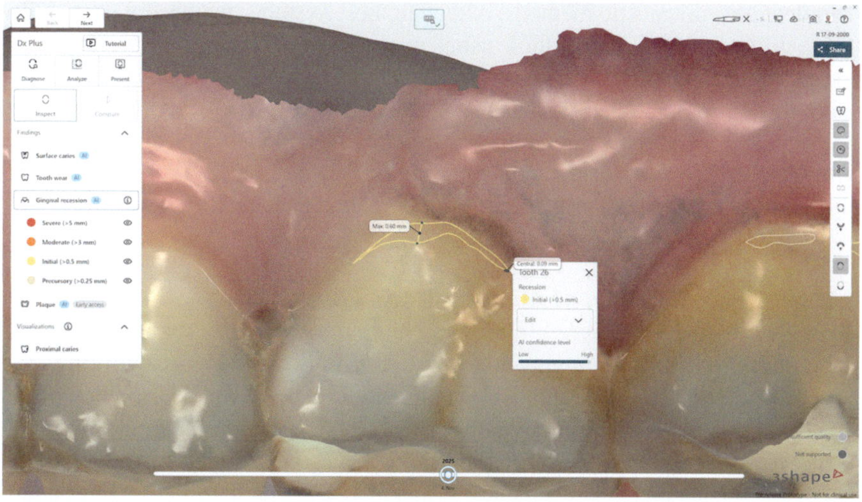

Fig. 4.4 Screenshot of the 3Shape Dx software showing AI-powered automated detection of gingival recession on an intraoral scan (Trios 6, 3Shape A/S). Note the high AI confidence level displayed by the software. (Courtesy of Dr. Jan Paulics)

present in sites affected by periodontitis and typically precedes its onset. This evidence supports the understanding that persistent gingivitis increases the risk of development of periodontitis, reinforcing the importance of early identification and monitoring of gingival changes in routine clinical practice.

A recent study investigated a deep learning approach for detecting early signs of gingivitis in orthodontic patients using intraoral images. The main advantage of this system lies in the use of standard intraoral photographs, which may reduce reliance on invasive periodontal probing. However, the approach showed limited sensitivity for mild inflammation, analyzed only a restricted gingival region, and did not assess disease severity or periodontitis. Overall, the findings suggest that AI-based gingivitis detection may serve as a complementary clinical tool for early monitoring, rather than a substitute for conventional periodontal examination [18].

Another investigation evaluated the use of fluorescence-based intraoral images as input for AI-assisted gingivitis detection. Using the modified gingival index as the clinical reference, the proposed system demonstrated a moderate ability to differentiate inflamed from non-inflamed gingival tissues, with overall performance around 67%. This approach highlights the potential of fluorescence imaging as a noninvasive tool to support gingival inflammation screening, particularly in contexts where conventional periodontal examination may be limited. However, the modest diagnostic performance reinforces the need for better reported datasets, standardized clinical reference criteria, and further refinement of AI models before such systems can be considered reliable for routine clinical application [19].

Overall, the current evidence suggests that AI-based approaches for gingivitis detection hold promise as supportive tools for early screening and monitoring rather than definitive diagnostic methods. Although these systems demonstrate the ability to identify gingival inflammation using noninvasive imaging, their performance remains influenced by image quality, limited anatomical coverage, and reduced sensitivity to mild inflammatory changes. Consequently, AI-assisted gingivitis detection should be regarded as complementary to conventional clinical examination, with future improvements depending on standardized reference criteria and technological advances that enhance clinical reliability and applicability [22].

4.3.3 Quantification of Alveolar Bone Loss

Periodontal bone loss represents a central hallmark of periodontitis, reflecting the progression from reversible gingival inflammation to permanent destruction of the supporting tissues. As the inflammatory process extends from the gingiva into the deeper periodontal structures, the host's immune response triggers resorption of the alveolar bone, leading to attachment loss and increasing tooth mobility. The pattern and extent of bone loss are therefore essential indicators of disease severity and play a key role in determining diagnosis, staging, grading, and treatment planning. Because these changes are irreversible and accumulate over time, early and accurate detection of bone loss is critical for preventing further deterioration and improving long-term periodontal stability [23].

Recent studies have demonstrated the feasibility of AI-based methods for the detection and quantification of alveolar bone loss using periapical radiographs [24]. One approach focused on automatically identifying bone loss areas through image segmentation techniques that combine intensity and texture features, allowing objective identification of affected regions and supporting estimation of disease extent [25]. Another study expanded this concept by proposing a fully automated system to measure the degree of alveolar bone loss based on clinically relevant landmarks, such as the cementoenamel junction, alveolar crest, and root apex [26]. By translating traditional radiographic measurements into automated workflows, these models showed promising agreement with dentist-defined reference standards. Despite encouraging results, both approaches were evaluated on relatively small datasets and were limited to two-dimensional radiographs, underscoring the need for further validation across larger and more diverse clinical scenarios before routine clinical implementation [25, 26].

A deep learning model was developed to detect periodontal bone loss on panoramic radiographs, demonstrating diagnostic performance comparable to that of experienced dentists. The system showed good overall accuracy and balanced sensitivity and specificity, suggesting that AI can reliably identify radiographic signs of bone loss across different tooth types. While the model did not outperform clinicians, it reduced examiner-related variability and required less manual effort, highlighting its potential as a supportive diagnostic aid. However, performance was influenced by image quality and tooth anatomy, and the study relied on two-dimensional panoramic images and a relatively limited dataset. Ultimately, the findings support the role of AI as a complementary tool to assist clinicians in screening and interpreting periodontal bone loss, rather than as a replacement for clinical judgment [27].

Due to the limitations of conventional radiographic methods discussed previously in this chapter, AI automated linear measurements of alveolar bone loss on 2D radiographs may be affected by inadequate positioning and technique (Figs. 4.5 and 4.6). Nevertheless, AI-driven dental software such as Diagnocat (Diagnocat Ltd.) can also be used to diagnose periodontal alterations such as calculus, furcation exposure (Fig. 4.7), and alveolar bone loss (Fig. 4.8) on CBCT images. Furthermore, virtual patients created from AI-driven segmentation and automated alignment of CBCT and digital optical scans combine information from hard and soft tissues and can also be used in 3D periodontal assessments (Figs. 4.9 and 4.10). The precision

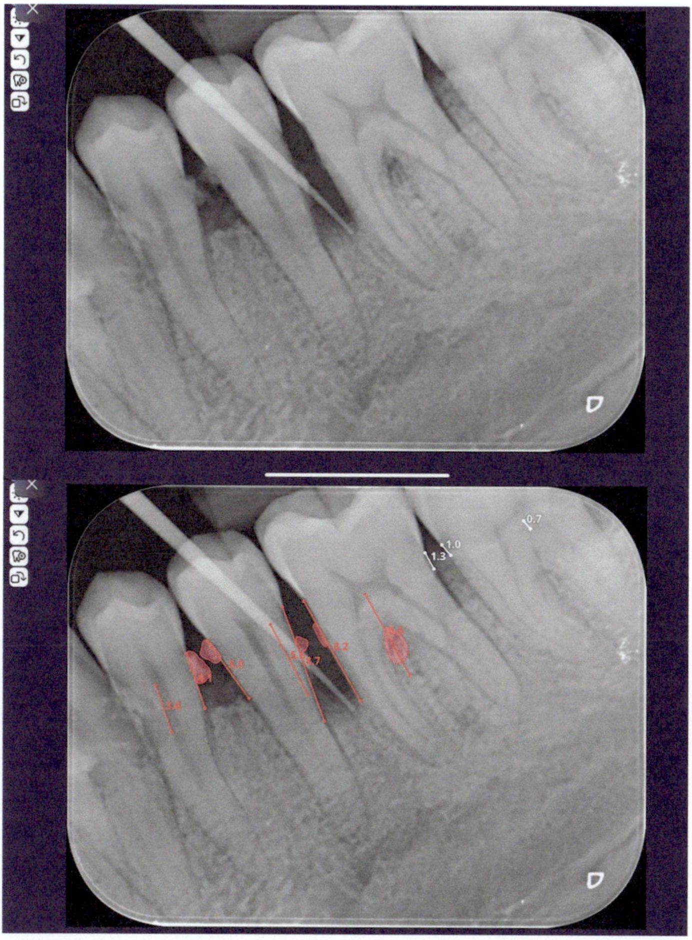

Fig. 4.5 Screenshot of the Diagnocat software showing AI-powered automated detection of periodontal calculus and marginal alveolar bone loss on a periapical radiograph

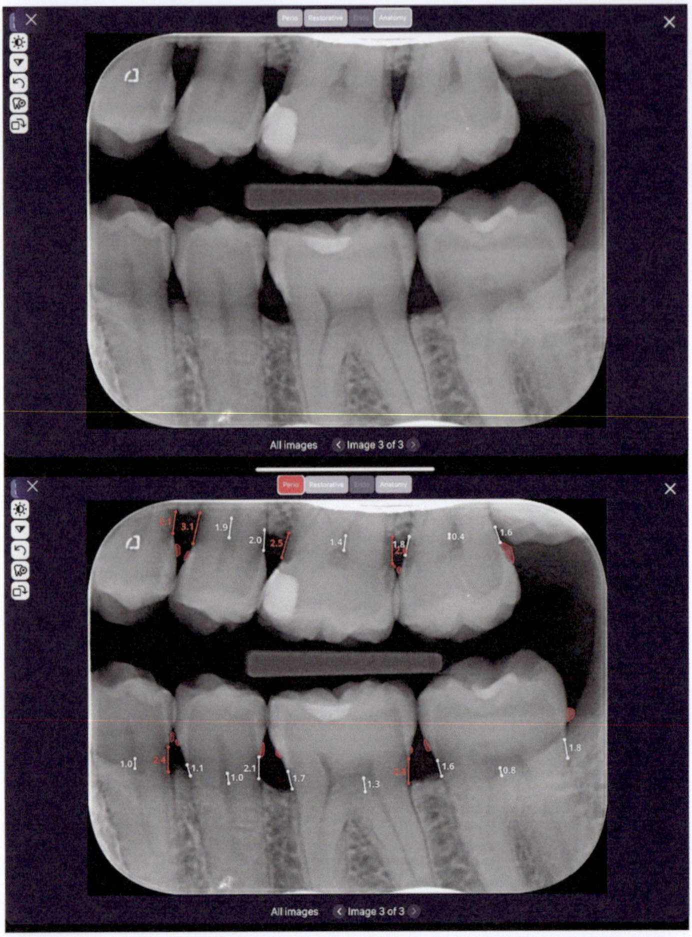

Fig. 4.6 Screenshot of the Diagnocat software showing AI-powered automated detection of periodontal calculus and marginal alveolar bone loss on a bitewing radiograph

and accuracy of the methods, however, are still to be determined by future laboratory and clinical research.

4.3.4 AI-Driven Assessment of Biomarkers in Periodontal Disease

As discussed above, periodontal biomarkers have gained increasing attention as objective indicators of disease activity and host response. These measurable biological signals found in saliva, gingival crevicular fluid, serum, or oral tissues reflect underlying inflammatory, immune, and microbial processes central to periodontal breakdown. Biomarkers such as cytokines, matrix metalloproteinases, and

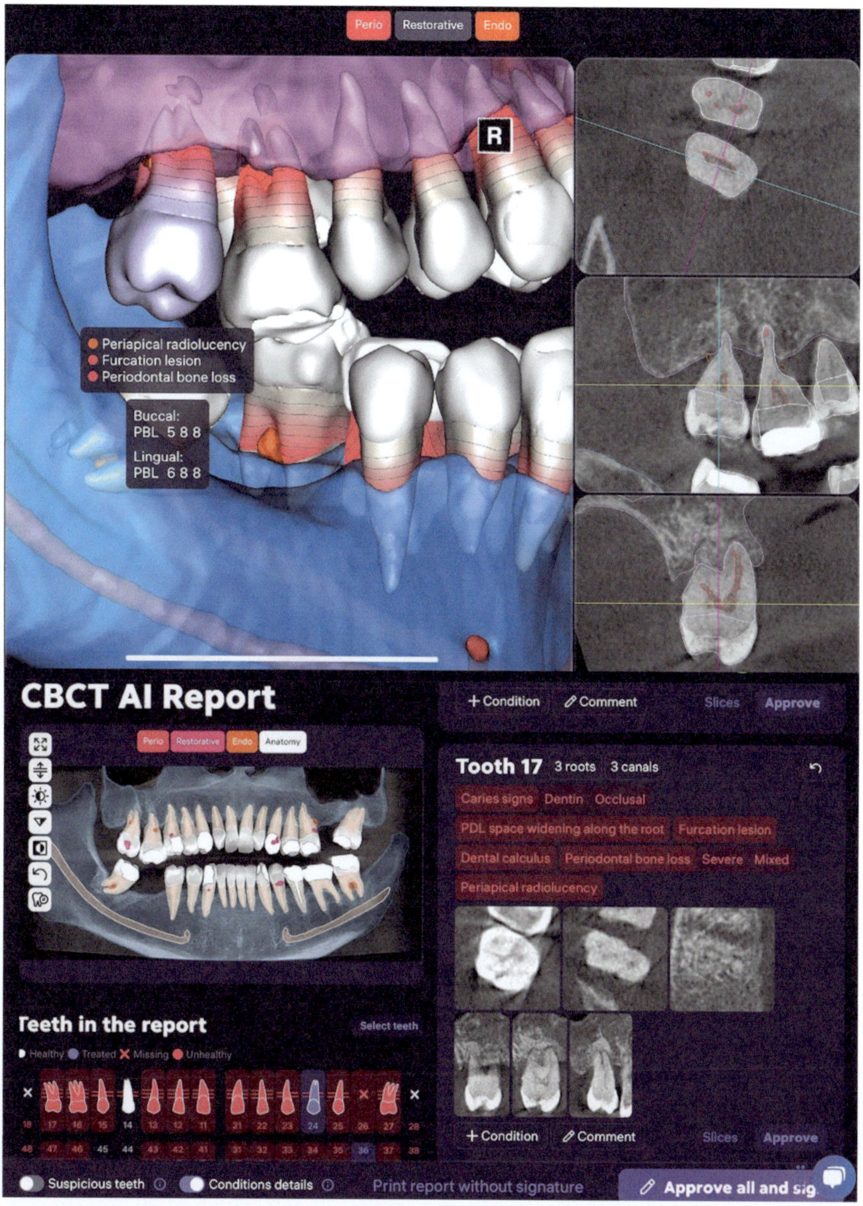

Fig. 4.7 Screenshot of the Diagnocat software showing AI-powered automated detection of furcation lesions and alveolar bone loss on CBCT. Note the lingual severe furcation exposure of tooth 37 (orange), visible on the 3D reconstruction through the edentulous space of tooth 46

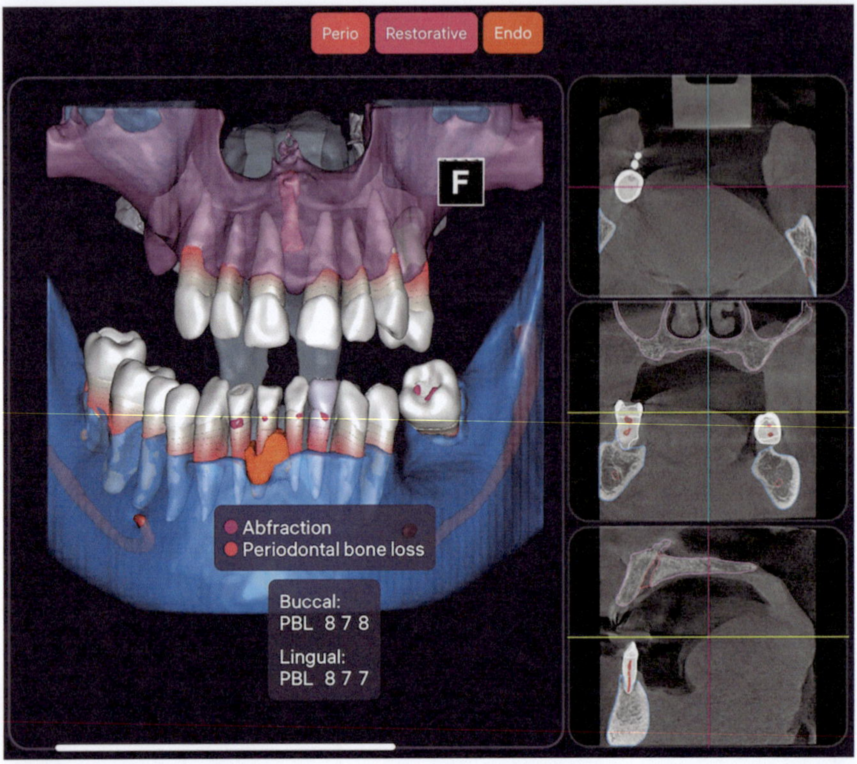

Fig. 4.8 Screenshot of the Diagnocat software showing AI-powered automated detection of anterior alveolar bone loss, which was associated with a periodontal abscess and an endo-perio lesion, on CBCT

tissue-destruction by-products can help identify active disease states, monitor progression, and evaluate responses to therapy. Because clinical parameters alone offer only a momentary snapshot of tissue status, integrating biomarker-based assessment provides a more dynamic understanding of periodontal pathology and supports earlier, more personalized intervention strategies.

Recent studies have shown that AI tools can support the diagnosis of periodontitis through the analysis of salivary biomarkers, offering a noninvasive and patient-friendly alternative to conventional examinations. By combining salivary metabolic profiles with machine learning algorithms, these approaches were able to distinguish individuals with periodontitis from healthy subjects with high diagnostic performance. Rather than relying on a single marker, the use of biomarker panels improved diagnostic reliability and better reflected the biological changes associated with active periodontal disease. From a clinical perspective, these findings highlight the potential of AI-assisted biomarker analysis as a complementary tool to identify disease activity, support early diagnosis, and monitor treatment outcomes,

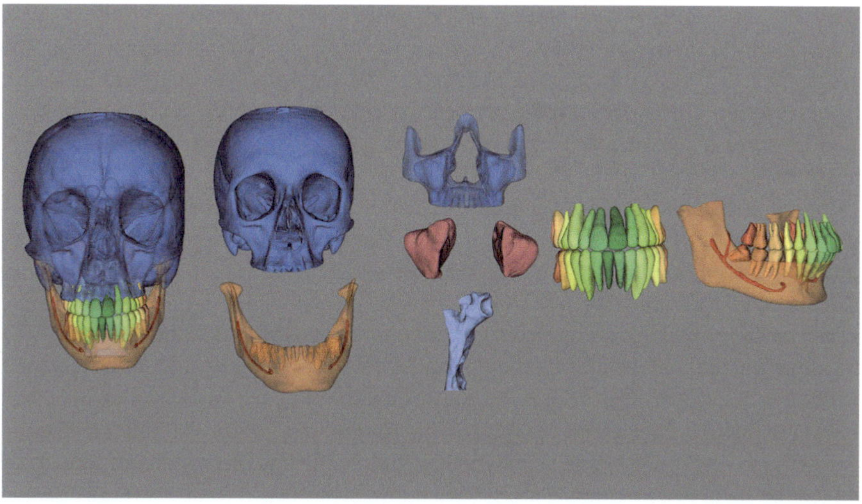

Fig. 4.9 Virtual patient generation of the different oral and maxillofacial structures (Relu creator, Leuven, Belgium) [20, 28, 29]. (Courtesy of OMFS-IMPATH Research Group (KU Leuven, Leuven, Belgium))

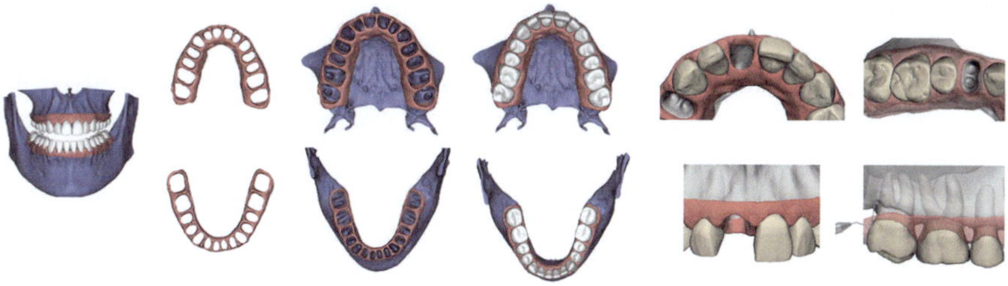

Fig. 4.10 Virtual patient creation for periodontal assessment (Relu creator, Leuven, Belgium). (Courtesy of OMFS-IMPATH Research Group (KU Leuven, Leuven, Belgium) and based on Fagundes FB/Papasratorn D et al. 2026 [21])

especially in situations where traditional clinical parameters may be limited or inconclusive [30, 31].

4.4 AI-Driven Assessment of Prognosis and Risk of Periodontal Disease

Periodontal disease is increasingly recognized as a multifactorial condition in which biofilm-induced inflammation interacts with host-related factors to determine disease onset, progression, and long-term outcomes. While microbial challenge initiates periodontal breakdown, epidemiologic and clinical evidence demonstrates that systemic, genetic, and environmental determinants—such as smoking, metabolic disorders, nutritional status, psychological stress, and inherited susceptibility—play a decisive role in shaping individual risk profiles [32, 33]. In this context, AI-based prognostic and risk assessment models have gained relevance by supporting a shift from reactive treatment toward preventive and personalized periodontal care, enabling earlier identification of patients at increased risk of disease development or progression [34].

Machine learning tools have been increasingly used to estimate risk of developing periodontitis by analyzing large sets of clinical and demographic information. Studies based on electronic dental records show that these systems can help classify patients into different risk levels with generally good accuracy. However, results vary considerably depending on the quality and size of the data used, the type of information included, and whether the models were properly tested in different patient populations. Approaches based on routine clinical data—such as age, systemic conditions, habits, and periodontal measurements—showed moderate to good performance, while models that included biological markers, such as genetic or molecular data, often achieved higher accuracy. Even so, differences in study design and patient samples make comparisons difficult, and the reduced performance observed when models were tested in new populations highlights the need for larger and more diverse clinical datasets [35–37].

Prospective studies have also explored the use of AI to predict how periodontal disease may progress over time, but with mixed reliability. Systems based on biological markers, such as proteins in gingival crevicular fluid or bacterial DNA in saliva, performed well in distinguishing healthy patients from those with advanced periodontitis. In contrast, identifying early or mild disease stages proved more challenging, likely because clinical and biological differences are less pronounced at these stages. Previous research methods relying mainly on patient history or routine clinical information showed lower predictive accuracy, emphasizing once again that AI-based risk prediction should be viewed as a supportive tool rather than a substitute for comprehensive clinical evaluation [37].

One large-scale study further expanded this concept by integrating human genetic data with oral microbiome profiles to predict periodontal-related conditions such as gingival bleeding and dental calculus. By combining genomic risk scores with salivary and tongue microbiome data, the AI models demonstrated good diagnostic performance, highlighting the dominant role of host genetics in individual susceptibility while showing that microbiome information adds complementary predictive value. Although this integrated approach reinforces the potential of AI to support personalized risk assessment in periodontal care, further validation in diverse populations and clinical settings remains necessary before routine clinical implementation [31].

Taken together, the available evidence suggests that AI-driven prognostic and risk prediction models could assist clinicians in identifying individuals at elevated risk and in guiding earlier preventive strategies. Nevertheless, their clinical impact is currently constrained by heterogeneity in study design, limited external validation, and variability in diagnostic criteria, underscoring the need for standardized methodologies, robust prospective datasets, and integration of comprehensive clinical and biological parameters before widespread adoption in periodontal practice.

4.5 Current Limitations and Future Directions

The integration of AI into routine clinical practice is a promising frontier, but its successful adoption hinges on a clear understanding of the current challenges. Recognizing these challenges is the first and most critical step toward developing more robust, reliable, and clinically validated AI solutions that can truly transform patient care in periodontology.

A critical assessment of the existing literature reveals several important limitations that need to be addressed. While current AI models for periodontal applications are promising, they are still in a developmental phase. Most systems remain exploratory, with limited prospective validation and insufficient evidence to support routine clinical use. Further refinement and validation are required before they can be considered powerful and indispensable clinical diagnostic tools.

Another challenge is the lack of standardization. The field of AI in periodontology currently lacks consistency in research methodologies, which makes it difficult to compare the performance of different AI models across studies. There is no consensus on data acquisition protocols, recording procedures, or performance metrics, making reproducibility and cross-study comparison particularly challenging. Establishing consistent protocols for data collection, labeling, and model evaluation is essential for advancing the science.

It is also important to note that several studies rely on retrospective data analysis. This approach can lead to the creation of smaller or imbalanced participant subgroups, which may inadvertently alter study results and limit the generalizability of the findings. Retrospective and controlled datasets commonly suffering from missing clinical variables, inconsistent follow-up, and heterogeneous diagnostic criteria may not reflect the variability encountered in routine periodontal care [38].

Finally, another significant limitation of many current AI models is their primary reliance on a single parameter, which is radiographic bone loss. Models trained exclusively on radiographic features fail to capture essential aspects of periodontal diagnosis, which is inherently multifactorial. To accurately determine disease severity and formulate a reliable prognosis, future AI systems must integrate a more comprehensive set of parameters. This includes important clinical data such as clinical attachment loss, tooth loss, general health status, smoking habits, and family history.

Collectively, these limitations underscore the need for large-scale prospective studies, standardized diagnostic frameworks, and multimodal datasets that reflect the biological and clinical complexity of periodontal disease. Future directions should prioritize real-world model testing, integration with electronic health records, and transparent reporting frameworks to ensure that AI systems are safe, equitable, and clinically interpretable.

Addressing these challenges is paramount for moving AI from the research bench to the clinical setting. Only with rigorous validation, standardized methodologies, and integration of comprehensive diagnostic parameters will AI evolve into a reliable clinical decision-support tool capable of enhancing but not replacing professional judgment in modern periodontology.

4.6 Conclusion

Current evidence demonstrates that AI can perform specific diagnostic tasks—particularly radiographic assessment of periodontal bone loss—with levels of accuracy and reproducibility that are comparable to expert interpretation under controlled conditions. However, technical performance alone is insufficient to justify clinical adoption. Robust validation, transparency, ethical governance, and demonstrable clinical benefit remain essential prerequisites.

The integration of AI into periodontal diagnostics should therefore be understood as an evolutionary process rather than a disruptive replacement of established practice. When aligned with biological principles, standardized diagnostic frameworks, and clinician oversight, AI has the potential to augment periodontal analysis by improving reproducibility, supporting risk-based decision-making, and enabling more personalized care. The challenge moving forward lies in translating technological capability into clinically meaningful innovation that strengthens, rather than complicates, periodontal diagnosis and patient management.

References

1. Chen MX, Zhong YJ, Dong QQ, Wong HM, Wen YF. Global, regional, and national burden of severe periodontitis, 1990–2019: an analysis of the Global Burden of Disease Study 2019. J Clin Periodontol. 2021;48(9):1165–88.
2. Botelho J, Machado V, Leira Y, Proenca L, Chambrone L, Mendes JJ. Economic burden of periodontitis in the United States and Europe: an updated estimation. J Periodontol. 2022;93(3):373–9.
3. Chapple IL, Van der Weijden F, Doerfer C, Herrera D, Shapira L, Polak D, et al. Primary prevention of periodontitis: managing gingivitis. J Clin Periodontol. 2015;42(Suppl 16):S71–A76.
4. Salvi GE, Roccuzzo A, Imber JC, Stahli A, Klinge B, Lang NP. Clinical periodontal diagnosis. Periodontol 2000. 2023.
5. Heitz-Mayfield LJA. Conventional diagnostic criteria for periodontal diseases (plaque-induced gingivitis and periodontitis). Periodontol 2000. 2024;95(1):10–9.
6. Genco RJ. Current view of risk factors for periodontal diseases. J Periodontol. 1996;67(10 Suppl):1041–9.
7. Kurgan S, Kantarci A. Molecular basis for immunohistochemical and inflammatory changes during progression of gingivitis to periodontitis. Periodontol 2000. 2018;76(1):51–67.
8. Meyle J, Chapple I. Molecular aspects of the pathogenesis of periodontitis. Periodontol 2000. 2015;69(1):7–17.
9. Tonetti MS, Greenwell H, Kornman KS. Staging and grading of periodontitis: framework and proposal of a new classification and case definition. J Periodontol. 2018;89(Suppl 1):S159–72.

10. Horner K, Eaton KA, editors. Selection criteria for dental radiography. 3rd ed. London: Faculty of General Dental Practice (UK); 2018. ISBN: 978–1–9999761-0-1.
11. Hausmann E, Allen K, Carpio L, Christersson LA, Clerehugh V. Computerized methodology for detection of alveolar crestal bone loss from serial intraoral radiographs. J Periodontol. 1992;63(8):657–62. https://doi.org/10.1902/jop.1992.63.8.657.
12. Jacobs R, Fontenele RC, Lahoud P, Shujaat S, Bornstein MM. Radiographic diagnosis of periodontal diseases—current evidence versus innovations. Periodontol 2000. 2024;95(1):51–69. doi: https://doi.org/10.1111/prd.12580.
13. Choi IGG, Cortes ARG, Arita ES, Georgetti MAP. Comparison of conventional imaging techniques and CBCT for periodontal evaluation: a systematic review. Imaging Sci Dent. 2018;48(2):79–86. https://doi.org/10.5624/isd.2018.48.2.79.
14. Lindhe J, Lang NP, Karring T. Tratado de periodontia clínica e implantologia oral. 7th ed. Rio de Janeiro: Guanabara Koogan; 2024. ISBN: 9788527740043.
15. Mansoor A, Patsekin V, Scherl D, Robinson JP, Rajwa B. A statistical modeling approach to computer-aided quantification of dental biofilm. IEEE J Biomed Health Inform. 2015;19(1):358–66. https://doi.org/10.1109/jbhi.2014.2310204.
16. Li S, Pang Z, Wenfeng S, Liu X, Zhang Y, Sun Y, Qin H. Low-shot learning of automatic dental plaque segmentation based on local-to-global feature fusion. In: 2020 IEEE 17th International Symposium on Biomedical Imaging (ISBI). 2020. https://doi.org/10.1109/ISBI45749.2020.9098741.
17. You W, Hao A, Li S, Wang Y, Xia B. Deep learning-based dental plaque detection on primary teeth: a comparison with clinical assessments. BMC Oral Health. 2020;20(1):141. https://doi.org/10.1186/s12903-020-01114-6.
18. Alalharith DM, Alharthi HM, Alghamdi WM, Alsenbel YM, Aslam N, Khan IU, et al. A deep learning-based approach for the detection of early signs of gingivitis in orthodontic patients using faster region-based convolutional neural networks. Int J Environ Res Public Health. 2020;17(22):8447. https://doi.org/10.3390/ijerph17228447.
19. Yauney G, Rana A, Wong LC, Javia P, Muftu A, Shah P. Automated process incorporating machine learning segmentation and correlation of oral diseases with systemic health. Annu Int Conf IEEE Eng Med Biol Soc. 2019;2019:3387–93. https://doi.org/10.1109/EMBC.2019.8857965.
20. Nogueira-Reis F, Morgan N, Nomidis S, Van Gerven A, Oliveira-Santos N, Jacobs R, et al. Three-dimensional maxillary virtual patient creation by convolutional neural network-based segmentation on cone-beam computed tomography images. Clin Oral Investig. 2023;27(3):1133–41.
21. Fagundes FB, Papasratorn D, Elgarba BM, Fontenele RC, Neves FS, Jacobs R. AI-driven gingival segmentation on CBCT: validation using delineation by intraoral scanning and CBCT-based cotton roll separation. J Dent. 2026 Jan;5:106331.
22. Erkul S, Özden YE, Özden İ, Kaya BD, Bal B, Kayahan ZÖ. The use of artificial intelligence in different dental applications. Cyprus J Med Sci. 2025;10(4):218–27. https://doi.org/10.4274/cjms.2025.2024-101.
23. Ghaffari M, Zhu Y, Shrestha A. A review of advancements of artificial intelligence in dentistry. Dent Rev. 2024;4(2):100081. https://doi.org/10.1016/j.dentre.2024.100081.
24. Lin PL, Huang PY, Huang PW. Automatic methods for alveolar bone loss degree measurement in periodontitis periapical radiographs. Comput Methods Prog Biomed. 2017;148:1–11.
25. Lin PL, Huang PW, Huang PY, Hsu HC. Alveolar bone-loss area localization in periodontitis radiographs based on threshold segmentation with a hybrid feature fused of intensity and the H-value of fractional Brownian motion model. Comput Methods Prog Biomed. 2015;121:117–26.
26. Lee SJ, Chung D, Asano A, Sasaki D, Maeno M, Ishida Y, et al. Diagnosis of tooth prognosis using artificial intelligence. Diagnostics(Basel). 2022;12:1422. https://doi.org/10.3390/diagnostics12061422.

27. Krois J, Ekert T, Meinhold L, Golla T, Kharbot B, Wittemeier A, Dörfer C, Schwendicke F. Deep learning for the radiographic detection of periodontal bone loss. Sci Rep. 2019;9(1):8495. https://doi.org/10.1038/s41598-019-44839-3.
28. Fontenele RC, Gerhardt MDN, Picoli FF, Van Gerven A, Nomidis S, Willems H, et al. Convolutional neural network-based automated maxillary alveolar bone segmentation on cone-beam computed tomography images. Clin Oral Implants Res. 2023;34(6):565–74.
29. Verhelst PJ, Smolders A, Beznik T, Meewis J, Vandemeulebroucke A, Shaheen E, et al. Layered deep learning for automatic mandibular segmentation in cone-beam computed tomography. J Dent. 2021;114:103786.
30. Kim HJ, Song Y, Lee HA, Kim S, Chung J. Metabolic phenotyping of saliva to identify possible biomarkers of periodontitis using proton nuclear magnetic resonance. J Clin Periodontol. 2021;48(9):1240–9. https://doi.org/10.1111/jcpe.13516.
31. Liu X, Tong X, Zhu J, Tian L, Jie Z, Zou Y, et al. Metagenome–genome-wide association studies reveal human genetic impact on the oral microbiome. Cell Discov. 2021;7(1):117. https://doi.org/10.1038/s41421-021-00356-0.
32. Genco RJ, Borgnakke WS. Risk factors for periodontal disease. Periodontol 2000. 2013;62(1):59–94. https://doi.org/10.1111/j.1600-0757.2012.00457.x.
33. Shimpi N, McRoy S, Zhao H, Wu M, Acharya A. Development of a periodontitis risk assessment model for primary care providers in an interdisciplinary setting. Technol Health Care. 2020;28(2):143–54. https://doi.org/10.3233/THC-191642.
34. Bashir NZ, Rahman Z, Chen SLS. Systematic comparison of machine learning algorithms to develop and validate predictive models for periodontitis. J Clin Periodontol. 2022;49(10):958–69. https://doi.org/10.1111/jcpe.13692.
35. Patel JS, Su C, Tellez M, Albandar JM, Rao R, Iyer V, et al. Developing and testing a prediction model for periodontal disease using machine learning and big electronic dental record data. Front Artif Intell. 2022;5:979525. https://doi.org/10.3389/frai.2022.979525.
36. Huang W, Wu J, Mao Y, Zhu S, Huang GF, Petritis B, et al. Developing a periodontal disease antibody array for the prediction of severe periodontal disease using machine learning classifiers. J Periodontol. 2020;91(2):232–43. https://doi.org/10.1002/JPER.19-0173.
37. Kim EH, Kim S, Kim HJ, Jeong HO, Lee J, Jang J, et al. Prediction of chronic periodontitis severity using machine learning models based on salivary bacterial copy number. Front Cell Infect Microbiol. 2020;10:571515. https://doi.org/10.3389/fcimb.2020.571515.
38. Pitchika V, Buttner M, Schwendicke F. Artificial intelligence and personalized diagnostics in periodontology: a narrative review. Periodontol 2000. 2024;95(1):220–31.

Current Limitations and Considerations 5

Hossam Dawa, Thomas Martin Grixti,
and Arthur Rodriguez Gonzalez Cortes

According to the current scientific evidence presented, AI holds the potential to revolutionize dentistry, promising to enhance diagnosis and treatment planning, as well as improve prognosis and patient outcomes. However, a significant gap still exists between the technical promise of AI and its limited, proven application in real-world clinical practice. Most published research describes what AI tools and algorithms can achieve under idealized laboratory conditions with curated datasets, controlled imaging parameters, and homogeneous patient populations. The favorable results in these controlled conditions, however, could be significantly different when these tools are deployed in heterogeneous, resource-constrained clinical environments. Ensuring that AI is adopted in safe, effective, and equitable conditions is not only as an implementation strategy but also as an ethical requirement to uphold patient safety, preserve clinical trust, and promote fairness in care [1].

5.1 Foundational Challenges: Data Quality, Availability, and Bias

High-quality and comprehensive data serve as the essential foundation for building robust and reliable AI models. The presence of data-related obstacles may therefore significantly hinder the development and widespread clinical validation of AI in dentistry, which have profound implications for model performance, generalizability, and equity [1].

H. Dawa
CESPU University, Porto, Portugal

T. M. Grixti
Private Practice, Msida, Malta

A. R. G. Cortes (✉)
Faculty of Dental Surgery, University of Malta, Msida, Malta
e-mail: arthur.nogueira@um.edu.mt

A. R. G. Cortes (ed.), *Dental Clinical Procedures using Artificial Intelligence*,
https://doi.org/10.1007/978-3-032-24895-4_5

The primary limitations regarding data availability and quality are multifaceted and interconnected:

5.1.1 Limited and Fragmented Datasets

Dental datasets are frequently incomplete, insufficient in size and diversity, and lack standardization. This fragmentation makes it difficult for researchers to construct strong and reliable AI models capable of covering a broad range of dental conditions and patient demographics.

5.1.2 Data Accessibility Challenges

Accessing comprehensive medical and dental data is significantly complicated by strict patient data protection regulations, such as the Health Insurance Portability and Accountability Act (HIPAA) in the United States and the General Data Protection Regulation (GDPR) in Europe. These legal frameworks, combined with organizational barriers and a lack of data-sharing infrastructure, severely restrict the availability of large-scale datasets for AI research and development [2].

5.1.3 Poor Generalizability

Many AI models in dentistry are developed using narrow datasets from specific populations. This practice can lead to overfitting, where a model performs well on its training data but fails to generalize accurately to new, unseen data from different clinical settings or patient demographics, representing a major obstacle to widespread clinical applicability.

A direct and dangerous consequence of these data limitations is the problem of algorithmic bias. When AI models are trained on imbalanced or nonrepresentative datasets, they can inherit and even amplify existing societal biases. This can introduce selection bias, leading to algorithms that underrepresent certain demographic groups. For example, in breast imaging, some commercial AI tools have demonstrated lower sensitivity in minority populations due to dataset imbalance, while others have shown performance variations in detecting cancer in dense breast tissue. Such disparities can create diagnostic tools that perform unequally across different patient populations, leading to significant inequities in patient care. These foundational problems related to data directly contribute to the technical and implementation hurdles that prevent AI from being effectively translated into clinical practice.

5.2 Technical Challenges for Implementation: From Algorithm to Clinical Practice

Overcoming technical barriers is of strategic importance to successfully translate AI models from controlled research environments into reliable clinical tools. It is important to identify and deconstruct the existing technical challenges that complicate the path from algorithm to clinical practice, including system interoperability, the inherent opacity of certain AI models, and a critical gap in rigorous clinical validation [3].

A primary challenge is the lack of interoperability. Numerous dental practices use varying software and imaging systems that are often incompatible with emerging AI platforms. This lack of integration hinders the smooth flow of data required for AI algorithms to function, thereby impeding the adoption and effective use of AI technologies in a typical clinical workflow.

A more conceptual but equally significant barrier is the "black box" problem. Many advanced AI systems, particularly those based on deep learning, operate in a way that is not easily interpretable by human users. This difficulty in understanding how a complex algorithm arrives at a specific recommendation creates a lack of transparency. As a result, this challenge may undermine the trust from clinicians, complicates accountability, and critically elevates medico-legal risk, as it undermines the ability to determine causation in the event of clinical errors and complicates the assignment of negligence.

Finally, there is a significant gap between the theoretical performance of AI models and their real-world application—a phenomenon often referred to as the "AI-chasm"—which is primarily defined by two issues, the lack of validation in clinical studies and unsatisfactory predictive performances of the AI algorithms.

5.2.1 Lack of Clinical Validation

As mentioned above, a substantial portion of AI models in dentistry are developed and tested outside of real clinical settings. There remains a deficit of rigorous, long-term scientific studies designed to validate their effectiveness, reliability, and applicability in routine dental practice.

5.2.2 Poor Predictive Performance

The disconnect between algorithmic design and clinical reality is highlighted by findings that some machine learning models have demonstrated poor performance in predicting tangible clinical outcomes. For example, certain models have failed to accurately predict the success of root canal treatments, underscoring that high theoretical accuracy does not always translate to clinical utility.

These technical challenges, combined with foundational data issues, are further complicated by the human and economic factors that influence the adoption of new technologies in professional practice.

5.3 Professional and Economic Barriers for Widespread Adoption

Beyond technical and data-centric issues, the successful integration of AI into the fabric of daily dental practice is heavily dependent on overcoming significant human, professional, and economic barriers. This section explores professional resistance, the skills gap, and the substantial resource constraints facing dental practices.

The primary human and professional challenges that hinder AI adoption include the following:

5.3.1 Resistance to Change

The dental profession, rooted in long-standing traditions, can exhibit resistance to disruptive technologies. This resistance stems not only from concerns about the reliability of AI but also from a deeper tension between professional identity and technological automation, including fears of an erosion of clinical judgment and a redefinition of professional roles.

5.3.2 Expertise and Training Deficit

There is a limited availability of AI expertise within the dental community. Bridging the gap between AI research and clinical dentistry requires focused education and training to equip dental professionals with the skills needed to use these technologies safely and effectively.

5.3.3 The Role of AI as a Supportive Tool

It is essential to clarify that AI is not a replacement for human expertise. Its intended role is to serve as a supportive tool to assist clinicians by automating routine tasks or providing diagnostic insights. The final clinical decision must always be made by the dentist, whose knowledge, skill, and judgment remain indispensable.

In addition to these professional challenges, economic and resource constraints present a major barrier to adoption. The high costs associated with acquiring AI systems, including hardware and software, can be prohibitive, particularly for smaller dental practices. Furthermore, the process of training staff and integrating AI technologies into existing clinical workflows is a time-consuming and costly endeavor. These practical barriers must be addressed alongside the deeper ethical dilemmas that arise once these systems are implemented.

5.4 Challenges and Ethical Implications in AI-Driven Dentistry

As artificial intelligence becomes more deeply integrated into clinical decision-making, it introduces complex ethical questions surrounding patient data, professional responsibility, and healthcare equity. It is critically important to address these ethical dimensions to ensure AI is deployed responsibly and in a manner that upholds the trust between patients and providers [4]. The main core ethical implications of AI-driven dentistry are the following:

5.4.1 Privacy and Data Security

The development of AI models relies on the collection and processing of vast amounts of patient health data, posing profound risks to confidentiality. Safeguarding this sensitive information requires strong data governance frameworks, rigorous security measures, and strict adherence to data protection regulations. Methodologies such as data encryption, which converts sensitive information into a coded format, represent a viable technical solution for providing an additional layer of security against unauthorized access.

5.4.2 Accountability and Liability

A significant ethical challenge is assigning responsibility when an AI system contributes to a diagnostic or treatment-related error. The integration of AI creates a shared decision-making paradigm where determining fault is no longer straightforward. This ambiguity may raise fundamental ethical questions about where responsibility lies: with the clinician who used the tool, the software developer who created the algorithm, the manufacturer, or the healthcare organization that implemented the system. Resolving this dilemma is essential for maintaining professional accountability and ensuring patients have recourse in the event of harm.

5.4.3 Fairness, Equity, and Patient Autonomy

Algorithmic bias, stemming from the use of nonrepresentative training data, can perpetuate and even amplify existing health disparities. If AI models are not trained on diverse datasets, they may underperform for minority populations, leading to inequitable diagnostic outcomes and reinforcing systemic biases in healthcare. Alongside this concern for fairness is the evolving paradigm of patient consent.

The traditional model of informed consent is being challenged as patients become more active participants in data stewardship. This shift requires new models for obtaining consent that allow for the ethical use of patient data in advancing AI while protecting individual autonomy and rights. The ethical principles governing AI in healthcare are inextricably linked to the legal and regulatory frameworks designed to enforce them.

This issue has also been raised in the literature, as these evolving consent paradigms raise questions about patient notification and choice regarding AI involvement in their care [5]. Patients may have preferences about AI use, and transparency about AI assistance may be ethically required. Practical implementation of AI-related informed consent remains undefined, with varying practices across jurisdictions and clinical settings.

5.4.4 Cybersecurity

AI systems introduce new cybersecurity vulnerabilities to dental practice environments [6]. Adversarial attacks can manipulate AI inputs to produce incorrect outputs, potentially affecting diagnostic recommendations. Cloud-based AI services create data transmission security requirements, and connected AI systems expand the attack surface for ransomware and other malicious actors. Many dental practices lack cybersecurity expertise to evaluate and mitigate these risks adequately.

5.5 Legal and Regulatory Guidelines

The rapid pace of artificial intelligence development has outstripped the creation of robust governance mechanisms, resulting in a fragmented and often ambiguous legal and regulatory landscape. As AI tools become more prevalent, navigating this environment becomes a critical challenge for clinicians, developers, and healthcare organizations. It is important to understand the current state of these evolving frameworks and their attempts to address the ethical problems of liability and oversight.

Traditional legal doctrines that place liability squarely on clinicians are ill-suited for the shared decision-making model of human-AI collaboration. This ambiguity of current legal frameworks is especially acute in radiology, where malpractice cases could arise involving FDA-cleared AI tools that failed to detect abnormalities, leaving courts to grapple with whether liability rests with the clinician, the hospital, or the software vendor. The opacity of "black box" algorithms further complicates the assignment of fault, creating legal uncertainty for all parties.

The current regulatory environment for AI in medicine varies significantly by region, with limited global harmonization. The European Union has adopted a precautionary, rights-centered approach, anchored by the GDPR and the new AI Act, which classifies medical AI as "high risk" and mandates strict conformity assessments, human oversight, and post-market monitoring. In contrast, the United States follows a more permissive, market-driven model where the FDA classifies AI tools as "software as a medical device" (SaMD) and emphasizes a "total product lifecycle" approach to ensure safety and efficacy. Canada has adopted a hybrid model, combining elements of both approaches to balance innovation with oversight.

To improve the quality and transparency of AI studies, there is a clear need for robust research and reporting standards. Researchers are strongly encouraged to follow established guidelines such as CONSORT-AI, SPIRIT-AI, and TRIPOD. Adherence to these standards is essential to ensure reproducibility and reliability of AI research, as well as its clinical relevance, thereby building a foundation of high-quality evidence to support the clinical effectiveness of AI applications. The need for clear standards and frameworks leads directly to the broader question of how to chart a responsible path forward for AI in dentistry.

5.6 AI Limitations: Clinical Case Studies

5.6.1 Bilateral Mandibular Fourth Molars

Supernumerary teeth are a developmental anomaly characterized by the presence of more teeth than the normal dental formula. While this condition is not unheard of, the presentation of supernumerary molars, specifically mandibular fourth molars (distomolars), represents a rare clinical manifestation [7]. The overall prevalence of supernumerary teeth in the deciduous dentition is reported to be between 0.3% and 0.8%, while in the permanent dentition, it ranges from 2% to 3.8% [8]. The occurrence of bilateral mandibular fourth molars is an especially uncommon finding, making each documented case a valuable contribution to clinical literature.

In the present case, an orthopantomography (OPG) was performed to assess general conditions, providing a panoramic view of the dentition surrounding bony structures. The OPG revealed as incidental finding the presence of unerupted bilateral mandibular fourth molars. The morphology of the germs closely resembled the shape of the ones of adjacent third molars. Nevertheless, only the one of the left side of the patient was identified by the AI software as a bone structure abnormality (Fig. 5.1).

The presence of supernumerary teeth, particularly when multiple, warrants careful clinical consideration. A comprehensive anamnesis is indicated to exclude underlying congenital abnormalities or syndromes which may have many other significant features. It is also important to note the controversial status of odontomas. Although morphologically similar to ST, odontomas are often excluded from studies on supernumerary teeth and are typically designated as evolutive odontogenic tumors.

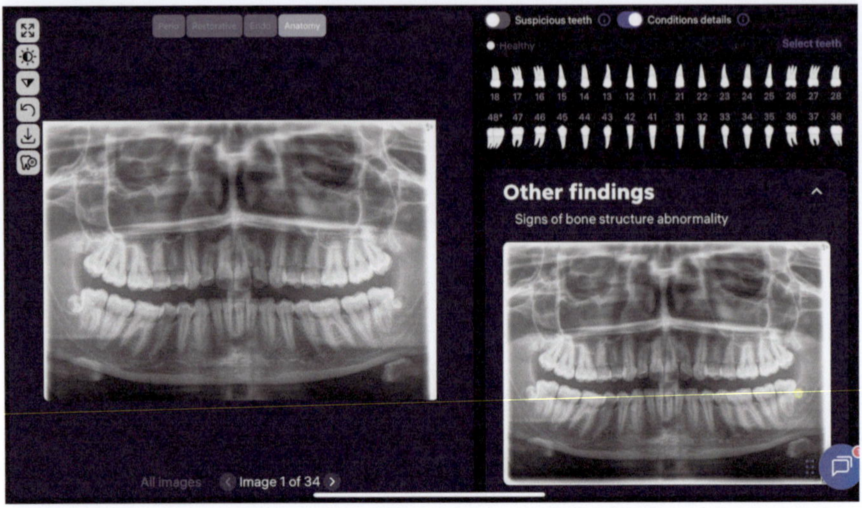

Fig. 5.1 Screenshot of an OPG AI report (Diagnocat) showing that only the left mandibular fourth molar was detected as a structural abnormality, whereas the right side one was not even included in the segmentation list

5.6.2 Teeth Overlapping on Bitewing Radiographs

A previous literature review described the main errors affecting bitewing radiographic images [9]. Wrong position of the film was a major issue, identified in 42.7% of cases. This error is precisely defined as the failure to make critical anatomical landmarks visible, including the distal surfaces of the maxillary canines, the mesial surfaces of the second molars, and the marginal bone crests. Such omissions defeat the primary purpose of the examination, which is to visualize these specific structures for the early detection of pathology.

On the other hand, overlapping of teeth can also significantly affect the diagnosis on a radiographic image (Fig. 5.2). This was present in 10.6% of the radiographs analyzed by the aforementioned study. It is caused by incorrect horizontal angulation of the central X-ray beam, rendering the detection of early-stage caries between the teeth difficult.

Further errors have also been resported, such as cone cutting. This occurred in 4.3% of the sample and shows as a clear and unexposed area on the film, creating a blind spot where diagnostic information is permanently lost. Other less frequent technique errors included were under/overaxial exposure (2.2%), caused by incorrect vertical angulation, and double image (0.3%), resulting from patient or cone movement during exposure.

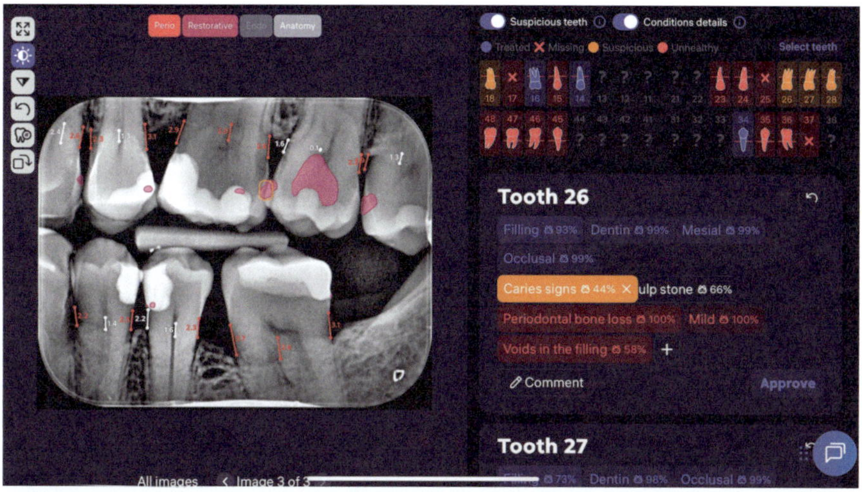

Fig. 5.2 Screenshot of an AI report of a bitewing radiography (Diagnocat) showing a low percentage of AI confidence in the diagnosis of caries on superimposed interproximal surfaces between teeth 26 and 27

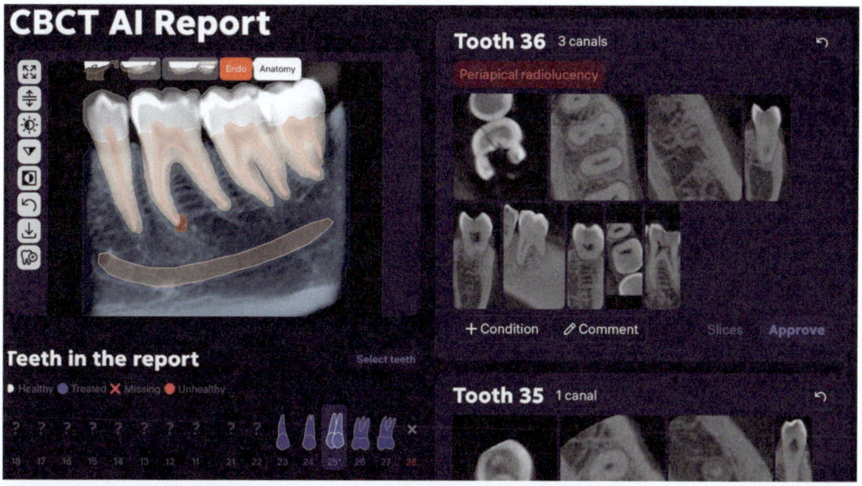

Fig. 5.3 Screenshot of a CBCT AI report (Diagnocat) showing an undetected crown fracture of the tooth 36, which extends cervically to the CEJ

5.6.3 Tooth Cracks and Fractures

One of the current clinically relevant flaws of most AI software programs is the lack of ability to detect and identify tooth fractures. While crown fractures are usually visible at clinical examination and CBCT (Fig. 5.3), root fractures usually lead to periodontal ligament space widening or even periapical radiolucencies, which can be usually detected by AI algorithms for CBCT scans (Figs. 5.4 and 5.5). The dental professional or oral radiologist should then carefully analyze every single radiolucent alteration highlighted by the software when suspecting of a tooth fracture (Fig. 5.6). In this context, CBCT scans with smaller voxels and fields-of-view inherently lead to higher diagnostic accuracy for root fractures. Given that smaller voxel settings require higher radiation doses, their routine use for general cases without fractures or with a clear diagnostic benefit is not clinically justified. Clinicians should therefore be guided by the ALARA principle and the European Guidelines on Radiation Protection in Dental Radiology to make the decision of radiographic scanning parameters on an individual basis.

5.6.4 Variation in the Percentages of AI Confidence

Despite the constant ongoing development and training of AI software systems, all conditions assessed are generally detected with a percentage of AI confidence. Some software manufacturers indicate that an AI confidence percentage greater than 50% for an alteration will classify the tooth as "unhealthy" or positive to possess that alteration. This is especially relevant for common alterations such as periapical lesions and caries.

A recent meta-analysis found a pooled sensitivity of 0.85 (95% CI: 0.83–0.93), indicating that the AI models correctly identified 85% of existing carious lesions [9]. This was complemented by a high pooled specificity of 0.90 (95% CI: 0.85–0.95), meaning the models correctly identified 90% of healthy tooth surfaces. The overall diagnostic accuracy was summarized by an area under the summary

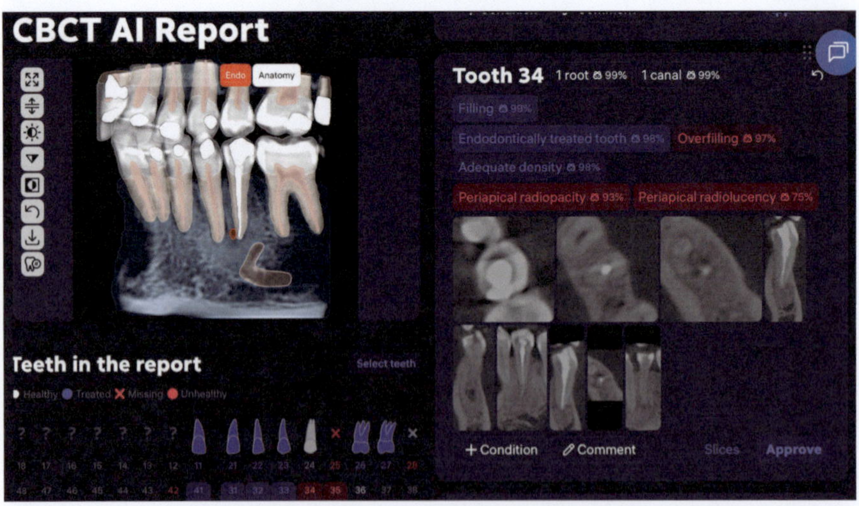

Fig. 5.4 Screenshot of a CBCT AI report (Diagnocat) showing alterations found for tooth 34, which was tender to percussion. Note that no additional, collateral or lateral root canals were detected by the Diagnocat

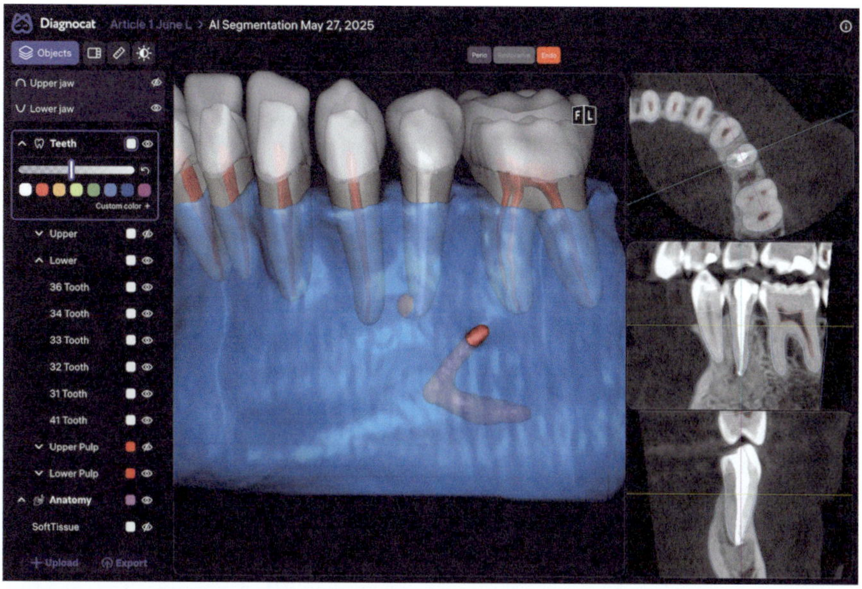

Fig. 5.5 Screenshot of a 3D AI model (Diagnocat) showing the presence of hypodense (radiolucent) area on the mesial aspect of the apex

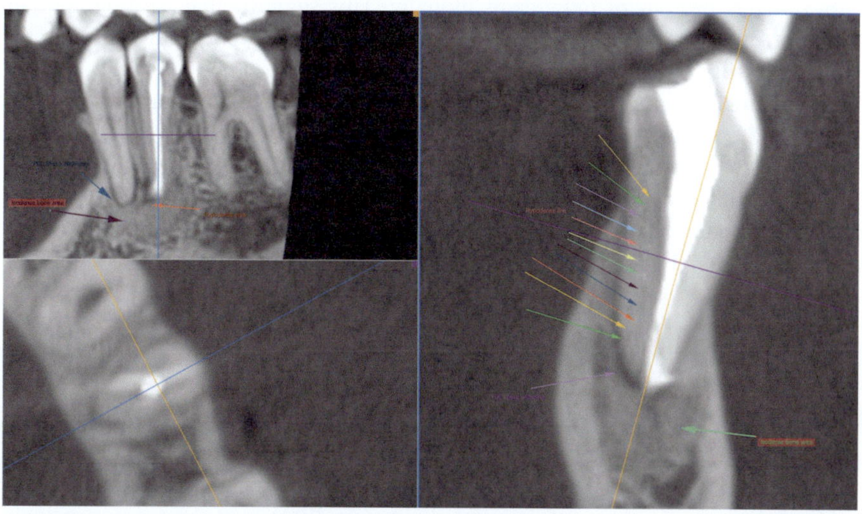

Fig. 5.6 Screenshot of the Horos software (The Horos Project), operated by an oral radiologist to assess the case of Figs. 5.5 and 5.4. Note the hypodense line suggestive of vertical root fracture leading to a widened periodontal ligament space contiguous with the periapical lesion

ROC curve (AUC) of 0.86, where a value of 1.0 represents a perfect test. A single combined measure, the pooled log diagnostic odds ratio, was 4.37 (95% CI: 3.16–6.27), with higher values indicating better discriminatory test performance.

To further interpret the clinical utility of these findings, the meta-analysis calculated likelihood ratios and posttest probabilities [9]. The positive likelihood ratio was 10.443, meaning a positive AI result is over ten times more likely to occur in a patient with caries than in one without. Conversely, the negative likelihood ratio was 0.168, indicating that a negative result is far more likely in a patient without caries. Clinically, this translates to a positive posttest probability of 79%; if a patient's test is positive, there is a 79% chance they genuinely have caries. The negative posttest probability was 6%; if the test is negative, there is a high degree of confidence (a 94% probability) that the patient is free of caries, making it a strong tool for ruling out disease.

These quantitative metrics indicate a high level of diagnostic accuracy for AI in this domain. However, it is important to explore how this performance varies under different conditions, such as the type of study experiment (in vitro or in vivo) and the type of dental imaging being analyzed. While the quantitative findings for AI in caries detection are promising, the aforementioned meta-analysis also identified significant heterogeneity among the reviewed studies [9]. A potential for selection bias in the datasets used to train and validate the AI algorithms was also described. The overall prevalence of dental caries in the analyzed datasets was 27.3%, a figure noted to be considerably lower than the prevalence in the real community, where caries affects billions of individuals globally. This suggests that the training data may not fully capture the spectrum of disease presentation, potentially limiting the generalizability of the AI models.

Furthermore, there is a lack of information regarding the accuracy of AI algorithms and software programs in detecting caries on CBCT images. As demonstrated below with the Diagnocat, clear caries lesions affecting the dentin could be presented with considerably different percentages of AI confidence (Figs. 5.7 and 5.8). On the other hand, in both cases, the affected teeth were classified and considered "unhealthy" by the software.

5.6.5 Quality of the Radiographs

Further then the factors reviewed before, two technical issues may alter the outcomes of an AI diagnostic report: radiographic superimpositions and the quality of the phosphorus plate and the corresponding radiographic image (Figs. 5.9, 5.10, and 5.11). A periapical radiograph is a two-dimensional image of a three-dimensional object. The projection of the X-ray beam can cause important anatomical structures such as root canals and surrounding anatomical landmarks to be superimposed to each other, leading to difficulties during interpretation. To address this issue, clinicians can control the X-ray projection angles to separate superimposed structures and gain substantial diagnostic benefits essential for achieving predictable and successful treatments.

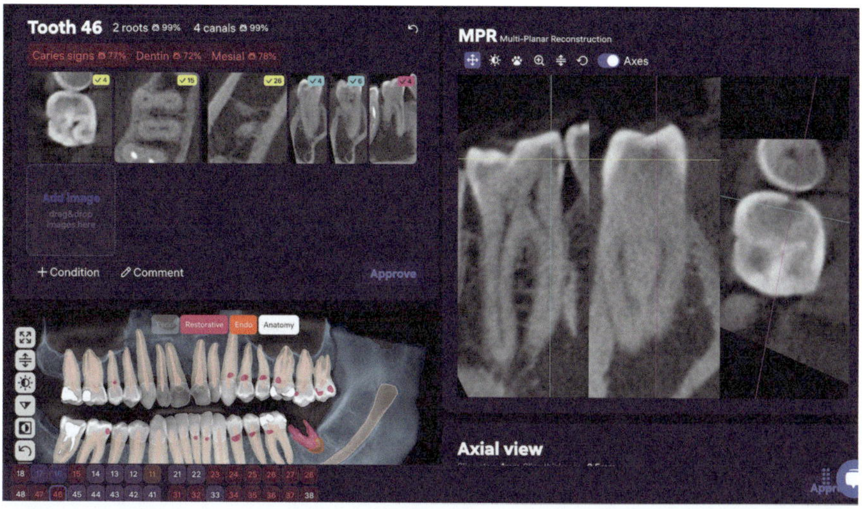

Fig. 5.7 Multiplanar reconstructed images of a CBCT AI report (Diagnocat) showing the presence of hypodense (radiolucent) crown area involving the dentin of tooth 46, despite a percentage of only 72% of AI confidence for such involvement reported by the software

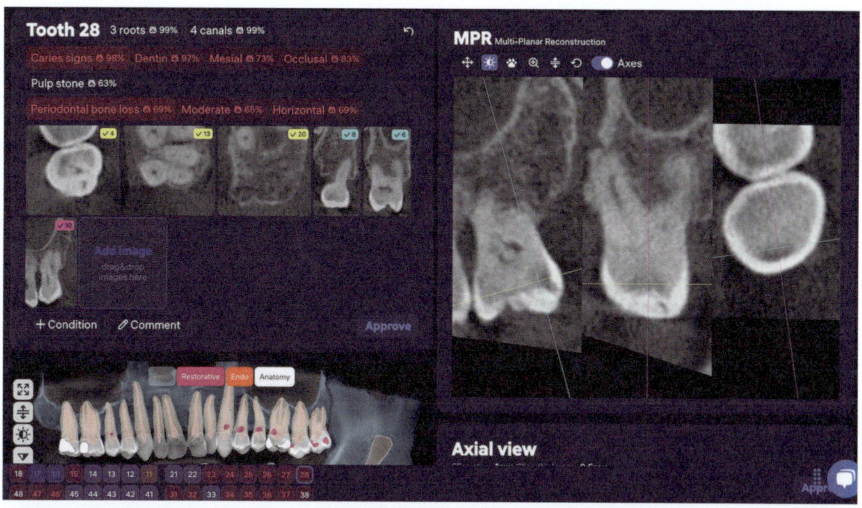

Fig. 5.8 Multiplanar reconstructed images of a CBCT AI report (Diagnocat) showing the presence of hypodense (radiolucent) crown area involving the dentin of tooth 28, with a percentage of 97% of AI confidence reported by the software

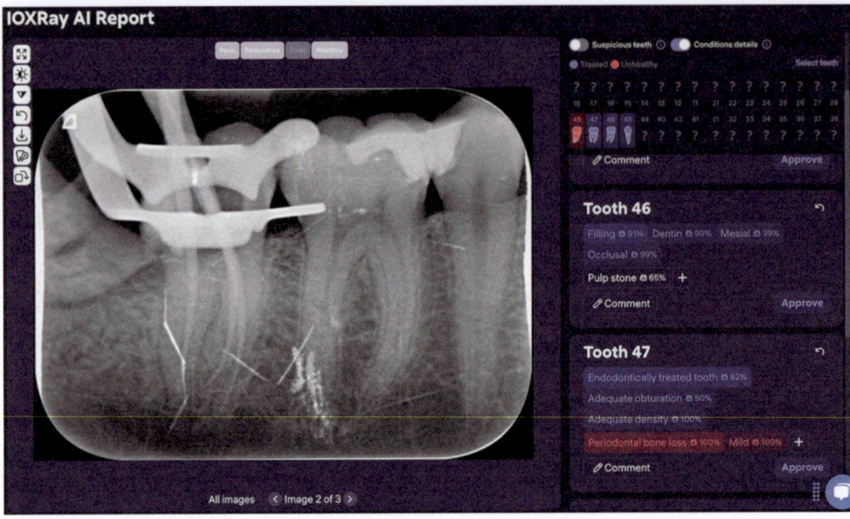

Fig. 5.9 AI report (Diagnocat) of a periapical radiography showing the situation during the endodontic treatment of tooth 47. Note the signs of damage on the phosphorus plate of this radiography and that the AI algorithm already considered the conditions of the obturation as satisfactory

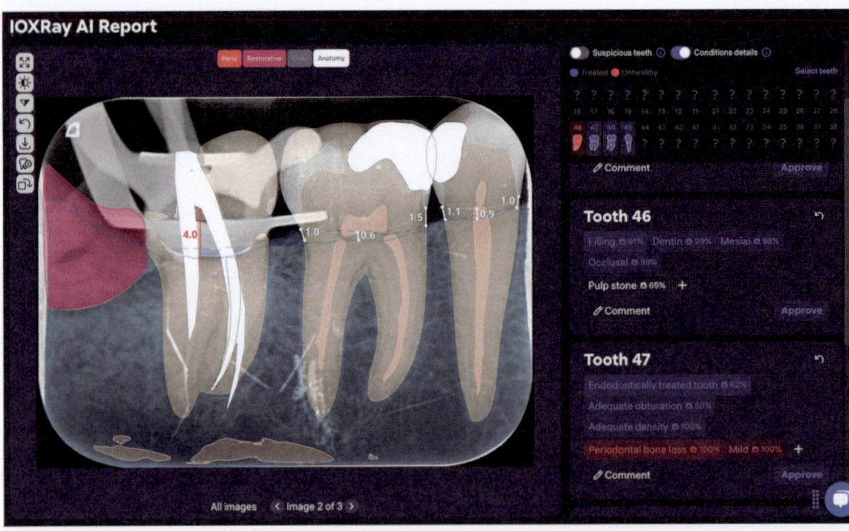

Fig. 5.10 AI report (Diagnocat) of the case of Fig. 5.9 with anatomical segmentation filter. Note that distal root canal could not be fully included by the segmentation, probably due to the conditions of the phosphorus plate used to obtain the image

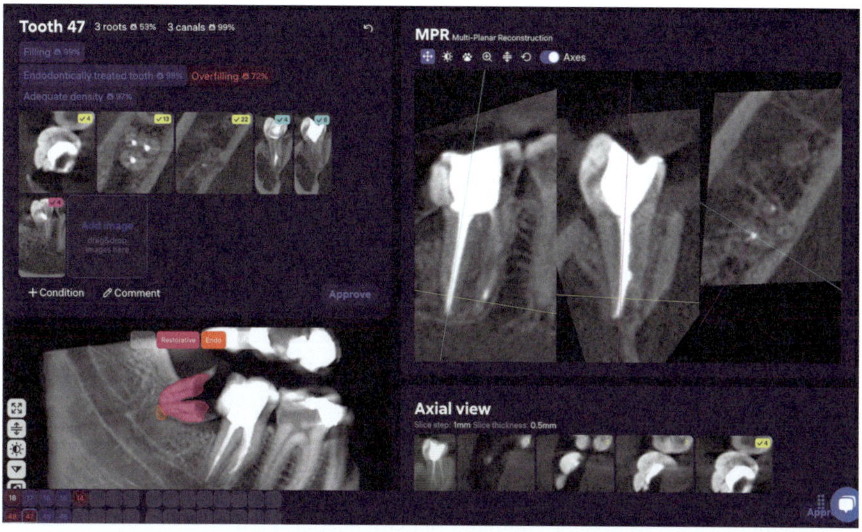

Fig. 5.11 AI report (Diagnocat) of a CBCT of the case of Figs. 5.9 and 5.10 taken after completion of the endodontic treatment for other reasons. Note that the distal root canal of tooth 47 was longer and could be adequately treated

Altering the vertical angulation of the X-ray beam provides solutions to several common diagnostic challenges in endodontics.

5.6.5.1 Visualizing Lingual Roots and Associated Pathology

When a clinician increases the vertical angulation, it causes a shortening of the tooth image on the radiograph. Because the buccal root is further from the film than the lingual root, it shortens more significantly. This differential shortening separates the root apices and produces a clearer, more accurate image of the lingual roots and any associated periapical lesions [10].

5.6.5.2 Distinguishing Anatomical Landmarks from Apical Pathology

Anatomical structures like nerve canals or foramina can be superimposed over a root apex, where they could be interpreted as a lesion of endodontic origin. Increasing the vertical angulation alters the vertical relationship between these structures and the root apices. For example, if the mandibular canal is located buccally to the roots of a mandibular molar, an increased vertical angle will cause the image of the canal to move vertically upward, superimposed on the roots. This principle can also be used to differentiate the mental and incisive foramina from adjacent root apices.

5.6.5.3 Reducing Superimposition of the Zygomatic Process

A common issue when radiographing maxillary molars is the superimposition of the dense, radiopaque zygomatic process over the root apices, which renders interpretation difficult. To overcome this, a cotton roll can be placed between the teeth and the film/phosphorus plate. This creates a more parallel relationship between the tooth and film, which in turn allows the clinician to reduce the vertical angulation. This change in projection angle effectively reduces the vertical angle, moving the image of the zygomatic process off the root apices and allowing for improved visualization.

While vertical shifts are powerful, the most versatile diagnostic tool comes from understanding the principles of horizontal angulation. The dental clinician should always ensure that the X-ray beam is completely parallel to the interproximal surfaces of the tooth/teeth to be diagnosed, especially for bitewing radiographs. Furthermore, one of the governing principles for interpreting horizontal angle shifts is a concept known as the buccal object rule, first described by Clark in 1916. The rule is based on the fact that an object's position on the film will shift based on its distance from the film when the X-ray beam angle is changed.

Specifically, a lingual object (closer to the film) will appear to move in the same direction as the X-ray beam shift, while a buccal object (further from the film) will appear to move in the opposite direction. This relationship is often remembered by the mnemonic "SLOB" (same lingual, opposite buccal) [10].

5.6.6 Clinically Relevant Issues Not Identified by the AI Algorithms

As mentioned in Chap. 1, anatomical variations and alterations such as impaction of a tooth may lead to issues on adjacent teeth and structures. However, the detection of unusual situations could be a challenge for AI algorithms due to the lack of training. One clinically relevant example is the unusual impaction of an upper third molar (Fig. 5.12), leading to important radiographic alterations on the adjacent second molar (Fig. 5.13), being contiguous with the maxillary sinus floor (Fig. 5.14).

5.7 Further Considerations on Current AI Systems

As previously discussed, the field of dentistry has been undergoing an important digital transformation, shifting from traditional analogue workflows to sophisticated, data-centric systems. This evolution is powered by technologies such as CBCT, intraoral scanners (IOS), and computer-aided design/computer-aided manufacturing (CAD/CAM), which enable highly detailed three-dimensional reconstructions and virtual treatment simulations. While these tools generate vast quantities of valuable clinical information, they also present a significant challenge: the sheer volume and complexity of this multimodal data increasingly exceed the capacity for consistent and comprehensive human interpretation.

This technological shift occurs within a critical global health context. The World Health Organization's 2022 Global Oral Health Status Report highlights that oral diseases affect an estimated 3.5 billion people worldwide, or nearly 45% of the global population. The report calls for the development of data-driven, standardized

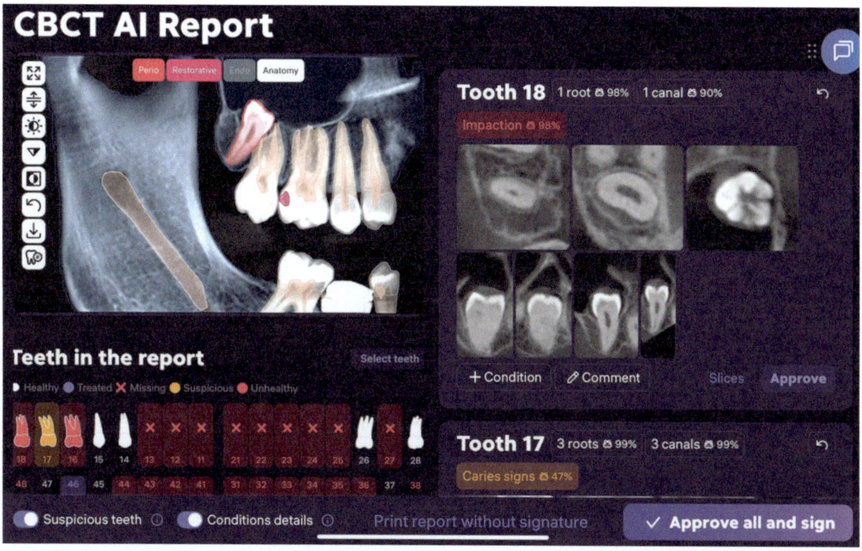

Fig. 5.12 CBCT AI report (Diagnocat) showing an ectopic maxillary right third molar. Note that the only alteration listed in the AI report was impaction

care pathways to help integrate oral health into universal health coverage and address widespread disparities in access to care. The sheer scale of this challenge demands solutions that can operate consistently and efficiently across diverse clinical settings, a requirement that has accelerated the turn toward artificial intelligence. AI has potential to provide an adequate solution to process this data and promote standardization, but its safe and effective integration into clinical practice is entirely dependent on a maturing landscape of methodological and regulatory governance.

Before evaluating AI as a potential solution, it is important to quantify the limitations of the current human-led interpretation within the data-rich environment of dentistry. The strategic importance of this diagnostic challenge becomes clear when we consider the scope and complexity of modern oral care.

Contemporary oral rehabilitation, as defined by the Glossary of Prosthodontic Terms (GPT-9), is a comprehensive field that encompasses the diagnosis and restoration of oral function and esthetics. Its domains include fixed and removable prosthodontics, implant-supported restorations, and occlusal therapy, which also addresses considerations related to the temporomandibular joint (TMJ). As previously discussed in this book, the diagnostic and treatment planning processes within these domains generate highly heterogeneous data streams, including radiographs, CBCT, intraoral scans, facial scans, jaw motion records with virtual articulator, and other types of data.

Synthesizing this diverse information into a coherent and reproducible treatment plan is a formidable task. The critical issue is observer variability, which remains substantial even among experienced professionals. Studies report only modest interobserver agreement ($\kappa = 0.4$–0.6) for a fundamental task such as early proximal

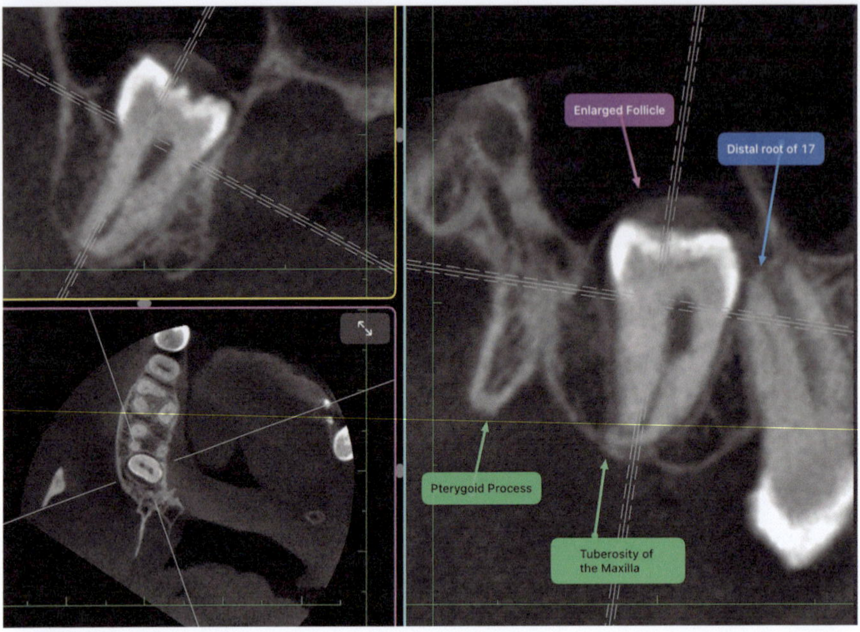

Fig. 5.13 Screenshot of the CBCT analysis of the case of Fig. 5.12, performed by an oral radiologist using the DICOM viewer software Falcon MD (iCAT solutions). Note the situation of tooth 18, being contiguous with the distal root of tooth 17

caries detection on bitewing radiographs, with even more notable disagreement among experienced clinicians on complex tasks like evaluating early peri-implant bone changes or subtle TMJ abnormalities.

This diagnostic inconsistency directly propagates into treatment planning, leading to unwarranted variations in care, from the initial indication for an intervention to the choice of a specific prosthetic or surgical modality. This reality underscores the urgent clinical need for more standardized and reproducible systems. The need for standardization has catalyzed parallel efforts to construct rigorous methodological and regulatory frameworks, ensuring that AI-driven solutions are developed responsibly from the outset (Fig. 5.15).

In response to the clinical need for greater consistency, parallel developments in AI methodology and regulation have created a robust framework designed to ensure that AI tools deployed in dentistry are safe, effective, and transparent. This governance structure is built upon two interconnected pillars: rigorous scientific standards for development and evaluation and legally binding regulatory pathways for market approval and surveillance (Fig. 5.16).

The maturation of medical AI has been guided by the establishment of updated reporting standards. These are not simply checklists but essential frameworks that promote transparent development and enable credible, independent evaluation of AI models. They provide a structured approach to ensure that research and clinical

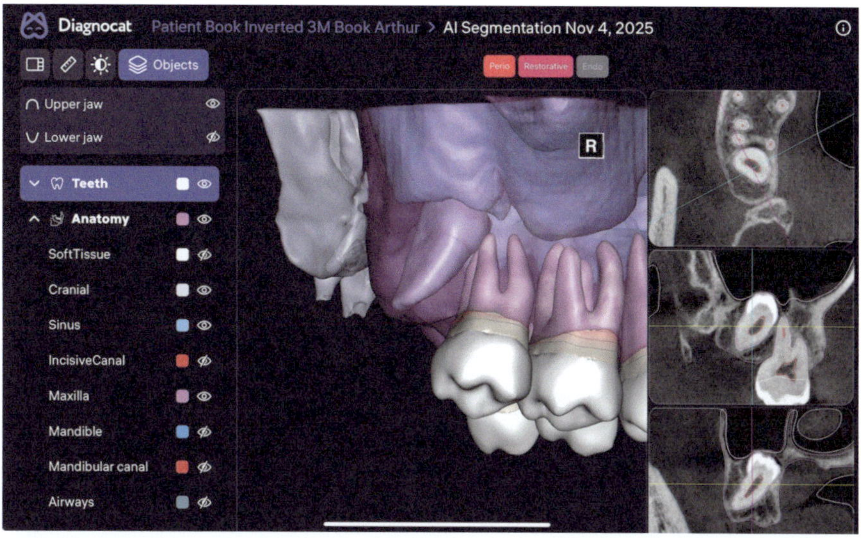

Fig. 5.14 CBCT 3D AI model (Diagnocat) of the case. Note that the shape of the maxillary sinus floor is incorrectly segmented, as its limits were only recognized on top of the ectopic crown of tooth 18

trials are conducted and reported with scientific integrity. Key standards include the following:

- TRIPOD-AI: An essential framework that guides the transparent reporting of how an AI prediction model was developed and validated, ensuring its claims can be critically and independently assessed.
- PROBAST-AI: A specialized tool designed to help researchers and clinicians systematically evaluate a study's risk of bias, thereby appraising the validity and credibility of its conclusions about an AI model.
- CONSORT-AI/SPIRIT-AI: Critical extensions to established guidelines that provide structured recommendations for reporting on clinical trials involving AI interventions (CONSORT-AI) and for developing robust protocols for such trials (SPIRIT-AI).

It is also noteworthy that formal regulatory pathways translate scientific best practices into mandatory legal requirements, ensuring that AI systems meet high standards before they can be used in patient care. These legal frameworks define clear expectations for safety, effectiveness, transparency, and post-market surveillance. The collective impact of these regulations is to create a predictable and trustworthy environment for both developers and clinicians. The leading frameworks governing dental AI include but are not limited to the US Food and Drug Administration's (FDA) software as a medical device (SaMD) framework, which outlines a risk-based approach to regulating software intended for medical

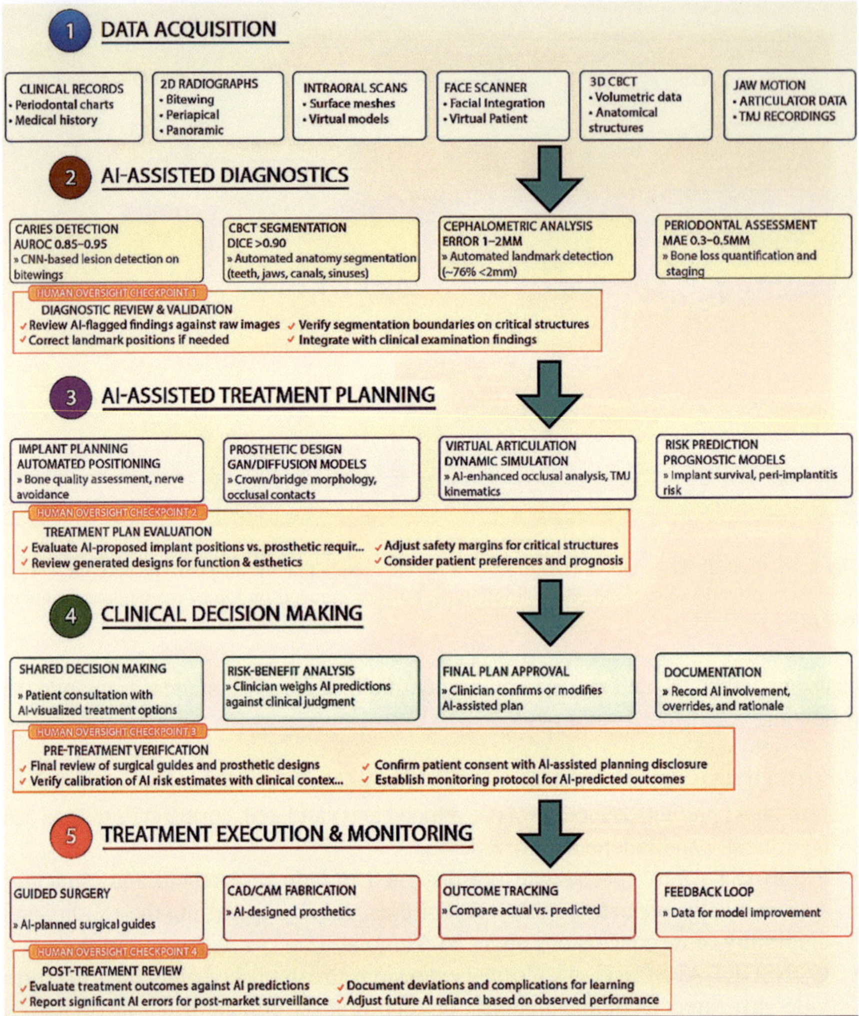

Fig. 5.15 Suggested characteristics of a standardized AI-powered clinical workflow

purposes, and the European Union's Medical Device Regulation (MDR), which establishes comprehensive rules for the safety and performance of medical devices, working in concert with the forthcoming AI Act that will introduce specific legal requirements for AI systems.

A recent review of 44 studies on dental AI reveals a heavy imbalance, with most research focused on validation rather than real-world deployment [4]. To understand this imbalance, one can use the Fryback and Thornbury model, a six-level framework for evaluating the efficacy of diagnostic technologies. The model provides a hierarchy for assessing a technology's impact, from its technical accuracy to its benefit to society as a whole:

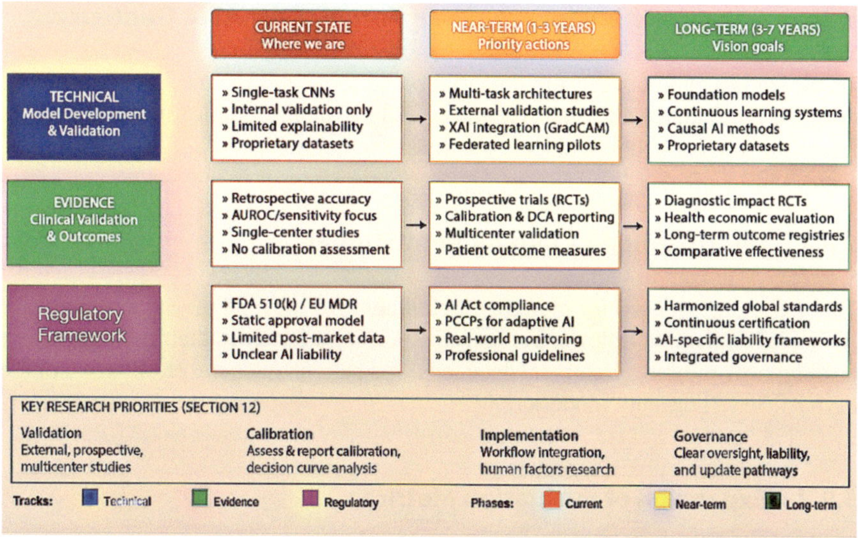

Fig. 5.16 Technical, scientific, and regulatory aspects of AI-powered clinical workflows

Level 1. Technical Efficacy: Focuses on the algorithm's accuracy, computational efficiency, and technical performance
Level 2. Diagnostic Accuracy Efficacy: Compares the sensitivity and specificity of AI to that of expert human dentists in controlled settings
Level 3. Diagnostic Thinking Efficacy: Assesses the effect of AI on clinician confidence and diagnosis
Level 4. Therapeutic Efficacy: Measures the influence of AI on actual treatment plans
Level 5. Patient Outcome Efficacy: Evaluates the direct impact on patient health (e.g., quality of life, morbidity)
Level 6. Societal Efficacy: Considers broad economic and public health benefits

The review of existing dental AI research showed a clear concentration at the bottom of this hierarchy. First, a total of 27 of the 44 studies only achieved Level 2, focusing solely on diagnostic accuracy in controlled, nonclinical environments. Another gap in clinical evidence can also be observed, as only one study reached Level 5 (Patient Outcome Efficacy) and only one study reached Level 6 (Societal Efficacy). Finally, orthodontics is the most explored field for AI applications, while other important fields of study such as prosthodontics and periodontics remain underrepresented.

5.8 Considerations on the Path Forward for AI in Dentistry

To bridge the gap between the potential of AI tools and the current practice, the research community and industry must adopt a more comprehensive approach. Important aspects to be considered are discussed below.

5.8.1 Prioritization of Deployment Studies

There is an urgent need for more research that moves beyond the lab and evaluates AI in real clinical workflows. This means focusing on studies that measure impact on diagnostic thinking, treatment decisions, and patient outcomes (Levels 3–6 of the Fryback and Thornbury model).

5.8.2 Expansion of Evaluation Metrics

Future assessments must look beyond simple accuracy. It is vital to include metrics that matter to patients and society, such as patient-centered outcomes (quality of life), equity (identifying and mitigating bias across demographic groups), and explainability (ensuring the AI's reasoning is transparent and understandable).

5.8.3 Support for Collaborations and Standardization

Developers, dental practitioners, and regulatory bodies must work together to establish clear guidelines and standards. Standardization in development, testing, and deployment will help ensure that AI tools are consistent and reliable and produce trustworthy results across different systems.

5.8.4 Assurance of Transparency

AI developers must be more transparent and provide opportunities for independent and rigorous assessment of their applications. Offering trials and collaborating with researchers will build confidence and allow dental professionals to make informed decisions about adopting new technologies.

Furthermore, based on all scientific evidence discussed, other important guidelines are recommended for education and clinical practice, as discussed below.

5.8.5 Development of AI-Centric Curricula

Dental schools and professional bodies must create and integrate standardized curricula that address the current educational gap. This training should equip future and current dental professionals with the knowledge to use, evaluate, and critically appraise AI tools.

5.8.6 Promotion of Clinician-AI Collaboration

Given the current performance variability, AI tools should be positioned to augment, not replace, clinical expertise and professional judgment. Current tools are not yet reliable enough to substitute for traditional diagnostic methods but can serve as a valuable supplementary aid.

5.8.7 Investment in Training and Technology

Dental clinics planning to adopt AI must anticipate the need for significant investments in both technology infrastructure and ongoing staff training to ensure successful integration into clinical workflows.

References

1. Aldhafeeri FM. Governing artificial intelligence in radiology: a systematic review of ethical, legal, and regulatory frameworks. Diagnostics (Basel). 2025;15(18):2300. https://doi.org/10.3390/diagnostics15182300.
2. Ghaffari M, Zhu Y, Shrestha A. A review of advancements of artificial intelligence in dentistry. Dentistry Review. 2024;4:100081. https://doi.org/10.1016/j.dentre.2024.100081.
3. Sitaras S, Tsolakis IA, Gelsini M, Tsolakis AI, Schwendicke F, Wolf TG, Perlea P. Applications of artificial intelligence in dental medicine: a critical review. Int Dent J. 2025;75(2):474–86. https://doi.org/10.1016/j.identj.2024.11.009.
4. Lal A, Nooruddin A, Umer F. Concerns regarding deployment of AI-based applications in dentistry—a review. BDJ Open. 2025;11(1):27. https://doi.org/10.1038/s41405-025-00319-7.
5. Vayena E, Blasimme A. Biomedical big data: new models of control over access, use and governance. J Bioeth Inq. 2017;14(4):501–13. https://doi.org/10.1007/s11673-017-9809-6.
6. Finlayson SG, Bowers JD, Ito J, Zittrain JL, Beam AL, Kohane IS. Adversarial attacks on medical machine learning. Science. 2019;363(6433):1287–9. https://doi.org/10.1126/science.aaw4399.
7. Banavar SR, Chippagiri P. Mandibular bilateral fourth molars—a rare and interesting occurrence. J Clin Diagn Res. 2014;8(5):ZJ01. https://doi.org/10.7860/JCDR/2014/7451.4209.
8. Luten JR. The prevalence of supernumerary teeth in primary and mixed dentitions. J Dent Child. 1967;34:346–53.
9. Arzani S, Karimi A, Iranmanesh P, Yazdi M, Sabeti MA, Nekoofar MH, Kolahi J, Bang H, Dummer PMH. Examining the diagnostic accuracy of artificial intelligence for detecting dental caries across a range of imaging modalities: an umbrella review with meta-analysis. PLoS One. 2025;20(8):e0329986. https://doi.org/10.1371/journal.pone.0329986.
10. Fava LR, Dummer PM. Periapical radiographic techniques during endodontic diagnosis and treatment. Int Endod J. 1997;30(4):250–61. https://doi.org/10.1046/j.1365-2591.1997.00078.x.

Part II

Dental Treatment Planning

Artificial Intelligence Tools for Dental Clinics

6

Newton Sesma, Lisya Vizotto de Barros, Marcelo Lucchesi Teixeira, Bruno B. R. Matias, Sergio Candido Dias, Angelica de Moura e Costa, Vinicius Dutra, Guilherme Saavedra, Tatiana Cursino Pereira, Fernando Antonio Reis Laurino, Lucas Rodrigues Pinheiro, and Arthur Rodriguez Gonzalez Cortes

6.1 Large Language Models (LLMs) in Dentistry

Large language models (LLMs) represent a significant advancement in generative artificial intelligence, trained on vast datasets to produce humanlike text and perform complex language-based tasks such as answering questions and providing recommendations [1, 2]. Their growing integration into various industries has spurred

Supplementary Information The online version contains supplementary material available at https://doi.org/10.1007/978-3-032-24895-4_6.

N. Sesma · L. V. de Barros · M. L. Teixeira · B. B. R. Matias
University of São Paulo, São Paulo, Brazil
e-mail: sesma@usp.br

S. C. Dias · L. R. Pinheiro
Private Practice, São Paulo, Brazil

A. d. M. e. Costa
MAC Radiology Institute, Curitiba, Brazil

V. Dutra
Department of Oral Pathology, Medicine, and Radiology, Indiana University, School of Dentistry, Indianapolis, IN, USA
e-mail: vidutra@iu.edu

G. Saavedra · T. C. Pereira · F. A. R. Laurino
São Paulo State University—UNESP, São Paulo, Brazil
e-mail: guilherme.saavedra@unesp.br

A. R. G. Cortes (✉)
Faculty of Dental Surgery, University of Malta, Msida, Malta
e-mail: arthur.nogueira@um.edu.mt

A. R. G. Cortes (ed.), *Dental Clinical Procedures using Artificial Intelligence*,
https://doi.org/10.1007/978-3-032-24895-4_6

significant investigation into their potential applications within healthcare and, more specifically, radiology. The ability of some LLMs to perform on par with clinicians in medical licensing and specialty examinations has underscored their potential as powerful analytical tools.

In healthcare, LLMs are being explored for a range of applications [3], from cloud-based systems assisting patients with initial medical inquiries to chatbots capable of simplifying complex radiology reports to improve patient comprehension without losing essential information [4]. A particularly innovative frontier is the development of vision-language models, which process and integrate information from both image and text inputs [5]. These multimodal systems are being designed to generate image captions, interpret report findings, and assist in diagnostic procedures, fundamentally enhancing how clinicians and patients interact with radiological data.

Evaluating LLMs against professional qualification examinations is a crucial, low-risk validation strategy. These benchmarks provide an objective measure of a model's foundational knowledge and reasoning capabilities before it can be considered for higher-stakes clinical decision support roles. This area of study provides critical insights into the current strengths and weaknesses of LLMs compared to human learners and practitioners.

6.1.1 LLM in Dental Education

Recent studies evaluating LLMs on dentomaxillofacial radiology (DMFR) qualification exams reveal a wide range of performance levels, often highlighting a significant gap between AI and human expertise, particularly in tasks requiring visual interpretation. A comparative study by Jeong et al. found that while dental students achieved an overall correctness of 81.2% on a DMFR exam, the ChatGPT Plus model scored 65.4%. The performance disparity was most pronounced in radiographic image interpretation, where students scored 78.5% while all tested chatbots scored below 35% [6]. Performance also varies significantly across different models, exams, and languages, which likely reflects the rapid evolution of the technology. A consistent finding across studies is that LLM performance is heavily influenced by question complexity and the degree of reliance on image analysis; models generally perform better on fundamental knowledge questions but struggle with the nuanced interpretation required for DMFR-specific radiographic images [6].

Beyond answering questions, LLMs are also being tested for their ability to generate educational content. A previous study found that GPT-4o could create board-style examination questions of a quality equivalent to those written by human experts [7]. However, some AI-generated questions were based on "hallucinations" or fabricated information. This finding underscores the indispensable need for human expert oversight to validate the accuracy and reliability of any AI-generated educational or clinical material. While these educational evaluations reveal the current knowledge base and reasoning limits of LLMs, their true clinical potential lies in their application to real-world diagnostic challenges, beginning with diagnosis and treatment planning.

6.1.2 LLM-Assisted Diagnosis and Clinical Decision Support

The potential for LLMs to augment clinical diagnostics represents one of their most promising applications in medicine. In DMFR, these models could theoretically assist clinicians by interpreting radiographic findings, generating differential diagnoses, and formulating treatment plans. However, the clinical utility of these tools is entirely dependent on their validated accuracy and reliability, which remains a key area of investigation.

When provided with text-based inputs such as patient symptoms and clinical findings, LLMs have shown some promising capabilities. A previous study found that GPT-3.5 generated outputs that received favorable expert ratings for differential diagnoses (mean 3.85/5) and treatment plans (4.13/5) [8]. However, performance is not uniform. Research by Hu et al. noted that while GPT-3.5 could produce well-structured outputs, its performance was variable and dependent on the complexity of the disease, and the model demonstrated a tendency to generate imprecise or "hallucinated" statements [9].

The direct interpretation of radiographic images is a more challenging task for LLMs, and current evidence shows highly inconsistent performance. The accuracy of vision-capable models varies significantly depending on the specific diagnostic task and, crucially, the model's level of specialization. The performance of general-purpose models on complex image tasks stands in stark contrast to the high performance achieved by specialized, fine-tuned models. This suggests that customization is a key driver of high performance.

Further analysis reveals specific limitations in image interpretation. A previous study observed that while GPT-3.5 could successfully describe general features of a pathology, such as its origin and periphery, it struggled to identify the precise shape of the lesion or accurately assess its effect on adjacent anatomical structures [10]. Similarly, Kahalian and collaborators found that providing specific diagnostic clues improved GPT-4.0's diagnostic performance, though the model's ability to generate a diverse and clinically relevant list of differential diagnoses remained limited [11]. While LLMs show nascent ability in interpreting clinical and image data, their most immediate utility may be in translating these interpretations into the primary clinical deliverable: the radiology report.

6.1.3 Automating the Generation of Radiology Reports Holds Strategic Value for Clinical Practice

This application of LLMs aims to reduce clinician workload, promote standardized reporting formats, and improve the efficiency of communication with referring colleagues and patients. Research in this area is exploring both text-based report generation from structured data and more advanced multimodal systems that interpret images directly.

Current evidence suggests that LLMs can effectively generate coherent and readable reports, though with some notable limitations in completeness. In a previous study, GPT-4 was tasked with generating radiology reports from structured checklists of findings. The resulting AI-generated reports were highly readable and free of grammatical errors but contained significantly fewer findings than reports written by dental students based on the same checklists. Importantly, because the task was constrained to the provided checklist data, no instances of hallucination were observed [12]. More advanced, specialized multimodal AI systems are also being developed. One such system, described by Dasanayaka and collaborators, combines computer vision with an LLM to generate reports from panoramic radiographs, achieving an overall diagnostic accuracy of 81.3% [13]. Similarly, a multilevel objective alignment transformer model was also developed to generate fine tooth-level reports from panoramic radiographs with reported accuracy of approximately 70%. Nevertheless, its ability to detect and describe jaw pathologies remains unknown.

LLMs also offer a promising avenue for improving how clinical information is communicated to patients. The multimodal system developed by Dasanayaka et al. included a feature for answering patient questions in multiple languages (English and Sinhala), demonstrating an accuracy of 74.1% and receiving an expert-rated quality score of 6.1/10 [13]. Other research has shown that commercially available chatbots can effectively simplify existing radiology reports for a lay audience without losing essential diagnostic information, thereby making complex medical findings more accessible to patients [4]. These developments signal a move toward more integrated AI tools in the radiology workflow, but their successful implementation hinges on addressing the significant challenges that currently limit their widespread adoption.

6.1.4 Practical Methodology for AI-Assisted Report Generation (Method by Dr. Angélica Costa)

The Foundational Principle of AI-assisted radiology reports are the creation of structured prompts to achieve quality outputs. The strategic implementation of AI in clinical documentation hinges on the principle of effective prompt engineering. In the context of generating radiological reports, a prompt is not a simple question, but a detailed, structured directive meticulously designed to elicit a precise, comprehensive, and clinically valuable response from the AI. This methodology ensures that the AI's computational power is channeled effectively, transforming raw human observations into a polished and professional report that adheres to the highest clinical standards. The quality of the output is directly proportional to the clarity and structure of the input command.

The sample prompt used in this methodology can be deconstructed into three main components, each serving a critical function in guiding the response of the AI model:

1. Persona definition: The instruction on the prompt "Act as an expert in Dental Radiology and Imaging ..." is an important first step. This command sets the context for the AI tool, instructing it to adopt a specific professional persona. This ensures that the response will utilize the appropriate technical vocabulary, adhere to the conventions of radiological reporting, and draw from a knowledge base relevant to the specialty.
2. Structural framework: The prompt explicitly details a multipart structure for the final report—description of the image, diagnostic hypotheses, and comments and recommendations. This rigid framework is essential for clinical utility. It forces the AI to organize the information logically, ensuring that the final document is not only comprehensive and descriptive but also clinically actionable, guiding the referring clinician toward a definitive diagnosis and appropriate patient management.
3. Data Input: The placeholder "[... INSERT THE DESCRIPTION OF THE ALTERATION HERE ...]" represents the critical junction between human expertise and AI processing. This is where the radiologist inserts their detailed, nuanced, and context-rich observations from the imaging study. This step perfectly illustrates the "garbage in, garbage out" principle, as the entire AI-driven analysis is built upon the foundation of this human-generated data. The accuracy and detail provided here directly determine the quality and relevance of the final report.

This structured approach transforms the AI from a general language tool into a specialized assistant for clinical documentation, ready for practical application in complex cases. The following two case studies using LLM received AI-driven radiology reports following the standards of oral radiology in Brazil (where this field is recognized as an official specialty of dentistry) but translated to English.

6.1.5 Case Study 1: Reactive Intra-sinus Bone Hyperplasia (Case by Dr. Angelica Costa)

- Patient profile: Female, 41 years and 3 months.
- Reason for examination: Routine tomographic study of the maxilla for follow-up.
- Initial radiologist's description: An extensive osteogenic reaction was observed, associated with an infectious-inflammatory process originating from teeth #25 and #26.

The alteration extends superiorly into the left maxillary sinus, presenting a heterogeneous, mixed-density pattern interspersed with areas of lower hyperdensity that suggest a chronic inflammatory response from the maxillary sinus to a persistent stimulus. Within the sinus cavity, a hyperdense mass is identified, delimited by denser, corticated margins and exhibiting a heterogeneous internal pattern. The

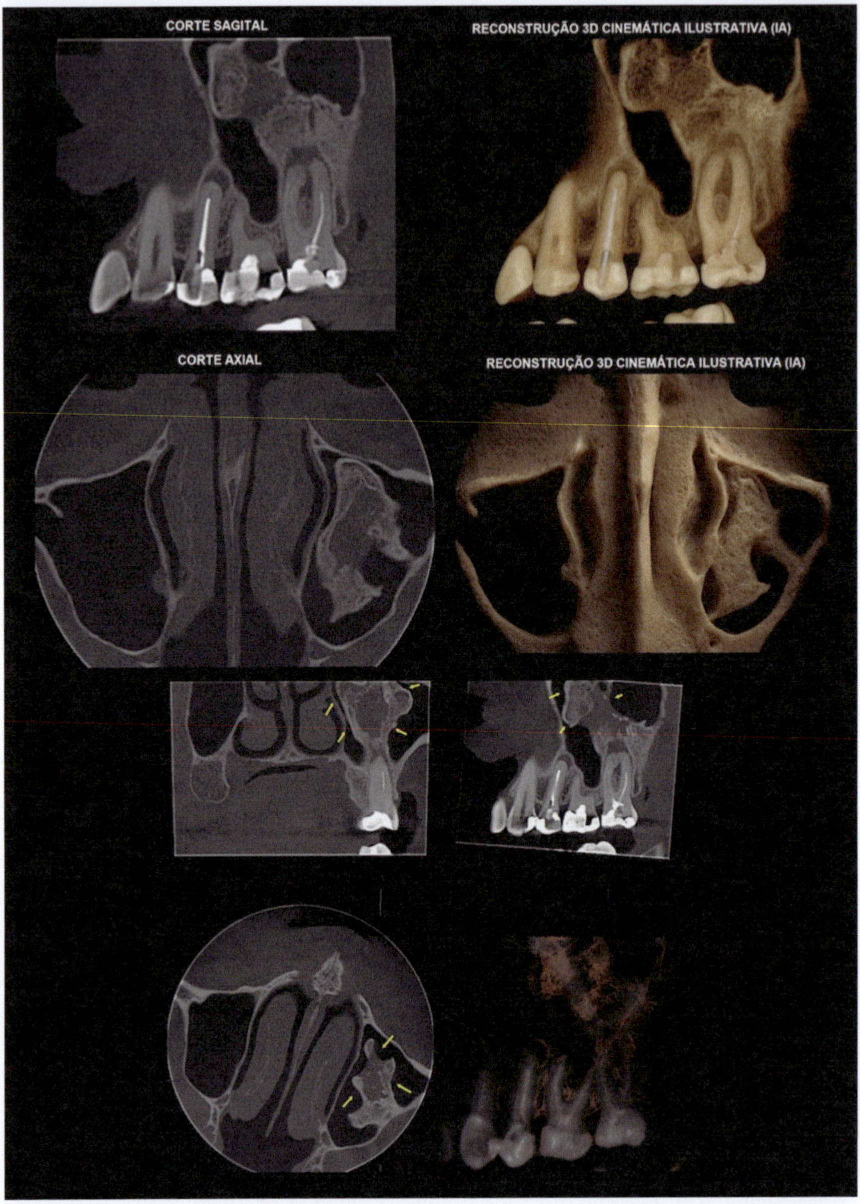

Fig. 6.1 Screenshot of the images from the LLM-driven radiology report showing two cinematic reconstructions in sagittal and axial views (top right quadrant of the figure) of the mixed periapical lesion projected into the left maxillary sinus

large formation alters the morphology of the sinus floor and occupies a considerable vertical extent of the cavity (Fig. 6.1). A channel establishing communication between the alveolar ridge crest and the sinus interior is also noted, consistent with a possible oroantral communication. Regional thickening of the sinus lining mucosa reinforces the secondary inflammatory nature of the condition. The collective findings are consistent with reactive intra-sinus bone hyperplasia resulting from a chronic, long-standing inflammatory stimulus directly associated with the involved teeth.

Final Hybrid Report: The tomographic study of the maxilla reveals, in the region of teeth #25 and #26—both affected by changes consistent with an infectious-inflammatory lesion at their apices (possible periapical lesion)—an extensive osteogenic reaction resulting from a chronic inflammatory process. The formation presents a heterogeneous, mixed-density pattern, extending superiorly and projecting into the left maxillary sinus. Within the sinus cavity, a voluminous hyperdense image is observed, peripherally delimited by a more densely corticated halo with well-defined borders. It exhibits a heterogeneous internal pattern and significant vertical projection, consistent with an adaptive response to a persistent inflammatory stimulus.

Associated with this condition, a channel communicating the alveolar crest with the interior of the sinus cavity is identified, compatible with a possible oroantral communication. The sinus lining mucosa shows irregular thickening in the adjacent region, reinforcing the chronic inflammatory behavior of the alteration. The collective findings configure a characteristic pattern of reactive intra-sinus bone hyperplasia secondary to a persistent odontogenic infectious stimulus related to elements #25 and #26.

The diagnostic hypotheses are as follows:

1. Primary hypothesis: Reactive intra-sinus bone hyperplasia associated with a chronic inflammatory process of odontogenic origin.
2. Differential diagnoses: Less likely possibilities include condensing osteitis with intra-sinus extension and chronic sinusopathy with reactive bone neoformation, although the volumetric behavior, morphology, and density pattern strongly favor the primary hypothesis.

Correlation with previous imaging studies for evolutionary assessment and integration with the clinical history is recommended, particularly regarding prior inflammatory episodes related to the involved teeth. Otorhinolaryngological and dental correlation are also suggested for a conclusive diagnosis and appropriate therapeutic planning.

This case demonstrates how the AI-assisted process refined the radiologist's core findings into a formally structured, highly detailed, and clinically coherent final report.

6.1.6 Case Study 2: Postradiation Maxillary Alteration (Case by Dr. Angelica Costa)

- Patient profile: Female, 50 years
- Reason for examination: Tomographic study of the maxilla for suspected osteoradionecrosis. Patient has a history of adenocarcinoma and received radiation therapy to the palate in 2021.

- Initial radiologist's description: In the posterior right maxilla, a well-delimited, hypodense area with regular margins and defined contours is observed, involving the medullary bone in the region of tooth #16. The pattern shows rounded bone resorption containing hypodense content consistent with gas accumulation. The alteration is not associated with cortical expansion or dehiscence but with thinning of the cortical bone of the right maxillary sinus floor (Fig. 6.2). Mild sinus membrane thickening is also present at the same side of the patient. No evident bone sequestra or periosteal changes suggestive of acute inflammation are identified at this time. This finding could represent a healing bone site (post-extraction or post-excision of a neoplastic lesion) or an active/recurrent osteolytic lesion.

Final Hybrid Report: In the posterior right maxilla, at the location of tooth #16, a well-delimited hypodense area with regular contours and defined margins is observed. It presents a pattern of rounded bone resorption involving predominantly the medullary bone, with the presence of gaseous content inside the lesion and slight cortical thinning of the right maxillary sinus floor. This is associated with a thin laminar thickening of the homolateral sinus mucosa. There is no tomographic evidence of bone sequestra, cortical rupture, or active periosteal reaction.

Given the patient's history of radiation therapy to the palate in 2021 for the treatment of adenocarcinoma, these findings may correspond to the following:

1. A healing bone site (post-extraction or post-excision of an osteolytic lesion)
2. A residual cavity with minimal sinus communication
3. A low-grade chronic inflammatory osteolytic condition
4. An initial manifestation of osteoradionecrosis

It is crucial to correlate these findings with clinical symptoms such as pain, dental mobility, or signs of bone exposure. A detailed recent local history is essential. Referral for evaluation by an oral medicine specialist or an oral and maxillofacial surgeon is strongly recommended to determine the need for biopsy, serial follow-up, or specific management to rule out recurrent osteolytic activity or progression consistent with osteoradionecrosis.

The hybrid report effectively balances the descriptive imaging findings with necessary clinical recommendations, showcasing a responsible and context-aware application of AI in a high-stakes clinical scenario.

6.1.7 AI in Visual Communication and Diagnostics

Beyond text-based report generation, AI offers powerful tools for visual communication, such as cinematic 3D reconstructions (Fig. 6.3). These advanced visualizations serve as a valuable aid for enhancing the understanding of complex anatomical relationships for both clinicians and patients. They are, however, intended for educational and illustrative purposes and must not be used for primary diagnosis. The

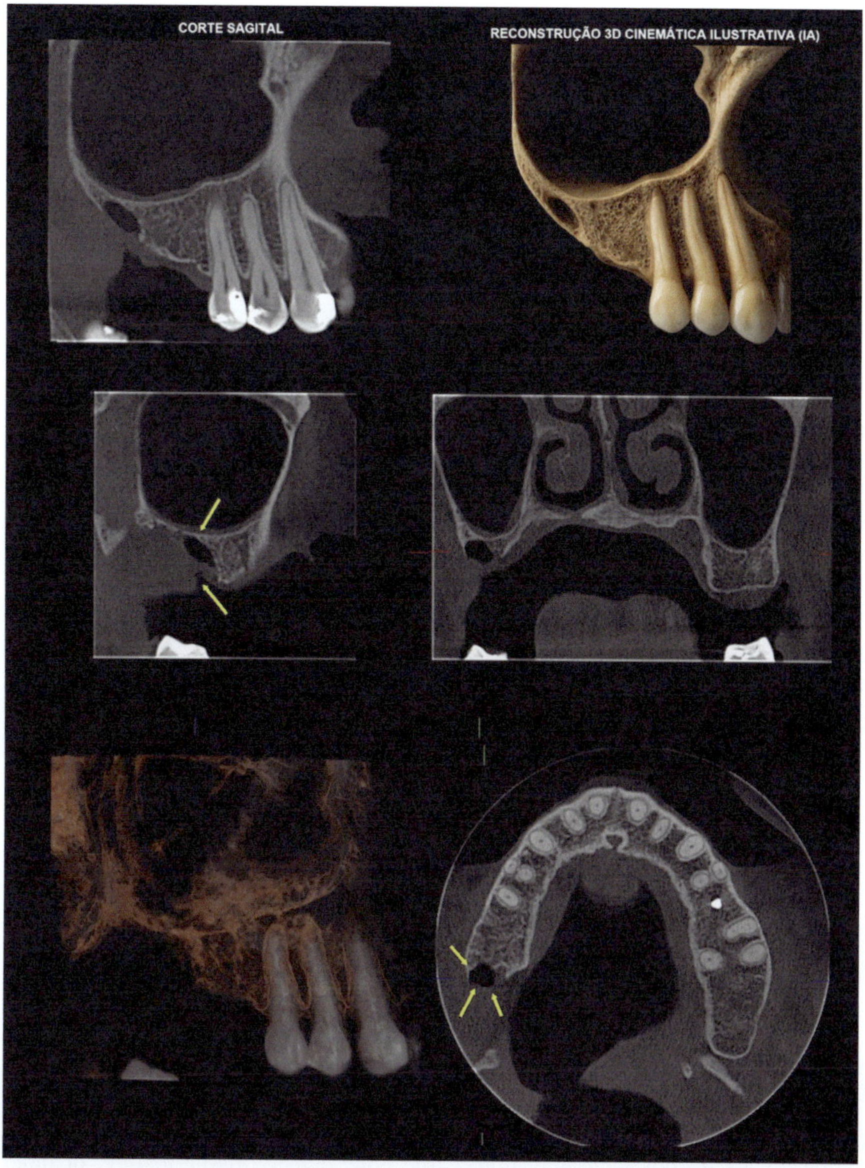

Fig. 6.2 Screenshot of the images from the LLM-driven radiology report showing an AI-driven cinematic reconstruction in sagittal view (top right corner) of the hypodense area on the alveolar crest at the right tuberosity of the maxilla

function and limitations of these AI-generated reconstructions are critical to understand their responsible use in a clinical setting.

AI-generated reconstructions aim to provide a high-quality, intuitive visual representation of complex anatomical and pathological structures. This facilitates

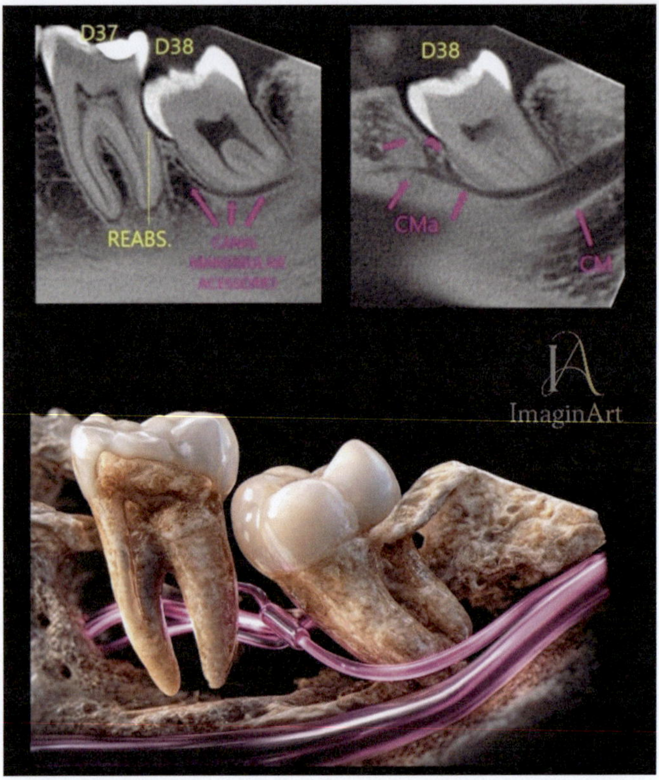

Fig. 6.3 Screenshot of the images from an LLM-driven radiology report showing sagittal slices (top) and the corresponding AI-driven cinematic reconstruction in sagittal view (bottom) of an impacted left mandibular third molar contiguous with a bifurcation of the mandibular canal

clearer patient education, enhances interdisciplinary communication, and assists in treatment planning discussions by making spatial relationships easier to comprehend. These reconstructions are generated using advanced algorithms that perform volumetric estimation, spatial modeling, and aesthetic rendering based on the original tomographic data.

It is important to recognize the limitation that these images are illustrative simulations. They do not accurately reflect true bone density, tissue texture, or other quantitative tomographic parameters. The visuals are constructed from computational inferences and rendering principles, not direct measurement. Therefore, they must never be used as a stand-alone basis for diagnostic decisions, which must always be made from the original, multiplanar tomographic slices.

These reconstructions enhance diagnostic communication by adding an interesting visual layer, which can also be performed for conventional 2D radiographs (Fig. 6.4). Nevertheless, the analysis remains firmly dependent and based on the radiologist interpretation of the source imaging data, as explained below.

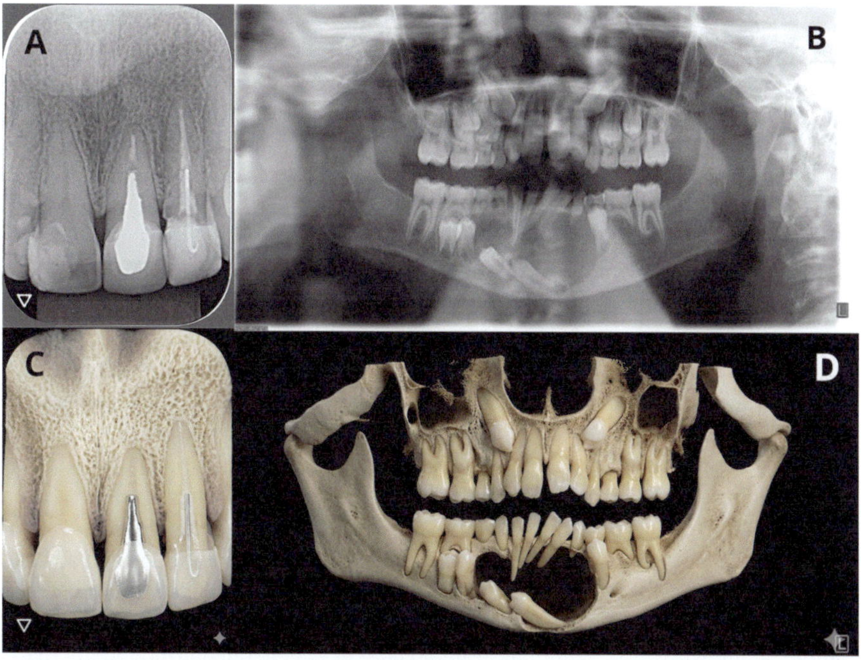

Fig. 6.4 Example of an AI-generated "cinematic" visualization derived from conventional dental radiographs (image-to-image workflow) using Gemini (Nano Banana Pro). (**a**) Grayscale periapical (intraoral) radiograph showing endodontic treatment and two intracanal retainers: a metallic post and a temporary post fabricated from orthodontic wire. (**b**) Grayscale panoramic radiograph demonstrating a radiolucent lesion in the anterior mandible consistent with an odontogenic keratocyst. (**c**) AI-generated "3D-like" (cinematic) rendering derived from the intraoral image in (**a**), applying a density-based color transfer function (CLUT/transfer function) and ray-tracing–like shading to enhance material appearance and interfaces while maintaining the original composition. (**d**) Perspective cinematic visualization derived from the panoramic image in (**b**), emphasizing depth cues and texture for communication and illustration. **Attention: This process does not convert a two-dimensional radiograph into a true 3D image**; it is an illustrative visualization based on the original projection. For illustrative/educational use only; not intended for diagnostic interpretation

6.1.7.1 Working Mechanism and Differences Among the Types of 3D Reconstructions

Three-dimensional (3D) reconstruction from radiographic and especially tomographic examinations (such as cone-beam computed tomography, CBCT) is one of the most powerful ways to "translate" volumetric information into human perception. When properly applied, it enhances spatial understanding, improves professional communication, facilitates planning, and makes teaching more intuitive. More recently, generative artificial intelligence (AI) tools have enabled "cinematic reconstructions" with a photorealistic appearance, using the tomographic slice itself as the basis and applying density mapping and virtual lighting. In the following sections, we present using a technical yet accessible approach the fundamentals of 3D reconstructions in CBCT, how generative AI can contribute to cinematic visualizations, how to structure reproducible prompts, and, most importantly, when to use (and when not to use) these images. Importantly, these visualizations are not intended for diagnostic purposes; they are meant exclusively for illustration, education, and communication, supporting the explanation of findings already present in the original examination.

In CBCT, the examination is not merely "an image": it is a set of voxels (pixels with depth) arranged in a volumetric matrix. Each voxel stores a value related to X-ray attenuation/absorption, which correlates with tissue density (air < soft tissues < trabecular bone < cortical bone < enamel < high-density materials). The first step in any 3D visualization is to recognize that volumetric data can be "read" in multiple ways and that many outputs remain two-dimensional representations of a volume (rather than a "true 3D object"). For this reason, the literature distinguishes "truly three-dimensional images" (e.g., stereoscopy/holography) from the 2D representations of volumetric data that are most commonly used in clinical practice.

Before discussing 3D data, it is worth noting that much of what is often referred to as "reconstruction" is, in fact, volume reformatting, such as multiplanar reconstruction (MPR) in axial/coronal/sagittal planes, as well as oblique, curved, and trans-axial reformations, previously mentioned in this book. The "reconstructed panoramic image," for example, is typically a curved reformation from the CBCT volume, along with cross-sectional (trans-axial) slices generated orthogonally to the selected curve. For this purpose, thickness and increment parameters can be adjusted according to the objective (for instance, simulating thicker projections or prioritizing detail with thin slices). A useful analogy is to think of the volume as a "block of information" and the reformations as different ways of slicing that block, each emphasizing specific anatomic relationships.

For a volume to become a visually interpretable image, voxel values must be mapped to visual properties. In practical terms, this is a transfer function: a set of rules that converts intensity (relative density) into color, opacity (transparency), and, when applicable, brightness/reflectance. In rendering workflows, this mapping can be understood as a type of CLUT (Color Lookup Table): a "table" that defines how each intensity range should appear in the final image (as shown in Chap. 3, Fig. 3.40). If the CLUT is well calibrated, high-density structures (cortical bone, enamel, restorative materials) remain visually more "prominent," while lower-density structures (medullary bone, soft tissues) appear more subtle, preserving the diagnostic hierarchy of the examination. If poorly calibrated, the rendering may look attractive but become misleading (contrast inversion, loss of interfaces, "blown-out" enamel, etc.).

For didactic purposes, the most common 3D visualizations can be grouped into three categories:

Surface rendering (indirect)

Also referred to in many contexts as indirect volume rendering, it is based on extracting a surface using an intensity threshold, generating a mesh that represents a tissue interface. A classic example is shaded surface display (SSD). It is

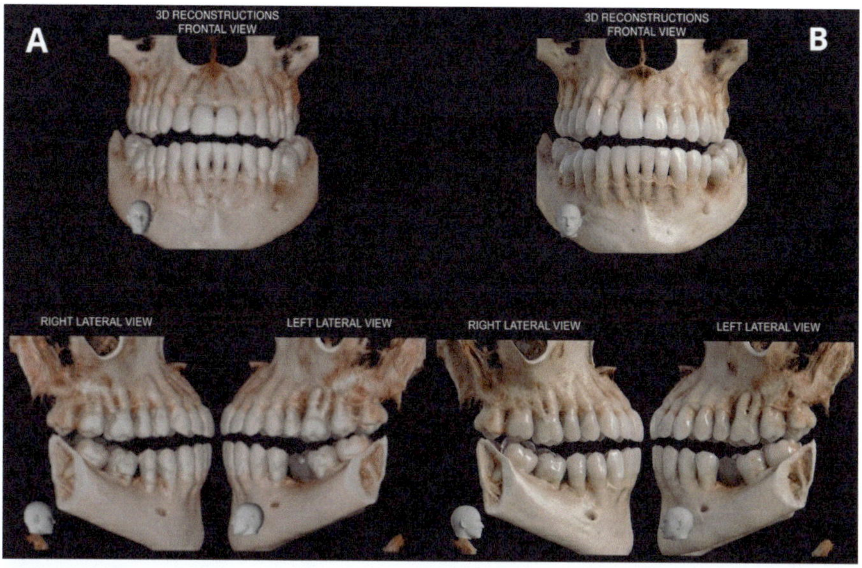

Fig. 6.5 Three-dimensional (3D) CBCT reconstructions of the maxillomandibular complex in frontal and lateral views, comparing conventional volume rendering with an AI-generated "cinematic" visualization. (**a**) Conventional volume rendering of the tomographic volume. (**b**) A set of three renderings (frontal, right lateral, and left lateral views) generated simultaneously from a single prompt, using (**a**) as the reference image, with lighting and material adjustments to enhance depth perception and surface detail of dental and osseous structures, while preserving the same volume, anatomy, and framing

useful for demonstrating contours and external relationships, but it is highly dependent on the selected threshold: thin structures may "disappear," and details may be oversimplified.

Volumetric rendering (direct)

In direct volume rendering (DVR), the entire volume contributes to the image. Rather than "peeling a shell" from the dataset, DVR integrates contributions along projected rays, weighting opacity, color, and other attributes. Conceptually, the volumetric-rendering pipeline is often described in three steps: volume projection, hidden-part removal, and shading. Variants such as maximum intensity projection (MIP) and slab techniques (greater thickness) can simulate projections and emphasize dense structures, but always at the cost of information overlap useful in some contexts and risky in others.

Cinematic reconstruction/visualization (cinematic rendering)

Cinematic rendering aims for a more photorealistic appearance through more complex illumination models, approaching ray-tracing–like behavior (richer light simulation, soft shadows, ambient occlusion, and depth cues) (Fig. 6.5). The goal is not to "reveal something new" within the volume, but rather to improve spatial perception and the communicative quality of the image. Studies using CT/CBCT data of the facial skeleton suggest that cinematic rendering can enhance 3D

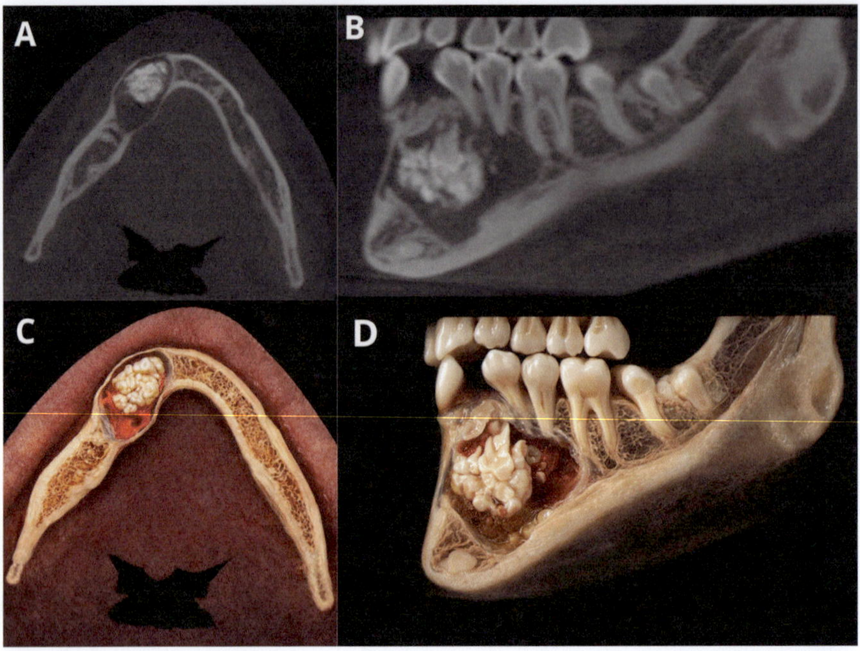

Fig. 6.6 Example of an AI-assisted "slice-to-cinematic" workflow from CBCT. (**a**) Axial grayscale CBCT slice (source image). (**b**) Sagittal multiplanar reconstruction (MPR) from the same dataset, demonstrating the spatial relationship of the odontoma with the mandible. (**c**) AI-generated cinematic visualization derived from the axial slice in (**a**), applying a density-based color transfer function (CLUT) and physically inspired, ray-tracing–like shading without altering the original slice geometry, field of view, or pixel resolution. (**d**) Perspective cinematic visualization from the same dataset, emphasizing material appearance, texture, and depth cues for communication and illustration. **For illustrative/educational use only; not intended for diagnostic interpretation**

perception and anatomic understanding compared with conventional volume rendering, with particular relevance for communication and visual comprehension.

This is where AI becomes relevant: when a tool can apply a coherent CLUT plus "cinematic" lighting without altering slice geometry, it can generate a more "realistic" 3D-looking visualization while still remaining based on the original data (Fig. 6.6).

Generative AI refers to a class of models trained to produce new outputs (text, images, audio) from patterns learned in large datasets [6, 7]. Traditional cinematic rendering often requires robust hardware and dedicated post-processing software. Cloud-based tools using generative AI have made this type of visualization far more accessible: any dentist can generate illustrative images within minutes, at lower cost and with a reduced learning curve. In practice, two AI systems have delivered satisfactory results in this workflow—Gemini (Google LLC, Mountain View, USA) and ChatGPT (OpenAI, San Francisco, USA)—although, in most cases, the best results depend on paid plans, which provide higher generation quality, greater stability, and fewer usage limitations.

It is important to note that this reflects the reality as of January 2026 and may change rapidly, as these platforms evolve continuously. Even so, the key counterpoint remains: because these models exhibit "creative" behavior, they may hallucinate (i.e., introduce changes not present in the data) when not strictly constrained by rules and a well-designed prompt [8]. In this context, different tool profiles can be observed: image-oriented multimodal systems such as Gemini often deliver fast outputs with high visual realism but may be more prone to "beautifying" the image and, at times, extrapolating anatomic details if strict constraints are not applied; in contrast, tools such as ChatGPT tend to provide greater structural consistency, although stability and visual "finish" may vary.

Accordingly, these tools can be excellent for enhancing communication between clinicians and with patients, enriching illustrations, and strengthening teaching making anatomic concepts and spatial relationships more intuitive provided they are used for educational and communicative purposes rather than diagnostic interpretation.

6.1.7.2 Steps to Create a Reproducible "Prompt" for AI-Driven Reconstructions (Technique by Dr. Lucas R. Pinheiro)

A reproducible prompt functions like a protocol: it reduces improvisation and increases predictability. The analogy is the examination itself: a CBCT scan without a protocol (FOV, voxel size, mA/kV, positioning) may seem to have a satisfactory appearance, but it will not be consistent. With generative AI, the prompt becomes the protocol.

Expectation versus reality: even with a very well-constructed prompt and strict rules, the realistic goal is to minimize errors not to eliminate them. Generative models may produce "hallucinations," which are creations and alterations of details in a plausible way that were not present in the original data. In imaging, this may be shown as "corrections," "enhancements," or "completions" that seem to make sense. However, such imaging changes are actually model-generated inventions. For this reason, one should always assume a residual risk that requires careful human oversight [6–8].

Below are the conceptually essential building blocks of the method.

Scope and mode definition (STRICT EDIT MODE)

Explicitly stating that the task is image-to-image and that the provided image is the "ground truth" prevents the model from treating the request as free generation. This reduces the risk of "reconstructing" a new anatomy. At this stage, it is also essential to specify what the input image will be, because it defines the boundary of what the AI is allowed to transform: it may be a two-dimensional radiograph (periapical/panoramic), a 3D reconstruction already exported from CBCT software, or a specific tomographic slice (axial, coronal, or sagittal). The more clearly the user defines the image type and the visualization goal, the more predictable the result tends to be and the lower the risk of the model attempting to "complete" or reinterpret structures beyond what is present in the original image.

Session isolation and a single source of truth
: Requiring that only the image from the current request can be used prevents contamination from prior examples. In practice, this reduces drift and pattern "blending."

Nonnegotiable rules (geometry, resolution, framing)
: This is the most critical element for responsible use: requiring the same resolution, the same slice, and the same framing "pixel by pixel" and prohibiting completion of truncated structures prevent the tool from performing "creative dentistry." This directly addresses a core behavior of generative AI: the tendency to complete patterns when gaps are detected.

CLUT and density hierarchy
: Specifying the hierarchy (air < soft tissues < trabecular < cortical < enamel < metal/high-density material) ensures that color and opacity mapping respects the original data, preventing unsafe visual inversions. This is consistent with how volumetric-visualization techniques rely on transfer functions to represent the volume.

"Cinematic" lighting with limits
: Allowing shading, ambient occlusion, and soft reflections (without "blowing out" details) seeks the communicative benefit of cinematic rendering while preserving slice integrity.

Noise/artifact handling with diagnostic priority
: Allowing mild reduction of non-anatomic noise and artifacts, while prohibiting smoothing that thickens cortical outlines, erases fine lines, or alters contours, is the difference between responsible post-processing and cosmetic editing.

Negative prompt (explicit prohibitions)
: Listing what must not happen (changing anatomy, adding a canal, removing a lesion, completing a root, etc.) is intentionally redundant: in this context, redundancy is a safety measure.

Here is a practical, step-by-step guide on how to use the tool (Fig. 6.7):

1. Open your preferred image-generation platform (e.g., Gemini or ChatGPT).
2. Whenever possible, select the most recent model/version available.
3. Enable the image-generation or image-editing mode (the feature that supports image-to-image).
4. Upload your source image (radiograph, CBCT slice, or an exported 3D view).
5. Paste your base prompt (your "protocol"), making sure it clearly states what must be preserved and what is allowed to change.
6. If needed, request targeted refinements until you reach the desired result with caution: the more iterative requests you make, the higher the chance of drift or hallucination, so prioritize minimal, well-specified adjustments.

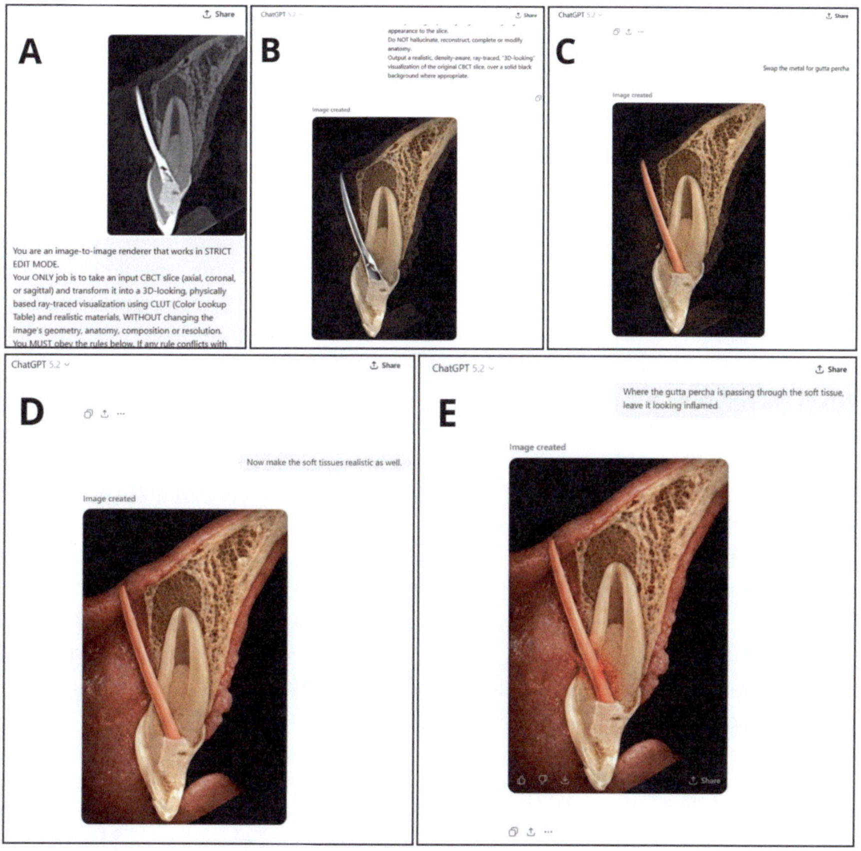

Fig. 6.7 Image-to-image workflow for AI-assisted cinematic 3D visualization derived from a CBCT slice demonstrating a root perforation, generated using ChatGPT 5.2 (Images), with iterative prompt-guided refinements. (**a**) Original cone-beam computed tomography (CBCT) slice. (**b**) First-pass "cinematic" 3D-like, physically based (ray-traced) rendering while preserving the original slice geometry, anatomy, and field of view. (**c**) Targeted material reassignment of a hyperdense intracanal structure, replacing an initially metallic-looking appearance with gutta-percha. (**d**) Refinement step to render soft tissues with greater realism while maintaining the original composition. (**e**) Localized adjustment to illustrate an inflammatory-appearing soft-tissue response at the site where gutta-percha extends through the perforation into the adjacent soft tissue. Note: AI-generated images are intended for visualization and communication only and are not suitable for diagnostic interpretation; side-by-side verification against the original examination is recommended

When to use (appropriate use)

Patient communication: a more realistic visualization can facilitate understanding, reduce anxiety, and improve adherence, provided you explain that it is a "way of visualizing" and not a new examination.

Education and training: lectures, presentations, case discussions, and anatomic demonstrations benefit from cinematic images, particularly for clinicians less familiar with interpreting slices.

Tip: use the AI itself (ChatGPT, Gemini, or another LLM) as a "prompt reviewer." Ask it to rewrite the prompt in a more objective, detailed, and less ambiguous manner, highlighting (1) what the input image is (radiograph, axial/coronal/sagittal MPR, 3D render), (2) what may change (only color/CLUT, lighting, shading), and (3) what is prohibited (changing anatomy, framing, resolution, completing structures). This tends to make the prompt more "readable" to the model and improves reproducibility by reducing room for creative interpretation. Illustration and didactic documentation: scientific marketing materials, internal manuals, preoperative guidance, and illustrative reports can benefit.

When not to use (ethical and technical boundaries):

Diagnosis and clinical decision-making: cinematic rendering (traditional or AI-based) should not be used to search for findings, "reveal" hidden features, or replace careful interpretation of MPR slices. It does not convert a 2D radiograph into true 3D, and it does not create information that is not already present in the original dataset. At most, it changes how existing information is displayed.

Any scenario in which the tool may alter anatomy: if strict constraints cannot be guaranteed (same geometry, same resolution, and no "completion" of structures), the risk of hallucination outweighs the benefit. The variability reported for LLM performance in dentomaxillofacial radiology and the need for supervision support this caution [9].

A helpful sentence to calibrate expectations is as follows: "this is a visualization lens, not a finding detector." Put simply: AI may improve how you show, not how you discover.

Data privacy and consent: an additional ethical issue that requires explicit discussion is whether patient images can be uploaded to generative AI platforms. Even when identifiers are removed, imaging data may still be considered personal health information, and cloud processing may create exposure risks depending on the platform's data-handling policies. In practice, clinicians should ensure robust de-identification and comply with local privacy regulations and institutional policies; however, in many settings, specific informed consent for AI-based processing and/or explicit authorization for external cloud tools may be advisable, particularly when the platform is not under institutional control. When in doubt, the safest approach is to treat AI-based rendering as a form of third-party data sharing and obtain patient permission or use solutions that guarantee confidentiality within a controlled environment.

In conclusion, CBCT-based 3D reconstructions rely on established principles of reformatting and volume rendering, in which density mapping (transfer functions/CLUT) and shading choices determine how the volume is perceived. Cinematic rendering adds realism and depth cues through more sophisticated illumination models, with evidence of communicative and perceptual gains compared with conventional volume rendering. Generative AI tools expand access to these visualizations but carry an intrinsic risk: generative models may extrapolate anatomic details if they are not strictly controlled. Therefore, the most important aspect of the responsible use of this method is a reproducible and protocol-like prompt, as it preserves geometry, maintains resolution and framing, respects density hierarchy, and constrains the output to a visual transformation of the original data. Under these premises, AI-assisted cinematic reconstructions have a clear role in dentistry: communication, education, and illustration, but never diagnosis.

6.1.7.3 Current Considerations and Limitations of AI-Driven Cinematic Images from CBCT (Analysis by Dr. Vinicius Dutra)

As explained in the previous subsection, the combination of artificial intelligence (AI) and conventional cinematic rendering techniques has recently enabled the generation of ultrarealistic images from CBCT data (Fig. 6.8). In this approach, AI-based image synthesis models transform conventional CBCT slices into visually enhanced renderings by learning complex appearance patterns from large-scale imaging datasets. Rather than relying on explicit physical reconstruction models or simple transfer functions, these systems infer lighting, shading, and material-like textures from the input data using deep neural networks. As a result, visual depth and surface realism are enhanced, while the original anatomical structures provided by the CBCT data serve as the primary spatial reference (Fig. 6.9).

The three-dimensional visualization effect is achieved through AI-driven neural rendering techniques that approximate global illumination and shading

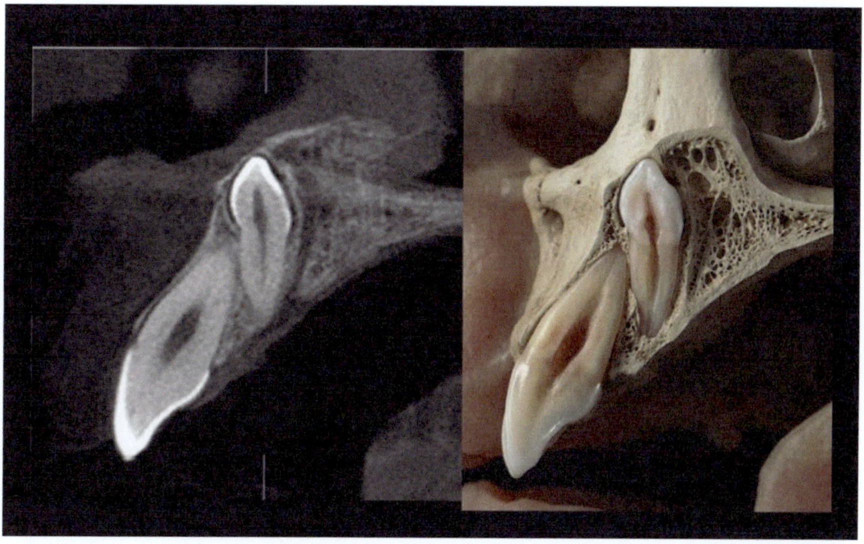

Fig. 6.8 Sagittal CBCT slice (left) and corresponding AI-based cinematic rendering (right) of a mesiodens (Nano Banana Pro, Google Gemini)

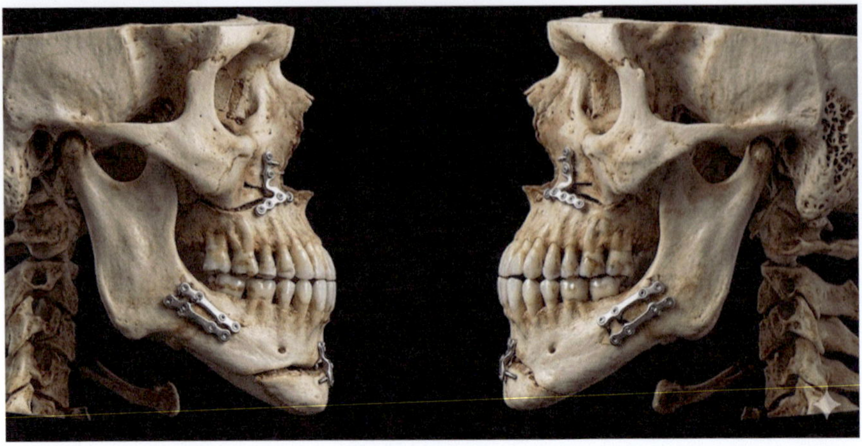

Fig. 6.9 Three-dimensional AI-based cinematic renderings of a postoperative orthognathic surgery case generated from CBCT data (Nano Banana Pro, Google Gemini)

phenomena commonly used in cinematic visualization. These models learn to reproduce complex visual cues—such as soft shadows, ambient occlusion, and surface texture variation—directly from grayscale CBCT inputs. While these effects improve depth perception and visual realism, they are generated through data-driven inference rather than explicit physical simulation. Importantly, AI-based cinematic rendering systems are designed to preserve the overall geometric structure of the original CBCT data. However, because the process involves probabilistic image synthesis, local visual distortions or artificial features may still be introduced, particularly in regions of pathology or high contrast. Consequently, these images should be interpreted strictly as visualization tools rather than diagnostic reconstructions.

Despite the impressive visual correlation with real anatomical structures, AI-based cinematic renderings currently lack scientific validation for diagnostic use. Upon closer inspection, subtle distortions may be observed, including instances in which pathology is artificially introduced or omitted (Fig. 6.10). Furthermore, repeated processing of the same input image can result in visually different outputs, reinforcing the nondeterministic nature of the technique. For these reasons, such images should presently be considered nondiagnostic. Nevertheless, they hold significant promise for educational purposes and patient communication. The outputs are highly sensitive to the prompts used, making detailed and precise prompt design—often including explicit material descriptions—critical for reproducible results.

These limitations should not discourage the use of AI-augmented cinematic renderings. Radiology has long recognized the inherent constraints of conventional three-dimensional renderings compared with original tomographic slices for image interpretation, and similar caveats apply here. However, with continued algorithmic

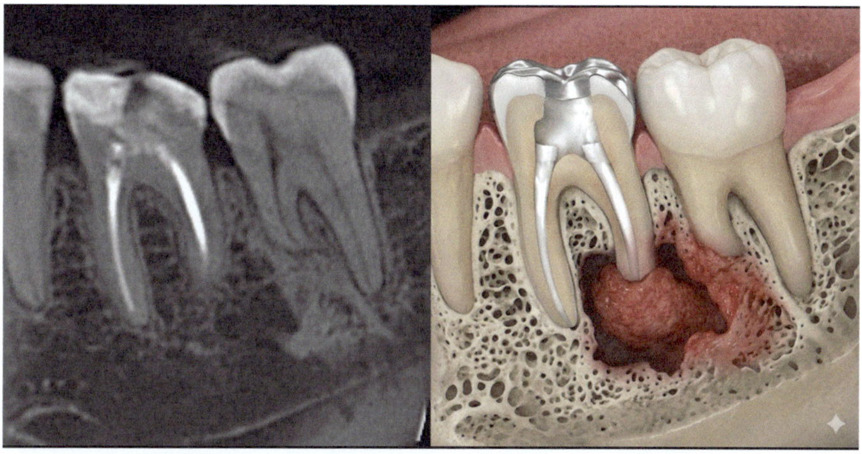

Fig. 6.10 Sagittal CBCT slice (left) and AI-based cinematic rendering (right) illustrating a false--positive periapical lesion artificially introduced by the AI model at the distal root of the mandibular left first molar. This example highlights the current limitations and nondiagnostic nature of AI-generated cinematic images (Nano Banana Pro, Google Gemini)

refinement, improved training datasets, and rigorous validation, AI-generated cinematic images may eventually acquire diagnostic relevance, potentially reshaping the future of radiologic visualization.

6.2 AI-Driven Commercial Dental Software Programs

As mentioned in the previous chapters, several dental software programs have AI-powered tools for oral diagnosis, such as Denti.AI Detect (Denti.AI), Second Opinion (Pearl), and Diagnocat AI (Diagnocat Ltd.). The latter was the choice of software to illustrate most of the cases of this book, for three main reasons. First, Diagnocat is one of a few current options of AI software that works with CBCT images. Moreover, it has tools for treatment and surgical planning, including the design of surgical guides, similarly to software programs such as Relu® Automate (Relu BV) and coDiagnostiX (Dental Wings). Finally, Diagnocat is the one with the highest number of diagnostic tools useful for the dental clinician, in the opinion of the editor of this book. It is also noteworthy that Diagnocat AI complies with important international standards and regulations for medical devices such as ISO 13485 and European Union Medical Device Regulation (MDR).

Diagnocat AI is a cloud-based web application. Its central function is to perform automated analysis of dental images by applying artificial neural network models (Fig. 6.11). However, the intended use of this platform is strictly as an adjunct tool, a point emphasized by both the manufacturer and the performance data. Clinicians

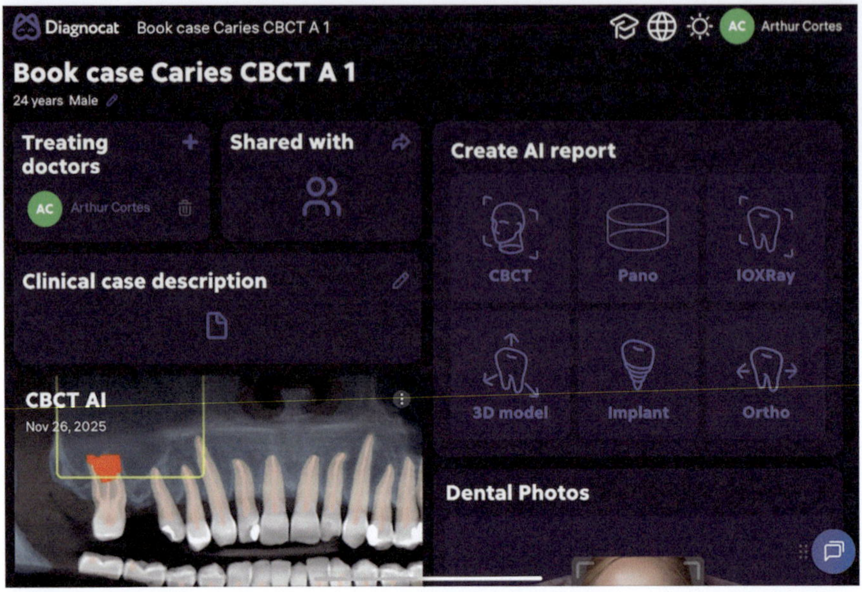

Fig. 6.11 Screenshot of the Diagnocat software showing the main AI tools to create reports. Note that the three tools on the top (CBCT, Pano, and IOXray) are the most important for diagnosis, while the three on the bottom (3D model, Implant and Ortho) are important tools for treatment planning

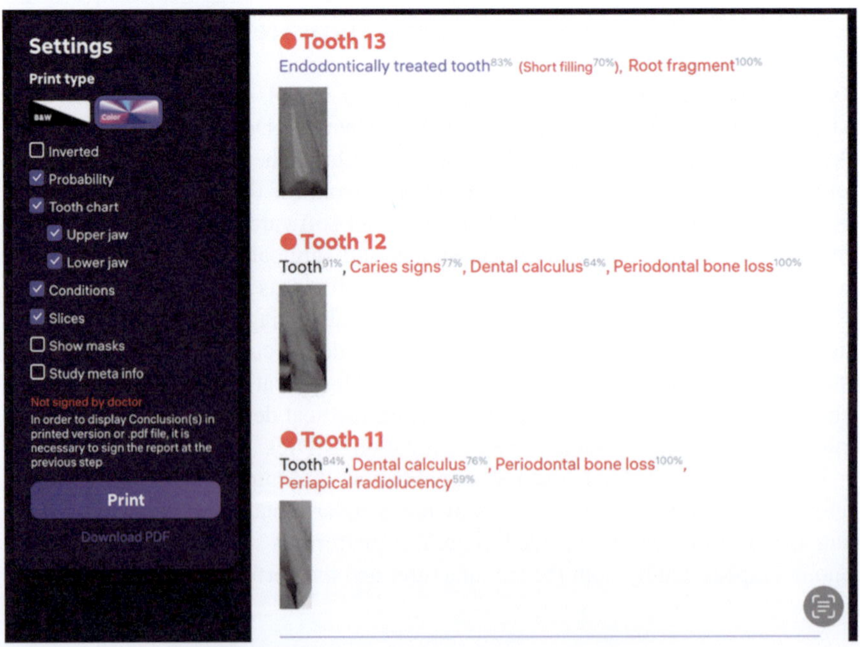

Fig. 6.12 Part of a diagnostic AI report exported as a PDF file (Diagnocat)

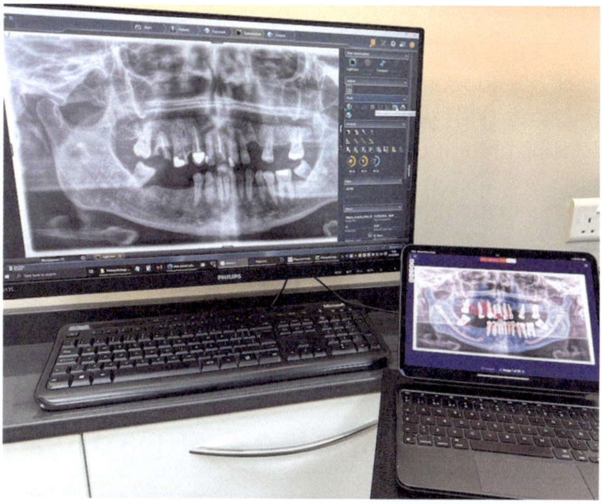

Fig. 6.13 Sidexis and Diagnocat software programs being used in a dental clinic

can export diagnostic reports as PDF files (Fig. 6.12) but should not use AI-generated output as the primary basis for interpretation.

One very important ability of these software programs is to communicate with dental imaging software of radiographic devices and/or dedicated to dental clinics, such as Sidexis (Dentsply-Sirona), by using specific dental software interfaces, such as SLIDA (Dentsply-Sirona) (Fig. 6.13). With this system, all radiographs taken during the daily routine of a dental clinic can be automatically uploaded to the platform of the Diagnocat system, ensuring a productive clinical and diagnostic workflow.

A recent scoping review consolidates findings on multiple convolutional neural network (CNN)-based models for detecting endodontic lesions, thereby offering a broader perspective on the technology's potential compared to the single-software focus of the report by the software program Diagnocat AI (Diagnocat, San Francisco, CA, USA) [14]. The review found that models such as U-Net and PAL-Net demonstrated high diagnostic performance, with reported sensitivity ranging from 67.3% to 97.1% and area under the curve (AUC) values as high as 0.98. However, the Diagnocat technical report revealed a critical limitation: the AI failed to detect any of the additional findings identified by the radiologists. These missed findings included complex pathologies such as endo-perio lesions, as well as anatomical variations like root canal bifurcations or calcifications. The system also struggled with rare anatomy, such as teeth with four roots or five canals, which powerfully illustrates the current limitations of such algorithms. It is noteworthy that the company always strive to update the technology of the AI-driven software, especially following important research findings such as the ones described herein.

Strengths and limitations of the Diagnocat software have also been discussed by a study using the software "radiological report" tool [15]. A comparison between the performance of this tool and reports from human radiologists identified topics of high agreement, such as teeth numbering and classification, number of roots and canals, presence of crown conditions such as restorations and caries, and the presence of endodontic treatment. On the other hand, topics such as the classification of the severity of periodontal bone loss, presence of intracranial posts, quality of endodontic obturations, and alterations of the periodontal ligament space were found to have low agreement.

The Diagnocat software undergoes frequent technological updates and improvements by the manufacturer, showing an increasing potential for overcoming the existing limitations. Furthermore, AI tools have also become available in implant planning software programs [16], as further discussed in this and the next chapters.

6.3 The Role of AI in Optimizing Digital Impressions

AI is also being integrated directly into data acquisition hardware, such as intraoral scanners (IOS), to improve the quality of digital impressions [17]. Its primary functions are to automatically fill minor defects in the 3D mesh and to remove unnecessary soft-tissue data, such as the tongue or cheek, from the scan. An in vitro study critically evaluated the impact of these AI features on the accuracy of complete-arch digital impressions by comparing scans taken with AI enabled (AI-ON) versus disabled (AI-OFF). To understand the results, it is essential to define the core metrics of scanner performance:

- Trueness: The closeness of a measurement to the actual, true value of the object being scanned
- Precision: The consistency and repeatability of measurements; how close multiple scans of the same object are to each other
- Accuracy: A combination of both trueness and precision, representing the overall reliability of the scan

The study found that while the AI-OFF setting tended to produce scans with slightly better trueness, the AI-ON setting delivered significant improvements in both precision and overall accuracy. The most notable benefit of the AI was its ability to reduce arch distortion in complete-arch scans, leading to a more consistent and reliable final model. This suggests that the AI's automated corrections, while perhaps introducing minute deviations from the absolute true surface, ultimately produce a more cohesive and repeatable digital impression, which is critical for clinical applications.

This leap in data acquisition fidelity, moving from raw point clouds to cohesive and accurate digital surfaces, provides the essential foundation upon which a high-fidelity virtual patient can be constructed.

6.4 The AI-Powered Tools to Create a Virtual Patient

The concept of the "virtual patient" represents the creation of a comprehensive, high-fidelity digital replica of an individual's anatomy and, increasingly, their interactive persona. Its strategic importance lies in its ability to serve as a platform for advanced diagnostics, meticulous treatment simulation, and immersive professional education. Artificial intelligence is a key enabling technology in this domain, automating the complex process of constructing these digital models and imbuing them with interactive capabilities [18, 19].

6.4.1 High-Fidelity Anatomical Models via Automated Segmentation

A virtual patient is created by integrating and aligning multiple digital data sources, including CBCT scans for hard tissues, intraoral scans (IOS) for teeth and gingiva, and 3D facial scans for soft-tissue esthetics. A pivotal and historically time-consuming step in this process is segmentation—the digital isolation of specific anatomical structures from a CBCT image.

Recent advancements have demonstrated the power of AI, specifically 3D U-Net type convolutional neural networks (CNNs), to perform automated, integrated segmentation of multiple craniomaxillofacial structures simultaneously [18]. This approach allows a clinician to generate a detailed anatomical model in a fraction of the time required by traditional methods.

The results of a previous study indicate that the CNN-driven approach is not only over 40 times faster but is also significantly more accurate and consistent in creating a CBCT-derived virtual patient. This radical improvement in efficiency and consistency effectively removes a significant bottleneck in digital workflows, making the routine creation of comprehensive virtual patients clinically feasible.

6.4.2 AI in Integrated Treatment Planning and Execution

The application of AI is maturing from performing discrete diagnostic tasks to serving as the central engine for integrated, interdisciplinary treatment workflows. This shift is strategically important, as it enables clinicians to achieve a high degree of predictability by seamlessly connecting different phases of care—from esthetic design to orthodontic movement and surgical execution. This integration facilitates clearer collaboration among dental specialties and ensures that the final clinical outcome remains faithful to the initial virtual plan.

An interdisciplinary rehabilitation case report illustrates how AI can guide treatment from the very first step. The process begins with the integration of patient data (photographs, CBCT, IOS) into an AI-powered software, Smile Cloud 3DNA [19].

(a) AI-powered esthetic analysis: The software analyzes the patient's unique facial and dental features to automatically suggest personalized esthetic arrangements for the final restorations.
(b) Motivational mock-up: This digital design is used to 3D-print a model for creating a motivational mock-up, allowing the patient to visualize and approve the proposed outcome before treatment commences.
(c) Prosthetically driven orthodontics: The final, AI-generated prosthetic plan becomes the blueprint for the subsequent orthodontic phase. In the reported case, this plan guided the treatment with ClearCorrect aligners, ensuring that every tooth movement was precisely calculated to create the ideal space and position for the future implant and crown.

    Once the orthodontic objectives were achieved, AI continued to guide the surgical and prosthetic phases of treatment.
(d) Implant planning: New CBCT and intraoral scans were superimposed in the AI planning software coDiagnostiX (Dental Wings). This allowed for the precise virtual placement of the dental implant, perfectly aligned with the prosthetically driven plan.
(e) Custom abutment design: In a novel application of AI, the software was used to digitally mirror the anatomy of the contralateral tooth. This mirrored profile was then used to design a 3D-printed custom healing abutment. This device helps guide the soft tissue during healing to form a correct and natural-looking prosthetic emergence profile.
(f) Integrated execution: From the 3D-printed surgical guide for implant placement to the final CAD/CAM fabrication of the crown, AI facilitated each step of the digital workflow.

This case demonstrates a near-ideal implementation of an AI-driven continuum of care; however, a broader critical appraisal is required to evaluate how these technologies perform across a wider range of clinical tasks and challenges.

6.4.3 Interactive Virtual Patients for Clinical Education from LLM

Beyond static anatomical models, generative AI is being used to create interactive virtual patients for clinical training. A recent study detailed the use of chatbots powered by GPT-4 to simulate authentic clinical encounters for dental students [20]. This educational tool was designed around a constructivist learning framework, where students actively build knowledge by engaging in realistic problem-solving.

The system comprises two interconnected AI personas: The AI Patient, which simulates a patient presenting with dental pain. It is programmed to replicate natural human interaction, providing information gradually and only in response to specific questions, compelling students to practice thorough and systematic history-taking; and the AI Clinical Supervisor, which acts as a "Socratic tutor." When students present their findings and proposed diagnostic plan, the AI supervisor probes them for justifications and fosters critical thinking rather than simply providing answers.

Student feedback on the AI role-play was highly positive, with 86% of final-year students strongly agreeing the activity aligned with real-world dental scenarios. They perceived the simulation as authentic, engaging, and relevant. However, the feedback also provided valuable nuance for future refinement; some students noted that the AI patient was "very keen to provide many details," suggesting that in real life, "clinicians often need to dig out all the details." This highlights an opportunity to program the AI to be less forthcoming, thereby better simulating challenging clinical encounters. The ability to create and interact with these virtual patients provides an ideal foundation for planning and executing real-world treatments.

6.5 AI-Empowered Immersive Technologies in Oral Rehabilitation (Methods by Prof. Newton Sesma, Dr. Lisya Vizotto de Barros, Dr. Bruno B. R. Matias, Dr. Sergio Candido Dias, and Dr. Marcelo Lucchesi Teixeira)

The incorporation of digital technologies has transformed both the practice and teaching of dentistry, particularly through the use of virtual reality (VR), augmented reality (AR), and mixed reality (MR). Originally developed in other scientific, commercial, and industrial fields, these resources have been successfully applied across various domains of dental knowledge, from academic training to clinical and surgical planning. Recent literature indicates that such technologies empowered by

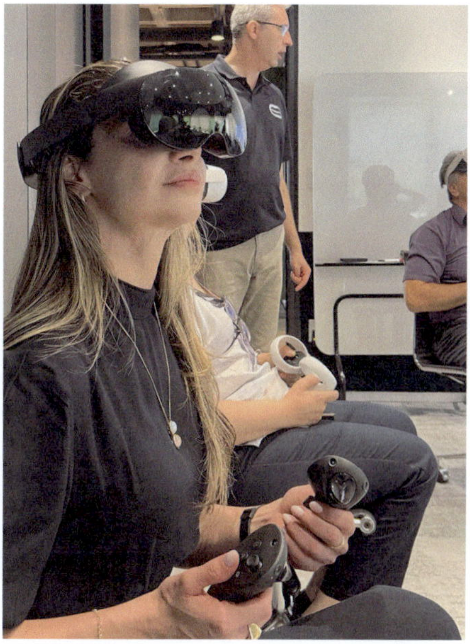

Fig. 6.14 Practical demonstration of VR in dentistry, using a headset and controllers for navigation and manipulation of virtual objects

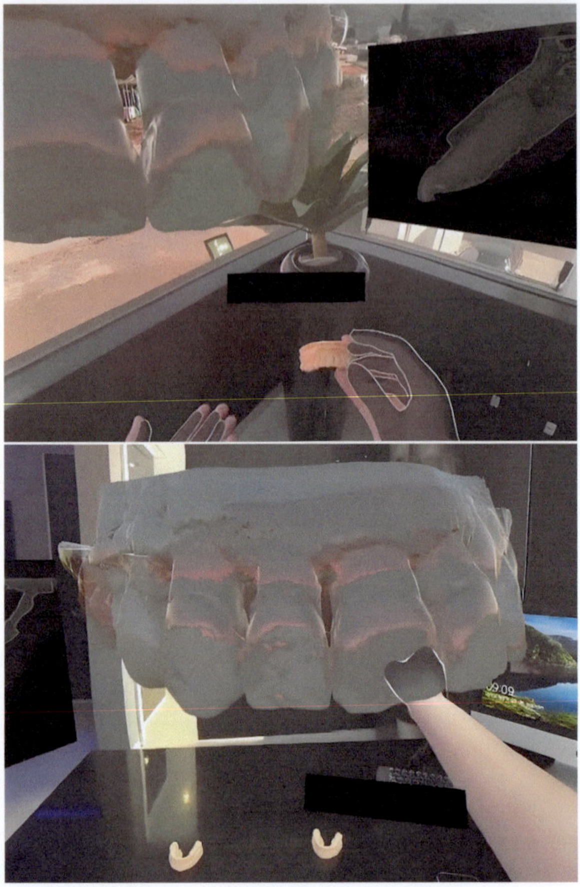

Fig. 6.15 Mixed reality visualization and manipulation of dental digital models. Top: digital model overlaid onto the real environment through mixed reality, integrating clinical data from different sources. Bottom: manual interaction with the enlarged dental arch, enabling a more precise and intuitive analysis

artificial intelligence (AI) enhance immersion, improve diagnostic accuracy, and offer new forms of interaction among professionals, students, and patients [21, 22].

6.5.1 Conceptual Foundations

VR consists of immersing the user in a fully digital environment, where it is possible to interact with three-dimensional objects and simulate procedures (Fig. 6.14). AR, in contrast, overlays digital elements onto the real environment, enabling the real-time superimposition of clinical information. MR combines both modalities, allowing the simultaneous manipulation of physical and virtual structures (Fig. 6.15), thereby creating highly promising scenarios for training and clinical practice [21, 23–26]. On the other hand, the term AI refers to a branch of computer science that leverages technology to mimic human behavior through machines capable of replicating human intelligence. AI reasoning evolves through data-driven machine

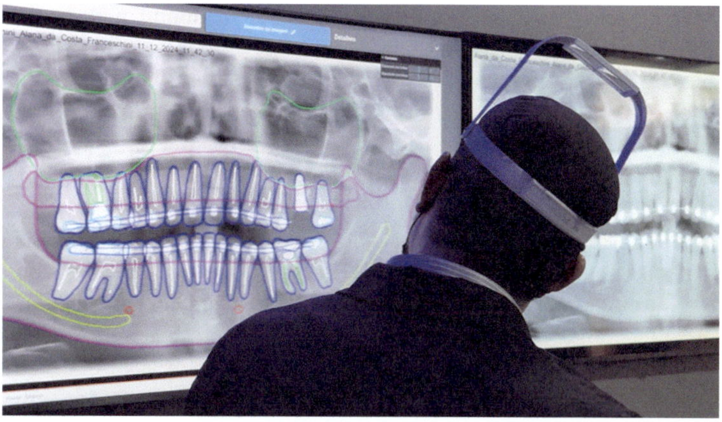

Fig. 6.16 Digital interface displaying radiographic analysis with anatomical contours generated by artificial intelligence, facilitating clinical interpretation

learning processes, enabling systems to construct algorithms and, consequently, solve prediction-based problems without the need for human intervention [27–29].

6.5.2 Applications in Dental Education

AI in dentistry refers to the use of algorithms capable of learning from large sets of clinical data, imaging examinations, and electronic health records to perform tasks such as lesion detection, diagnostic support, and therapeutic planning. Machine learning models—and particularly deep learning architectures—have demonstrated performance comparable to or even exceeding that of specialists in specific tasks, especially in the analysis of radiographs, cone-beam computed tomography, and intraoral photographs (Fig. 6.16). AI has the potential to reduce diagnostic variability among clinicians, standardize clinical workflows, and enhance decision-making, provided that it is validated using large, representative, and ethically structured datasets [29, 30]. Besides this, the image diagnostic can improve the efficiency by the differentiation of gray scale by algorithms, when compared to human vision.

Recent studies report significant progress in the clinical application of AI across orthodontics, endodontics, implant dentistry, and digital prosthodontics. AI-driven tools can detect caries and periodontal disease, identify root canals with greater accuracy, suggest optimal orthodontic positioning, plan guided implant placement, and personalize prosthetic rehabilitation based on individual morphological profiles. Within integrated digital workflows, AI already operates in conjunction with intraoral scanning, jaw-tracking devices, CAD/CAM systems, and 3D printing, supporting processes ranging from diagnosis to the delivery of the final prosthesis or surgical guide [31, 32].

The relevance of AI also extends to the field of dental materials science. Evidence shows that algorithms can predict mechanical properties, fracture resistance, color stability, and the longevity of restorative materials such as composite resins, ceramics, and implants [33]. This advancement enables the personalization of material selection and restorative planning based on each patient's functional and esthetic profile, representing a meaningful step toward precision dentistry.

When combined with immersive technologies, AI further amplifies the clinical and educational potential of these systems. VR can reproduce complex clinical scenarios for training and simulation, whereas AR can project clinical information directly into the surgeon's field of view during procedures, supporting guided surgeries, implant path planning, and real-time visualization of anatomical structures. AI functions as the intelligent layer within these environments, adjusting simulations, recognizing anatomical patterns, and providing personalized recommendations [34].

Dental education, traditionally based on repetitive practice under instructor supervision, has benefited greatly from the integration of immersive technologies. Digital simulators empowered by AI enable standardized training, objective assessment, and immediate feedback, significantly reducing the time required for motor skill acquisition when compared to conventional methods [26]. In addition to enabling unlimited patient and procedural scenarios, extended realities (XRs) makes it possible to experience rare or high-cost situations, assess errors in real time, and quantify manual movements with millimetric precision [21]. These tools also promote self-assessment and reflective learning, helping students identify their limitations and improve their performance.

6.5.2.1 Training in Restorative Dentistry

The use of immersive technologies in prosthodontic education has shown significant benefits in the acquisition and assessment of clinical skills. AR-based self-assessment methods reduce training time and yield scores comparable to those assigned by human evaluators, making them reliable tools for both students and instructors [35]. Moreover, the integration of haptic simulation—stimulation of tactile sensations such as pressure and vibration—and continuous feedback given by AI improves the quality of tooth preparations compared with evaluations performed exclusively by instructors [36]. Virtual navigation approaches have also been shown to reduce excessive material removal, increasing the safety and predictability of prosthetic outcomes [37]. The use of VR empowered by AI for introductory procedures, such as caries removal and cavity preparations, provides a safe environment for beginners, minimizing the risk of irreversible damage and enabling students to consolidate dental anatomy knowledge prior to practice on physical models and/or patients (Figs. 6.17 and 6.18) [38].

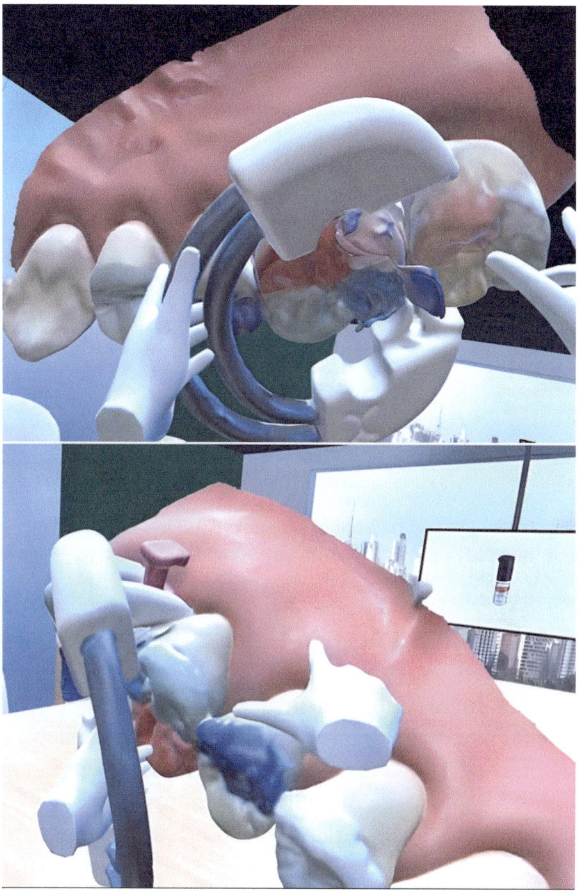

Fig. 6.17 Clinical simulation in virtual reality demonstrating the training of rubber dam clamp positioning from an occlusal view (top) and a buccal view (bottom)

6.5.2.2 Training in Implantology and Surgery

In implantology, virtual simulation with haptic technology, 3D spatial perception, and high-resolution imaging has proven effective in improving students' manual dexterity and self-assessment skills—essential competencies in surgical procedures [39]. The literature indicates that ERs enhance surgical training by achieving higher levels of competence, better professional perception, and lower postoperative complication rates [21, 23, 39]. Thus, AR/VR technologies represent high-impact tools in both undergraduate and postgraduate education, offering safe, interactive practice environments with strong potential for transfer to clinical practice (Figs. 6.19 and 6.20).

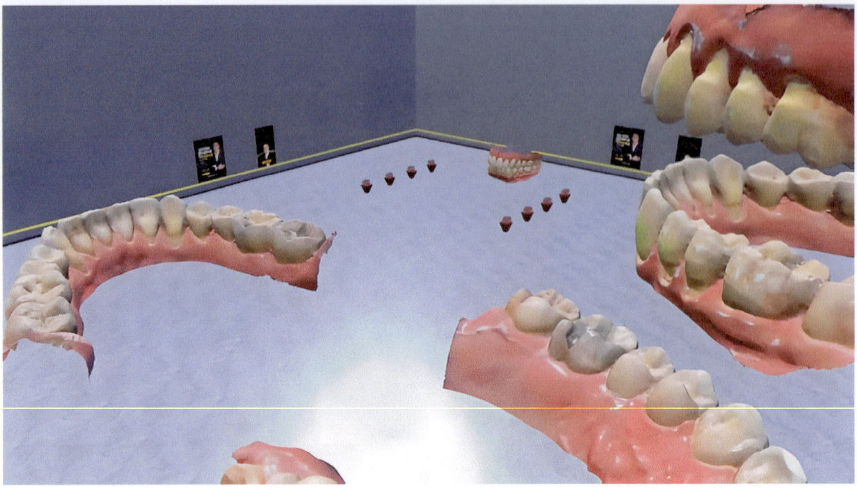

Fig. 6.18 Three-dimensional anatomical models displayed in a virtual reality environment to support the study of dental anatomy in restorative dentistry

6.5.3 Clinical Applications

6.5.3.1 Intraoral Scanning

Digital intraoral scanning (IOS) has become an increasingly integrated tool in dental practice, allowing for the gradual replacement of conventional impressions. The use of AR glasses can significantly improve workflow by projecting already-scanned areas in real time, thereby preventing the operator from having to alternate their view between the clinical field and the computer screen (Fig. 6.21) [40]. Consequently, AR-assisted IOS enhances ergonomics, increases scanner tracking, and simplifies orientation, although it may require a greater number of images and longer processing time in certain stages [41, 42]. Another advantage of IOS is the ability to generate a virtual model based on the actual clinical case for study, diagnosis, or even virtual interventions.

6.5.3.2 Esthetic Planning

Digital esthetic planning has greatly benefited from XR technologies, enabling the immediate visualization of different prosthetic scenarios. The use of virtual mock-ups and wax-ups facilitates communication between the clinician and dental technician, optimizing data integration within the team, improving esthetic predictability, and reducing errors during the restorative process [43, 44]. VR enables full-result simulations, while AR allows real-time interactions, including the superimposition of three-dimensional models directly within the oral cavity, thereby increasing patient engagement and confidence in the

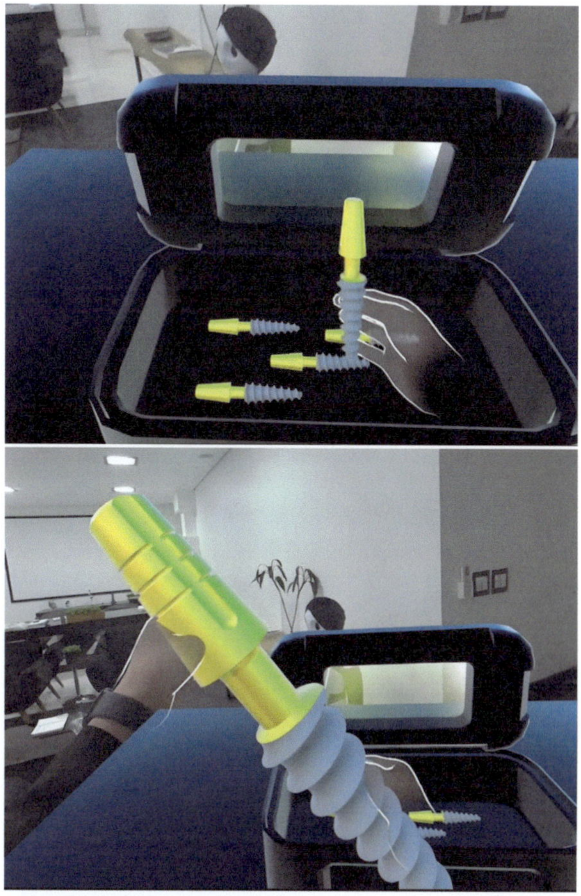

Fig. 6.19 Virtual reality environment illustrating (top) the presentation of implant components and (bottom) their detailed manipulation to facilitate subsequent clinical recognition

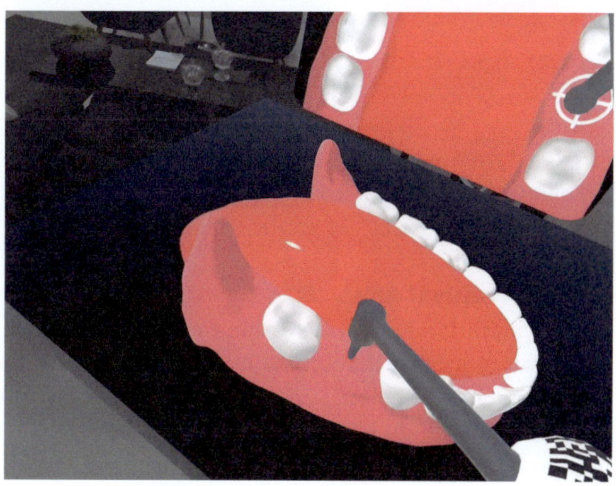

Fig. 6.20 Immersive virtual reality simulation enabling controlled practice of bone drilling for dental implant placement

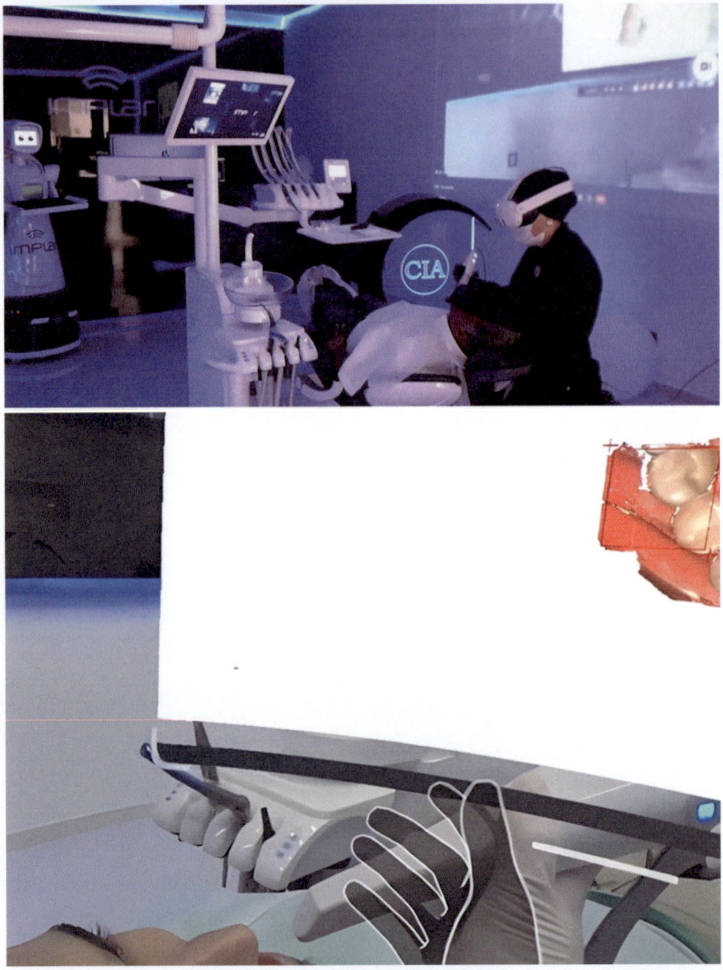

Fig. 6.21 Intraoral scanning procedure assisted by virtual reality glasses, showing the external clinical environment (top) and the operator's immersive field of view (bottom)

proposed treatment (Fig. 6.22) [45]. Avatars representing the esthetic project in 3D can be interacted with in VR or MR environments. This is an emerging trend with significant practical applications.

6.5.3.3 Occlusal Analysis

Digital methods have transformed occlusal analysis, making it more accurate and less subjective than conventional techniques. These tools allow real-time measurement of occlusal contacts and masticatory forces with high reliability [46]. Recent studies demonstrate that digital analysis is also effective in implant-supported rehabilitations, offering better control over force

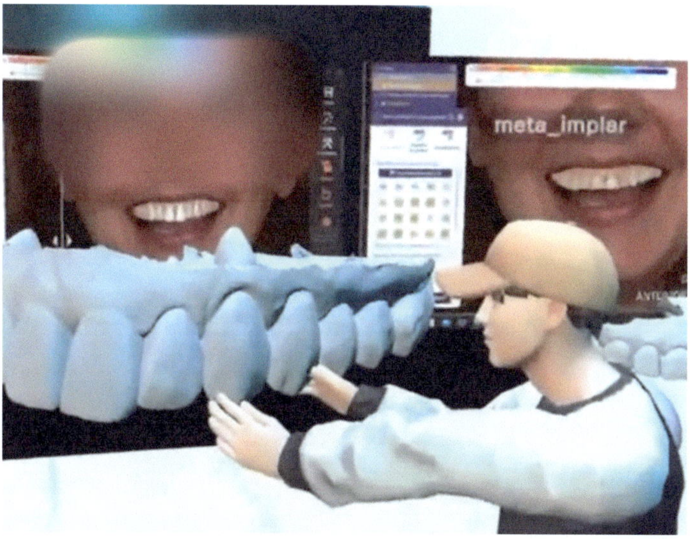

Fig. 6.22 Use of immersive technologies to analyze, manipulate, and compare digital wax-up options in aesthetic smile planning

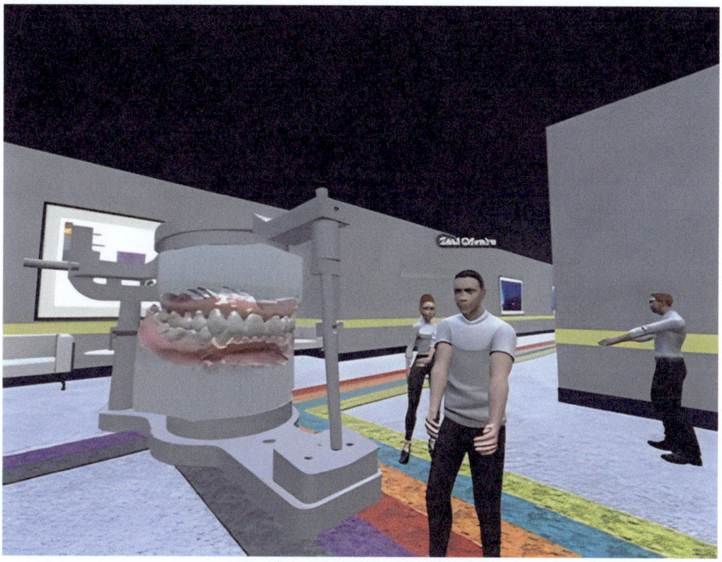

Fig. 6.23 Occlusal analysis on a semi-adjustable articulator performed in an immersive environment, enabling collaborative discussion among professionals

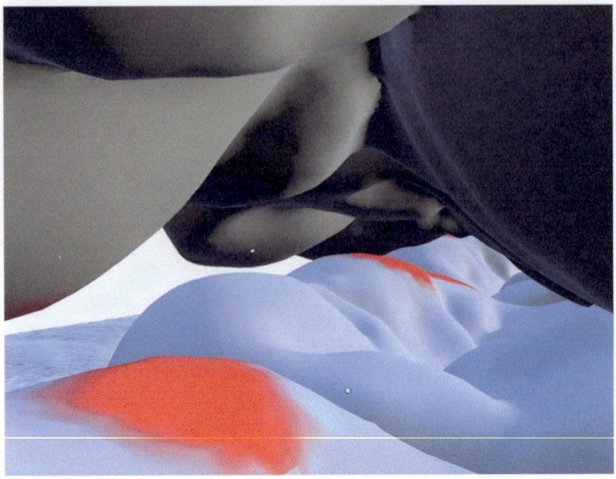

Fig. 6.24 Intrabuccal perspective in a virtual environment showing the distribution of occlusal contacts on a scanned digital model

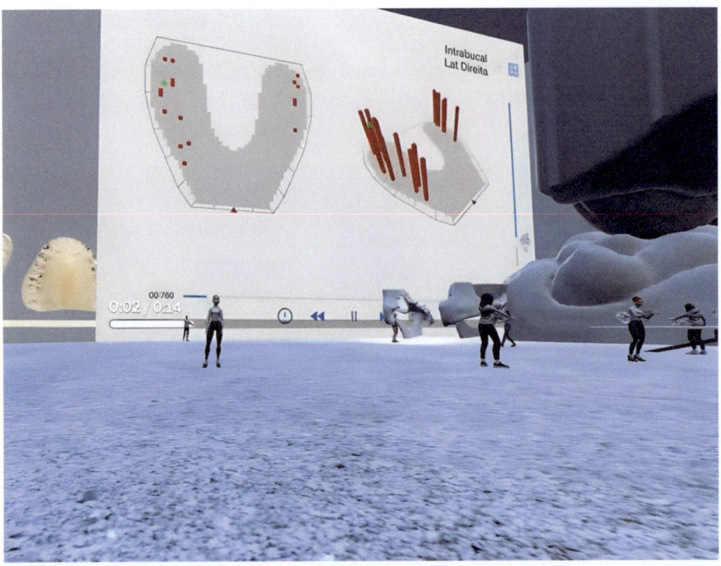

Fig. 6.25 Immersive virtual reality visualization of the occlusal analysis performed with the OccluSense® (Bausch), displaying the distribution and intensity of contacts

distribution [47]. Moreover, comparisons between clinical and virtual records show strong agreement, reinforcing the validity of digital models for clinical use [48, 49]. In this context, immersive technologies add a three-dimensional visualization layer, enhancing clinical interpretation and integration with digital planning [50, 51]. This entire process can be brought into VR environments, providing improved visualization and understanding of each patient's functional system (Figs. 6.23, 6.24 and 6.25).

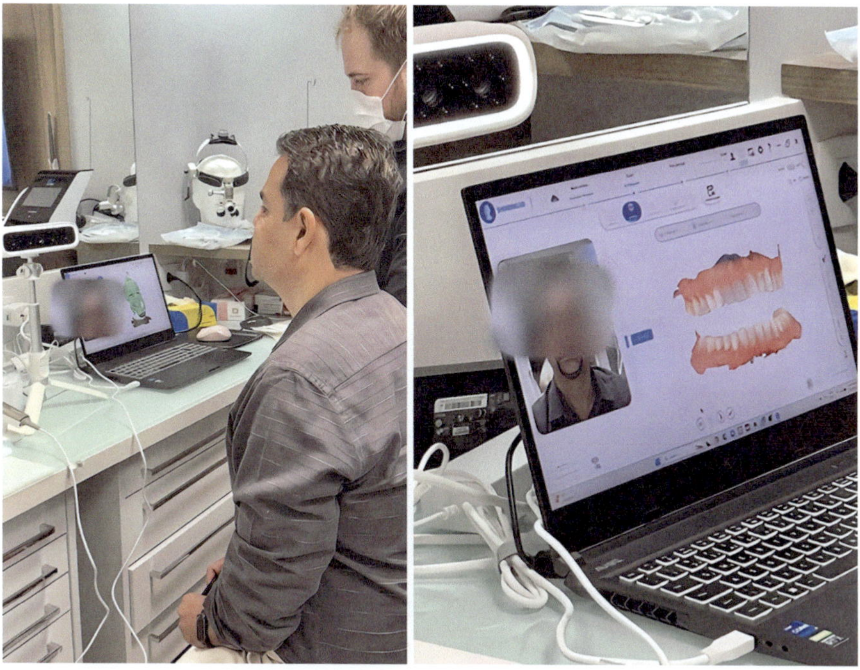

Fig. 6.26 3D facial scanning obtained with the MetiSmile® (Shining 3D), a device that records facial morphology and expression with high resolution and enables data fusion with intraoral scan and CBCT files, ensuring a more predictable digital planning workflow

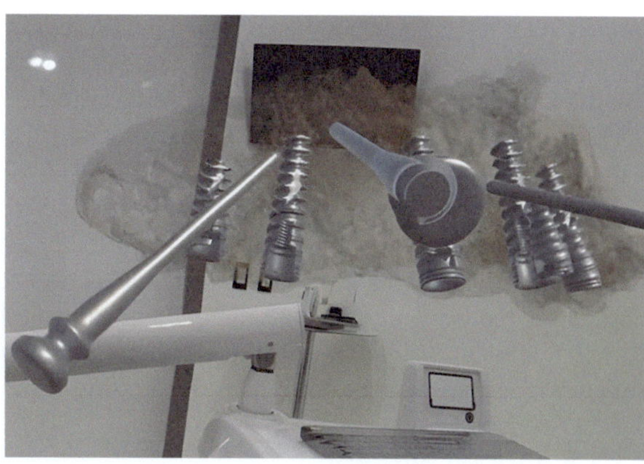

Fig. 6.27 Augmented-reality representation of digital implant planning, allowing precise 3D analysis before surgery

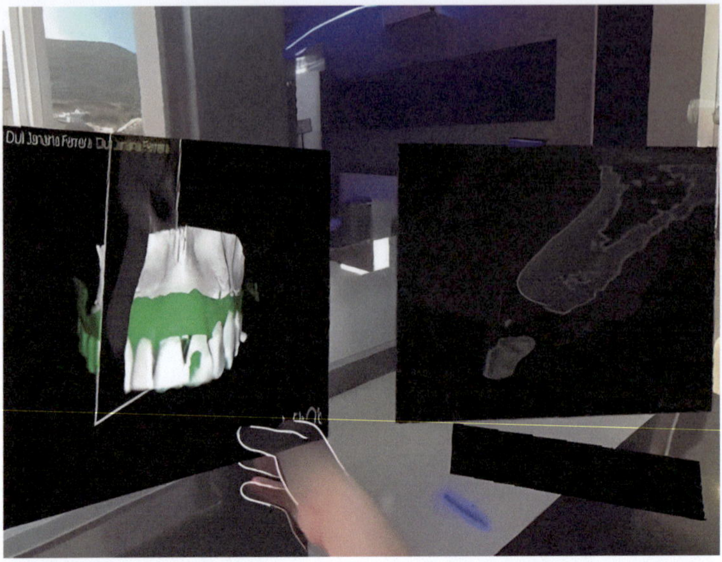

Fig. 6.28 Manipulation in VR of digital models and tomographic slices for precise analysis in implant planning

6.5.3.4 Virtual Implant Planning

Beyond education, these technologies have proven valuable in preoperative planning, allowing realistic simulations, outcome prediction, and precise intraoperative navigation, thereby reducing surgical risks [21]. Virtual implant planning represents an essential stage of modern implantology, traditionally performed using dedicated software that integrates cone-beam computed tomography (CBCT) data, IOS, facial scanning (Fig. 6.26), and diagnostic wax-ups, which can also be combined with jaw-tracking software. The accurate superimposition of these digital models enables safer and more predictable definition of implant position, angulation, and depth (Fig. 6.27) [52].

Recent advances have made it possible to perform this planning in three-dimensional holographic environments, supported by artificial intelligence for automatic model segmentation and alignment across different imaging sources, eliminating the need for conventional implant software [53, 54]. This more intuitive approach allows the operator to virtually manipulate implants using hands or controllers, storing the files for subsequent 3D printing of surgical guides (Fig. 6.28) [55].

6.5.3.5 Implant Surgery

Implant surgery is one of the fields most benefited by immersive technologies. The use of MR-based dynamic navigation has shown results comparable to those of static guided surgery techniques [56]. AR glasses allow real-time projection of the

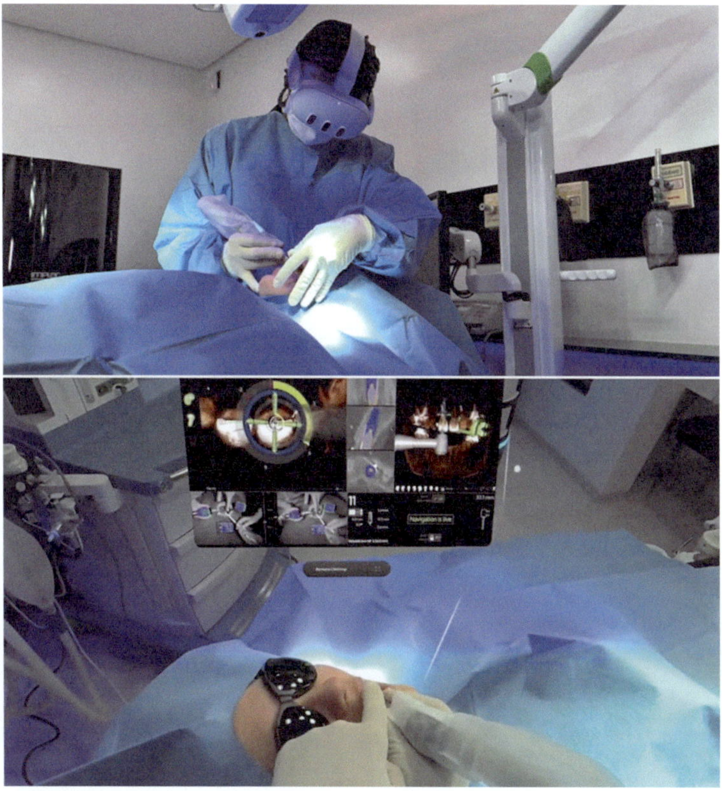

Fig. 6.29 Navigated implant surgery in the esthetic area guided by a system integrated with VR glasses, showing the external view of the procedure (top) and the digital interface with 3D feedback to the operator (bottom)

CBCT-based surgical plan directly onto the operative field, highlighting critical structures and enhancing procedural safety (Fig. 6.29) [40].

Conventional dynamic navigation, although highly accurate (with a mean error of 0.35 mm and an angular deviation below 4°), presents certain limitations, such as high costs, a steep learning curve, and the risk of interruptions due to sensor failures [39, 57]. In this context, the incorporation of AR into dynamic navigation systems has emerged as a promising alternative, allowing the surgeon to simultaneously visualize the operative field and the overlaid digital information, thereby improving real-time surgical performance (Video 6.1) [25, 55, 58–60].

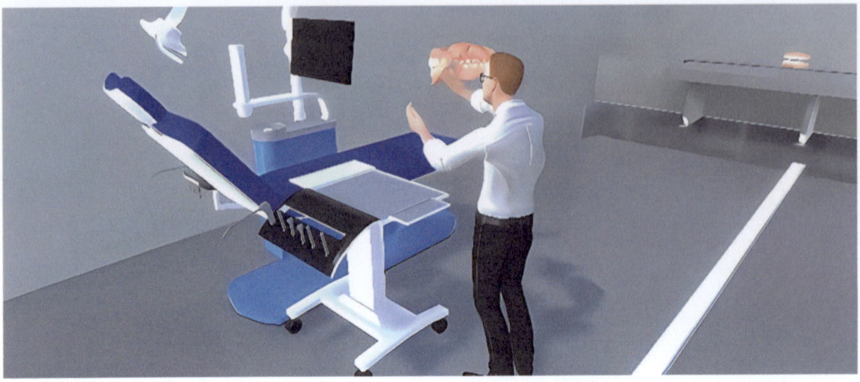

Fig. 6.30 Avatar performing inspection of a dental model in a fully virtual operatory within the metaverse

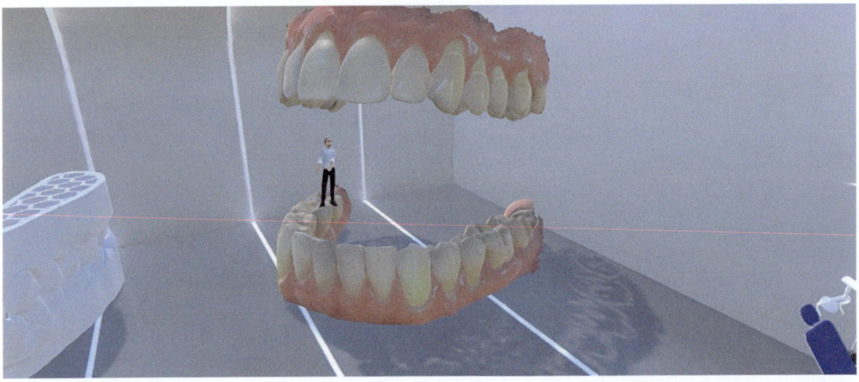

Fig. 6.31 Immersive experience in the metaverse, where an avatar walks among enlarged dental structures for detailed analysis

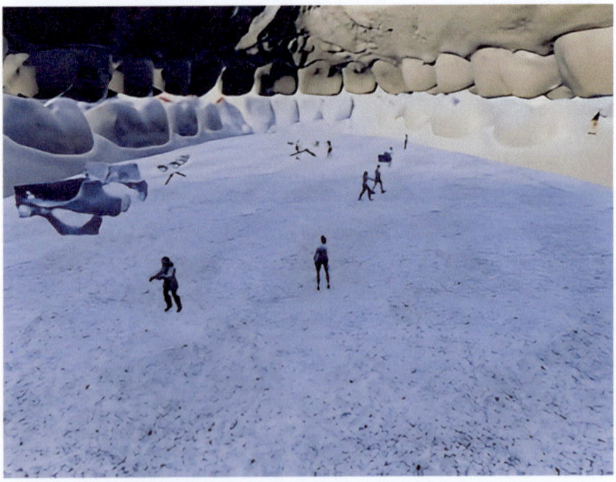

Fig. 6.32 Large-scale dental simulation in the metaverse, allowing multiple avatars to share observations inside a virtual oral cavity

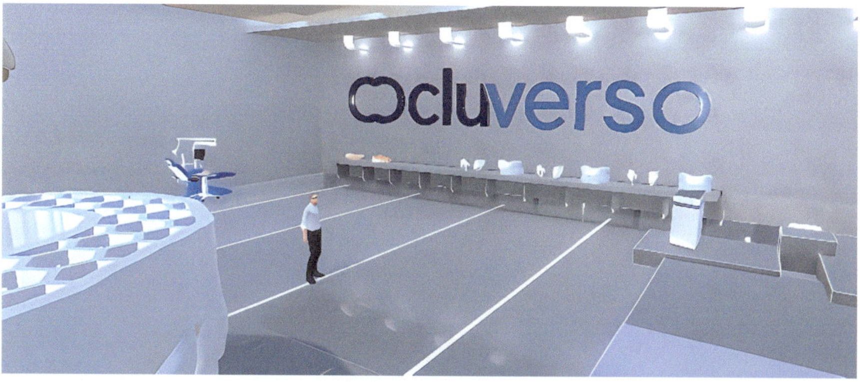

Fig. 6.33 Fully customizable virtual dental environment within the metaverse, allowing the integration of clinic logos, visual identity elements, and digital models tailored to specific educational or demonstrative needs

6.5.4 Metaverse

The metaverse, defined as a collective, immersive, and persistent virtual universe that integrates VR, AR, and MR technologies [61], has been increasingly incorporated into dentistry as both an educational and clinical tool. Its applications include virtual classrooms with continuous and personalized access [40, 62], real-time interdisciplinary interaction for treatment planning [63], and the use of digital twins—dynamic virtual replicas of anatomical structures—capable of simulating procedures and predicting individualized outcomes (Figs. 6.30, 6.31, 6.32 and 6.33) [64].

Among its advantages are immersion in high-fidelity scenarios; enhanced communication among professionals, technicians, and patients in teledentistry; and the development of immersive platforms that expand remote collaboration and real-time case discussion [36]. Additionally, it enables the standardization of educational experiences, although challenges related to cost, interoperability, and system reliability still persist [45, 65]. Future perspectives suggest that the metaverse will likely consolidate as an integrated environment for education, research, and clinical practice in dentistry.

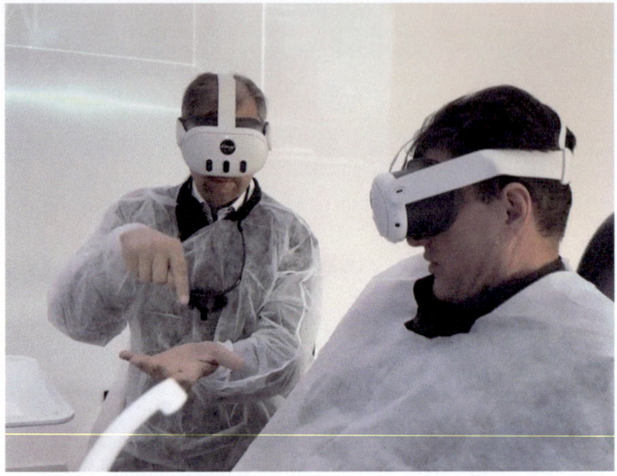

Fig. 6.34 Patient education using VR headsets, where the clinician and the patient view the treatment together in an immersive way

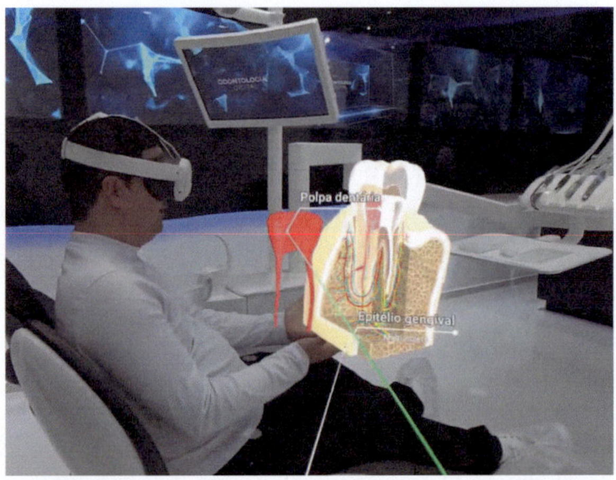

Fig. 6.35 Immersive virtual reality demonstration that allows the patient to visualize anatomical structures and better understand the proposed treatment

6.6 Other Applications

Beyond education and clinical applications, immersive technologies have increasingly consolidated as complementary tools in dentistry, impacting multiple domains. In therapeutic applications, the metaverse can support physiotherapy for temporomandibular disorders by guiding mandibular exercises aimed at reducing pain and functional limitation [45, 66, 67], within the broader concept of teledentistry.

These technologies also strongly influence the patient experience by transforming technical concepts into accessible visual representations that enhance understanding, reduce anxiety, and improve therapeutic adherence [45]. XR tools enhance clinical communication by turning technical concepts into intuitive representations, strengthening patient trust and supporting the management of dental phobias through immersive desensitization (Video 6.2) [36, 45]. The patient thus shifts from being a passive recipient of information to an active co-participant, capable of visualizing treatment scenarios, understanding risks and benefits, and even experiencing real-time simulations (Figs. 6.34 and 6.35). This immersive, multisensory journey brings dental practice closer to contemporary marketing trends, in which experience becomes the main competitive differentiator and determinant of satisfaction [61].

Furthermore, patient experience can be significantly enhanced through the use of the metaverse during dental procedures, diverting the patient's focus from the treatment itself to leisure experiences such as virtual museum visits, sports events, or immersive performances (Video 6.3).

6.7 Methods Based on Dynamic Virtual Patients and Multidisciplinary Integration (Methods Presented by Dr. Fernando Antonio Reis Laurino, Dr. Tatiana Cursino Pereira, and Prof. Guilherme Saavedra)

The virtual patient has evolved from a static three-dimensional (3D) digital model into a dynamic, functionally driven representation capable of integrating morphology, occlusion, facial information, and mandibular motion. This transition reflects the growing need for treatment planning systems that incorporate patient-specific functional behavior rather than relying solely on geometric alignment. Contemporary literature positions the virtual patient as a central digital infrastructure for complex restorative, orthodontic, and implant workflows, particularly when multimodal datasets are coherently integrated [68, 69].

Within this framework, the dynamic virtual patient represents a significant advancement by unifying morphological, functional, biomechanical, and esthetic information in a single environment. Unlike static 3D models, dynamic systems enable simulation of integrated dental, skeletal, and joint behavior, improving predictability in interdisciplinary planning. This approach is particularly indicated in cases requiring modification of the maxillomandibular relationship followed by esthetic restorative treatment [70–72].

Construction of a dynamic virtual patient relies on the integration of heterogeneous digital data, including intraoral scans, facial scans, cone-beam computed tomography (CBCT), and mandibular motion records. CBCT typically serves as the spatial reference, enabling accurate superimposition of surface-based datasets while maintaining consistent 3D coordinates across software platforms. Once aligned, these datasets can be transferred between restorative design, implant planning, and simulation environments without repeated registration, ensuring workflow continuity [68, 69].

Beyond anatomic representation, the dynamic virtual patient incorporates an individualized kinematic model capable of reproducing real mandibular motion and occlusal interactions. AI is central to this process, supporting multimodal data integration, automated segmentation and registration, detection of inconsistencies, and prediction of clinical outcomes. These capabilities reduce reliance on subjective interpretation and streamline complex manual procedures [29, 73].

An important step in transforming the virtual patient into a functional planning tool is the incorporation of occlusal information and virtual articulator parameters. Accurate registration of centric relation, vertical dimension of occlusion, and face-bow data enables virtual mounting and occlusal simulation before irreversible clinical procedures. Evidence shows that digital and AI-assisted articulation systems can determine the maxillomandibular relationship with precision comparable to optimized intraoral scanner workflows, reinforcing their suitability for restorative and interdisciplinary planning [74].

Dynamic functionality is further enhanced by integrating mandibular motion data. Hardware-based and video-based jaw-tracking systems allow reconstruction of individualized mandibular trajectories, including protrusive and lateral movements. This enables functional simulations that more closely approximate clinical reality, particularly in extensive rehabilitations or occlusally sensitive cases. Consequently, the virtual patient becomes a structured repository of static and dynamic information that can be reused across diagnostic, planning, surgical, and restorative phases [75, 76].

Clinical implementation requires an integrated digital ecosystem, typically centered on Exocad for design and supplemented by AI modules for analysis, simulation, and predictive modeling. The workflow involves synchronizing CBCT data, intraoral scans, digital photographs, and dynamic facial records, following a sequence that mirrors real clinical procedures and emphasizes steps requiring clinical verification.

The development of the dynamic virtual patient aligns with the broader evolution of the digital twin concept in dentistry. Initially limited to static anatomic representations, digital twins now incorporate patient-specific functional and kinematic variables, enabling virtual assessment of occlusal interferences, biomechanical stability, and esthetic outcomes. AI has accelerated this expansion by enhancing data processing, simulation accuracy, and predictive capabilities [40, 64].

The dynamic virtual patient should be regarded as a digital infrastructure rather than a final product. Its value lies in providing a coherent, multimodal representation of the patient that becomes clinically meaningful when combined with artificial intelligence (AI) tools capable of analyzing, simulating, and optimizing treatment outcomes. In this model, the virtual patient supplies high-quality input data, while AI functions as the analytical and generative engine acting upon this integrated dataset [64].

The protocol is fundamentally based on the integration of multiple complementary data sources. Computed tomography contributes volumetric information on osseous and dental structures, intraoral scanning provides high-resolution surface detail, and three-dimensional facial registration situates dental and skeletal changes within the patient's facial proportions. AI facilitates this integration by automating registration across distinct coordinate systems, reducing acquisition-related discrepancies, and extracting functional information from dynamic records [68].

Construction of the dynamic virtual patient begins with standardized multimodal data acquisition. The reliability of the final model depends on protocols that minimize artifacts and ensure compatibility across datasets [69]. CBCT serves as the primary volumetric component, offering three-dimensional information on maxillomandibular structures, while intraoral scanning complements it with detailed surface models of teeth and soft tissues, enabling precise capture of occlusal morphology and gingival contours [70, 71].

Three-dimensional facial scanning adds an essential esthetic dimension by contextualizing planned dental and skeletal modifications within the patient's facial framework. Structured-light and photogrammetry-based systems allow noninvasive capture of static and dynamic facial morphology, including expressions relevant to esthetic and functional validation. Following acquisition, datasets undergo preprocessing: tomographic volumes are segmented to isolate key anatomic structures, with deep learning algorithms accelerating segmentation while still requiring clinical oversight. Intraoral scans are cleaned and optimized to correct noise and capture defects.

A critical step is the fusion of tomographic and surface data. Differences in acquisition methods and coordinate systems necessitate precise registration to ensure the accuracy of the integrated model. AI-enhanced registration methods improve reliability by aligning datasets based on surface correspondence and correcting systematic discrepancies. Facial scans are then incorporated through overlapping regions between dentition and perioral structures, completing the multimodal integration required for a coherent dynamic virtual patient [72, 73].

Following acquisition and preprocessing, all datasets undergo spatial registration and multimodal fusion to generate a unified virtual model. This step is technically demanding because each modality—CBCT, intraoral scanning, facial scanning, and mandibular motion capture—operates within its own coordinate system. Differences in scale, orientation, and spatial origin can produce mismatches between tomographic bone surfaces and optical scan-derived dental surfaces, potentially compromising subsequent planning. Earlier registration methods relied on manual landmark identification, which introduced variability and limited precision.

Contemporary workflows employ AI-based registration algorithms that use surface correspondence and iterative optimization to achieve submillimetric accuracy. These systems typically perform an initial coarse alignment based on shared anatomic features, followed by fine refinement that minimizes intersurface distances. AI is particularly valuable for compensating systematic discrepancies between modalities, such as the lower resolution of tooth surfaces in CBCT compared with optical scans. Deep learning models help differentiate true positional discrepancies from acquisition-related artifacts, improving the reliability of fusion.

Integration of three-dimensional facial scans adds further complexity, requiring overlap regions between dentition and perioral structures to enable automated registration and geometric validation. Mandibular motion data are then incorporated to construct an individualized kinematic model. AI algorithms interpolate continuous trajectories from discrete motion records, reduce noise, and identify patient-specific

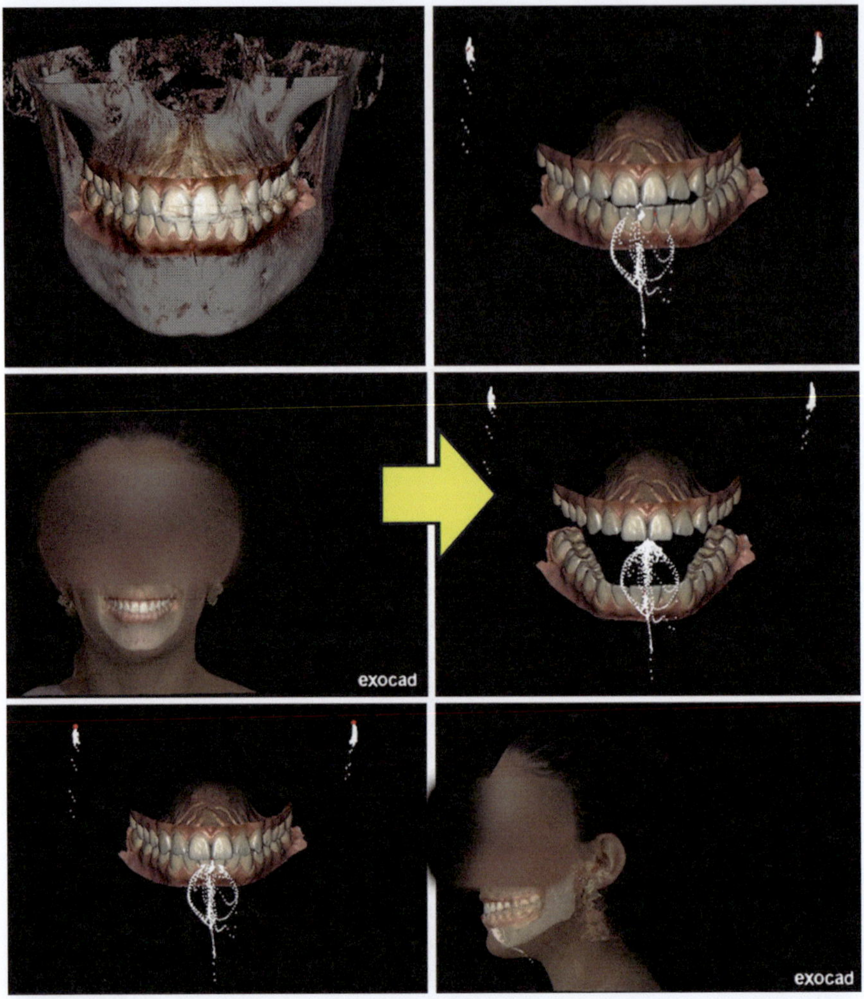

Fig. 6.36 In this case, intraoral scans (iTero Lumina) were superimposed onto a CBCT imported to the Chemnitz 3.3 software (Exocad GmbH, Align Technology). The patient's facial scan was then incorporated, before registering centric relation (left side column). From these data, mandibular movements (right side column) such as lateral excursion, opening, and protrusion were captured using an axiograph (SDI Matrix, Poland), imported into the software, and integrated into the digital planning process. This step allowed personalization of the patient's mandibular motion patterns, thereby characterizing the dynamic virtual patient concept

functional patterns, completing the multimodal fusion required for a dynamic, functionally representative virtual patient [19, 68].

Once multimodal registration is complete, the kinematic model is used to simulate mandibular movements and dynamic occlusal interactions (Fig. 6.36). This model captures the functional behavior of the stomatognathic system, surpassing static representations by enabling prediction of occlusal performance during mastication, speech, and swallowing. Real temporomandibular joint trajectories define the mandible as a moving body relative to the maxilla under specific joint and occlusal constraints. AI algorithms analyze movement patterns, fill incomplete trajectories, correct artifacts, and expand the functional envelope available for simulation. Dynamic occlusal simulation identifies contacts and critical proximities throughout mandibular excursions, allowing early detection of interferences and evaluation of force distribution and biomechanical stability. Integration with dynamic facial records enables visualization of the functional and esthetic consequences of planned interventions. Before clinical use, the model is validated against occlusal records, axiographic data, and facial images to ensure accuracy [68, 69].

After validation of the dynamic virtual patient, AI-assisted diagnostic analysis begins. Algorithms trained on large datasets automatically identify anatomic landmarks, compute cephalometric parameters, and compare them with individualized normative values, reducing interobserver variability and improving diagnostic accuracy [29, 70].

Dynamic occlusal analysis within the virtual patient environment enables automated detection of tooth contacts along functional trajectories, identifying interferences and contact patterns that may compromise stability or longevity. AI systems compare the patient's occlusion with idealized models, quantify deviations, and assess occlusal stability based on contact distribution at maximum intercuspation. In parallel, AI-assisted facial analysis evaluates proportions, symmetry, and smile characteristics, supporting esthetic decision-making. Advanced predictive models can also estimate soft-tissue changes resulting from planned dental or skeletal movements. Together, these analyses generate a structured and objective diagnostic report that guides interdisciplinary planning in complex cases [29, 71].

The transition from diagnosis to therapeutic planning occurs within the dynamic virtual patient environment, where objective findings are translated into coordinated, sequenced clinical interventions. Predictive simulation enables virtual testing of alternative strategies before irreversible procedures, improving safety and treatment predictability. Planning establishes the target maxillomandibular and dento-occlusal relationships based on functional, esthetic, and biomechanical criteria, supported by multiobjective optimization algorithms. Different therapeutic scenarios can be compared quantitatively and visually, facilitating clinical decision-making and shared planning with the patient. Simulation of intervention sequencing further verifies the technical feasibility of each step and anticipates intermediate conditions, ensuring coherence and predictability throughout the treatment plan.

Virtual orthodontic planning integrated into the dynamic model allows precise definition of tooth movements required to achieve final positions compatible with prosthetic objectives. Biomechanical simulations determine safe and efficient movement trajectories, while AI algorithms estimate individual tissue responses to proposed orthodontic forces. Integration with restorative planning ensures that post-orthodontic tooth positions meet spatial, alignment, and angulation requirements for predictable prosthetic rehabilitation.

Virtual restorative design represents the final stage of integrated planning. Within the Exocad environment linked to the dynamic virtual patient, definitive tooth morphology is developed by simultaneously considering functional, esthetic, and biomechanical requirements. Restorative design is informed by antagonist occlusal anatomy, patient-specific mandibular motion trajectories, principles of anterior guidance and canine disclusion, esthetic proportions derived from facial analysis, and minimum material-specific thickness requirements. AI-based generative algorithms can propose tooth morphologies that satisfy these parameters concurrently, accelerating the design process while maintaining adherence to principles of ideal occlusal function.

Functional validation is performed through complete kinematic simulation, confirming the absence of interferences, the stability and distribution of occlusal contacts, the effectiveness of occlusal guidance, and the maintenance of loads within physiologic limits. Automated verification algorithms identify discrepancies requiring refinement, while sensitivity analysis evaluates the robustness of the plan against predictable clinical variations. This phase concludes with standardized, comprehensive documentation that consolidates the approved plan and supports communication among clinicians, specialists, and laboratory teams [72, 73].

Execution of the virtual orthodontic plan involves direct conversion of the three-dimensional setup into clinical devices, reducing intermediate steps, cumulative errors, and fabrication time. Clear aligners are particularly suited to this workflow, with sequential tooth movements determined by biomechanical algorithms that respect biological limits and enhance predictability. AI optimizes movement sequencing, attachment design and placement, and quality control of fabricated aligners to ensure dimensional accuracy. Integration with restorative planning guarantees compatibility between final tooth positions and prosthetic requirements. Serial intraoral scans enable objective monitoring of treatment progress and early detection of deviations, while digital visualizations enhance communication, informed consent, and patient engagement [75, 76].

The restorative design phase is the stage in which definitive dental morphological changes are developed, integrating functional and biomechanical requirements with individualized esthetic goals and the technical constraints of contemporary restorative materials. Exocad, when integrated with the dynamic virtual patient, provides a comprehensive computational environment that allows these dimensions to be addressed simultaneously. AI-assisted tools further accelerate the design process while maintaining adherence to established principles of occlusal function and dental esthetics [75].

The workflow begins by importing the finalized orthodontic setup into Exocad, establishing the precise three-dimensional position of each tooth after orthodontic correction. Restorative designs are then developed within the spatial boundaries defined by interproximal relationships and maxillomandibular alignment. Integration with the dynamic facial model ensures continuous facial contextualization, allowing decisions regarding crown length, incisal edge position, and buccal surface morphology to be evaluated in harmony with adjacent soft tissues and overall facial characteristics.

Exocad's automated facial analysis, enhanced by computer vision algorithms, identifies facial reference points in two-dimensional photographs or three-dimensional models, calculates validated esthetic proportions, and compares them with normative standards adjusted for patient demographics. These objective analyses complement clinical judgment and support decisions regarding ideal tooth dimensions in anterior rehabilitation. The Smile Creator module enables development of an initial two-dimensional esthetic project by virtually positioning anterior teeth within the patient's smile. Once approved, this 2D mock-up is converted into three-dimensional structures using algorithms that infer morphology from 2D projections and tooth libraries. AI accelerates this conversion by selecting library morphologies that best match the patient's facial characteristics.

After esthetic requirements are met, attention shifts to functional occlusal surfaces—an especially critical step in extensive rehabilitations. Exocad provides tools for defining supporting cusps, fossae, guiding inclines, and contact areas according to mutually protected occlusion or canine guidance. Integration with the dynamic kinematic model allows occlusal design to be evaluated during function rather than solely at maximum intercuspation. Continuous simulation of mandibular movements enables automatic detection of interferences during excursions. AI algorithms further refine occlusal morphology by generating optimized surfaces based on ideal occlusion patterns, ensuring stability at maximum intercuspation, effective posterior disclusion, and balanced force distribution.

Minimum thickness verification is essential, particularly for ceramic restorations, where insufficient material thickness increases fracture risk. Exocad provides automated thickness analysis through color-coded maps that identify areas below material-specific thresholds and guide design or preparation adjustments. Consideration of insertion paths is another key technical requirement, especially in multiunit rehabilitations intended for simultaneous cementation. Exocad's automated path-of-insertion analysis identifies a common insertion direction and highlights areas requiring modification to ensure passive seating.

Exporting the final design marks the conclusion of the digital restorative workflow. Exocad generates STL files for CAM milling or 3D printing, and virtual manufacturing simulations help identify potential technical limitations or tool collisions, improving predictability and feasibility.

Biomechanical validation extends beyond geometric verification by assessing the predicted mechanical behavior of restored structures under physiologic functional loads. This step is particularly important in extensive rehabilitations, where changes in occlusal morphology or maxillomandibular relationships may redistribute forces and create stress concentrations. Integrating finite element analysis (FEA) with the dynamic virtual patient enables quantitative prediction of stresses on teeth, restorations, and supporting structures under various loading scenarios. Construction of FEA models begins with converting surface meshes from the virtual patient into three-dimensional volumetric models, forming the basis for accurate biomechanical simulation.

Direct intraoral mock-up serves as an additional transfer tool for esthetic validation before definitive preparations. It enables patients to directly experience the proposed changes in appearance, phonetics, and tactile perception, supporting final refinements before irreversible procedures. Once approved, the mock-up can be digitized and compared quantitatively with the original digital design to verify transfer fidelity and identify discrepancies requiring correction.

The clinical installation phase represents the culmination of the digital workflow, during which fabricated components are definitively positioned intraorally, translating the virtual plan into functional reality. Despite extensive digital planning, this phase requires meticulous execution to preserve the precision achieved in earlier steps. Digital planning documentation functions as a continuous reference, allowing verification that each clinical action conforms to the approved virtual design.

Occlusal adjustments are often necessary during installation, even with highly accurate digital workflows, due to minor discrepancies arising from manufacturing tolerances, cementation dynamics, or material deformation. Digitally guided occlusal adjustment uses dynamic occlusal simulation as a reference to differentiate planned contacts that must be preserved from unplanned interferences requiring selective correction. AI-based optimization can further refine this process by determining the most efficient sequence of adjustments. Because modifying one contact may alter force distribution and create new interferences, algorithms evaluate alternative adjustment pathways and select those that achieve ideal occlusal balance with minimal material removal and fewer iterations.

Esthetic evaluation is essential before definitive cementation, as real clinical perception may reveal nuances not fully captured in digital simulations. Provisional restorations are assessed under various functional conditions with active patient participation. Standardized clinical photographs allow objective comparison with the digital plan, and image-based analysis can quantify esthetic concordance, guiding refinements or remanufacturing when necessary.

Post-installation photographic and radiographic documentation establishes a baseline for longitudinal monitoring, capturing the immediate posttreatment condition before tissue adaptation or material wear occurs. These baseline records are compared with subsequent follow-up examinations to detect early deviations and assess the stability of outcomes over time.

Long-term follow-up is essential to maintain the functional, biologic, and structural integrity of rehabilitations. Contemporary protocols combine individualized clinical evaluations with serial digital documentation, including intraoral scans, periodontal assessments, radiographic examinations, and AI-assisted analyses. These tools enable early detection of subtle changes such as occlusal wear, tooth migration, periodontal inflammation, or early prosthetic complications. AI algorithms support identification of pathologic patterns, risk stratification, and development of personalized preventive strategies. Integrating clinical findings, digital data, and patient-reported outcomes supports a proactive, longitudinal care model focused on preventing complications and maximizing the longevity and predictability of completed treatments.

6.8 Benefits of AI Integration in Dental Treatment Planning

Across the diverse applications reviewed, several consistent benefits of integrating AI tools into clinical workflows emerge. These advantages are grounded in the evidence presented in the source literature.

6.8.1 Enhanced Efficiency

As previously discussed, AI tools reduce the time required for complex and laborious tasks. One of the most important instances is the anatomical segmentation, which an AI-driven approach completed in 1.1 min whereas a semiautomated method needed 48.4 min, representing a more than 40-fold increase in speed [18].

6.8.2 Improved Accuracy and Consistency

The potential of AI from the research raised herein suggests that AI tools contribute to more reliable and repeatable outcomes. In intraoral scanning, AI-ON settings significantly improved the precision and overall accuracy of complete-arch impressions [17]. Similarly, automated segmentation achieved a 99.6% similarity (dice similarity coefficient) to an expert-refined reference, far surpassing the 88.3% achieved by the semiautomated method and effectively reducing interobserver variability.

6.8.3 Predictable and Integrated Workflows

AI can serve as a digital thread connecting multiple treatment phases. The interdisciplinary case report demonstrated how AI-assisted planning—from esthetics and orthodontics to surgery and prosthodontics—led to a final clinical result that was highly faithful to the initial virtual design, maximizing predictability.

6.8.4 Advanced Simulation and Education

AI enables the creation of sophisticated and scalable training environments. The use of generative AI chatbots to simulate patient and supervisor interactions provides students with authentic, on-demand opportunities to practice clinical reasoning and communication skills in a low-risk setting.

6.8.5 Improved Patient Communication

Further than the use of digital workflow with prosthetically driven treatment plans, AI-generated visualizations make treatment plans more tangible and understandable for patients. The use of simulations and 3D-printed mock-ups derived from AI-assisted esthetic planning increases patient engagement and treatment acceptance. This advantage has also been previously observed in methodologies using digital workflow with CAD-CAM technology in oral rehabilitation and prosthodontics.

6.9 Identified Challenges and Limitations

Despite its significant potential, the current generation of AI tools is not without its limitations. The reviewed literature highlights several key challenges that must be addressed for responsible and effective implementation.

6.9.1 Variability in Performance

The reliability of AI is not uniform across all clinical tasks. For instance, in radiological interpretation, AI showed excellent agreement for objective tasks like tooth identification but only "slight" agreement for more subjective assessments such as bone loss classification. Furthermore, studies noted a risk of overdiagnosis in evaluating endodontic treatment outcomes, where AI demonstrated higher sensitivity than clinicians but at the cost of lower specificity, creating a potential for false positives.

6.9.2 Need for Human Oversight

Current AI tools are promising assistive technologies, but definitely not replacements for professional expertise. AI algorithms can miss complex, rare, or incidental findings that fall outside their training data. The Diagnocat report noted that radiologists identified numerous additional findings (e.g., endo-perio lesions, calcifications, root canal bifurcations) that the AI report had overlooked, underscoring the continued necessity of human clinical judgment.

6.9.3 Data Dependency and Generalizability

The performance of an AI model is fundamentally limited by the data on which it was trained, which directly relates to the need for human oversight described above. Because AI struggles with "rare anatomical configurations," such as teeth with four or five canals, it is clear the tool "has not yet learned to identify this anatomical variation." Models trained on small, homogenous, or scanner-specific datasets may lack external validity, meaning their performance may degrade when applied to different patient populations or images from different devices. This limitation affects their generalizability to diverse, real-world clinical scenarios.

6.9.4 Technical and Interpretive Challenges

AI systems can exhibit unique failure modes. As previously discussed in Chap. 5, generative AI chatbots can suffer from "hallucinations," producing incorrect or nonsensical responses. In imaging, AI can struggle to detect rare anatomical configurations or interpret lesions affected by image artifacts from restorative materials, which can impede accurate segmentation and diagnosis.

References

1. Su MC, Lin LE, Lin LH, Chen YC. Assessing question characteristic influences on ChatGPT's performance and response-explanation consistency: insights from Taiwan's Nursing Licensing Exam. Int J Nurs Stud. 2024;153:104717.
2. Le Guellec B, Lefevre A, Geay C, et al. Performance of an open-source large language model in extracting information from free-text radiology reports. Radiol Artif Intell. 2024;6:e230364.
3. Hirosawa T, Harada Y, Yokose M, Sakamoto T, Kawamura R, Shimizu T. Diagnostic accuracy of differential-diagnosis lists generated by generative pretrained transformer 3 chatbot for clinical vignettes with common chief complaints: a pilot study. Int J Environ Res Public Health. 2023;20:3378.
4. Jeblick K, Schachtner B, Dexl J, et al. ChatGPT makes medicine easy to swallow: an exploratory case study on simplified radiology reports. Eur Radiol. 2024;34:2817–25.
5. Siepmann R, Huppertz M, Rastkhiz A, et al. The virtual reference radiologist: comprehensive AI assistance for clinical image reading and interpretation. Eur Radiol. 2024;34:6652–66.
6. Jeong H, Han S-S, Yu Y, Kim S, Jeon KJ. How well do large language model-based chatbots perform in oral and maxillofacial radiology? Dentomaxillofac Radiol. 2024;53:390–5.
7. Hak-Sun K, Gyu-Tae K. Can a large language model create acceptable dental board-style examination questions? A cross-sectional prospective study. J Dent Sci. 2025;20:895–900.
8. Uranbey Ö, Özbey F, Kaygısız Ö, Ayrancı F. Assessing ChatGPT's diagnostic accuracy and therapeutic strategies in oral pathologies: a cross-sectional study. Cureus (Palo Alto, CA). 2024;16:e58607.
9. Hu Y, Hu Z, Liu W, et al. Exploring the potential of ChatGPT as an adjunct for generating diagnosis based on chief complaint and cone beam CT radiologic findings. BMC Med Inform Decis Mak. 2024;24:55.
10. Silva TP, Andrade-Bortoletto MFS, Ocampo TSC, et al. Performance of a commercially available generative pre-trained transformer (GPT) in describing radiolucent lesions in panoramic radiographs and establishing differential diagnoses. Clin Oral Investig. 2024;28:204.

11. Kahalian S, Rajabzadeh M, Öçbe M, Medisoglu MS. ChatGPT-4.0 in oral and maxillofacial radiology: prediction of anatomical and pathological conditions from radiographic images. Folia Med (Plovdiv). 2024;66:863–8.
12. Stephan D, Bertsch A, Burwinkel M, et al. AI in dental radiology-improving the efficiency of reporting with ChatGPT: comparative study. J Med Internet Res. 2024;26:e60684.
13. Dasanayaka C, Dandeniya K, Dissanayake MB, Gunasena C, Jayasinghe R. Multimodal AI and large language models for orthopantomography radiology report generation and Q&A. ASI. 2025;8:39.
14. Karobari MI, Adil AH, Mathur A, Snigdha NT. Applications and clinical translation of artificial intelligence in CBCT-based detection of endodontic lesions: a scoping review. Oral Radiol. 2025; https://doi.org/10.1007/s11282-025-00876-5.
15. Feltraco LT, Rossetto C, Yeung AWK, Soares MQS, Oenning AC. Utility of the radiological report function of an artificial intelligence system in interpreting CBCT images: a technical report. Dentomaxillofac Radiol. 2025;54(3):20240404.
16. Ayres AP, Correa DS, de Moura e Costa AJ, Pradíes G, Cortes ARG. The use of artificial intelligence to create a virtual patient for oral and maxillofacial surgical planning. Sci Lett. 2024;1(1):6. https://doi.org/10.48797/sl.2024.124.
17. Róth I, Géczi Z, Végh DC, Hegedüs T, Pál A, Hermann P, Schmalzl J. The role of artificial intelligence in intraoral scanning for complete-arch digital impressions: an in vitro study. J Dent. 2025;156:105717. https://doi.org/10.1016/j.jdent.2025.105717.
18. Nogueira-Reis F, Morgan N, Suryani IR, Tabchoury CPM, Jacobs R. Full virtual patient generated by artificial intelligence-driven integrated segmentation of craniomaxillofacial structures from CBCT images. J Dent. 2024;141:104829. https://doi.org/10.1016/j.jdent.2023.104829.
19. Fonseca FJPO, Matias BBR, Pacheco P, Muraoka CSA, Silva EVF, Sesma N. Artificial intelligence-assisted treatment planning in an interdisciplinary rehabilitation in the esthetic zone. J Esthet Restor Dent. 2025; https://doi.org/10.1111/jerd.70034.
20. Jones B, Desu A, Honig CDF. Artificial intelligence chatbots as virtual patients in dental education: a constructivist approach to classroom implementation. Eur J Dent Educ. 2025; https://doi.org/10.1111/eje.13135.
21. Joda T, Gallucci GO, Wismeijer D, Zitzmann NU. Augmented and virtual reality in dental medicine: a systematic review. Comput Biol Med. 2019;108:93–100. https://doi.org/10.1016/j.compbiomed.2019.03.012.
22. Puleio F, Tosco V, Pirri R, Simeone M, Monterubbianesi R, Lo Giudice G, Lo Giudice R. Augmented reality in dentistry: enhancing precision in clinical procedures—a systematic review. Clin Pract. 2024;14(6):2267–83. https://doi.org/10.3390/clinpract14060178.
23. Blanchard J, Koshal S, Morley S, McGurk M. The use of mixed reality in dentistry. Br Dent J. 2022;233(4):261–5. https://doi.org/10.1038/s41415-022-4451-z. Epub 2022 Aug 26.
24. Dzyuba N, Jandu J, Yates J, Kushnerev E. Virtual and augmented reality in dental education: the good, the bad and the better. Eur J Dent Educ. 2025;29(3):497–515. https://doi.org/10.1111/eje.12871. Epub 2022 Nov 20.
25. Sadilina S, Balmer M, Joda T. Implementation of augmented, mixed and virtual reality in implant dentistry. ITI Forum Implantologicum. 2024; https://doi.org/10.63580/iti.fi.45746.
26. Huang TK, Yang CH, Hsieh YH, Wang JC, Hung CC. Augmented reality (AR) and virtual reality (VR) applied in dentistry. Kaohsiung J Med Sci. 2018;34(4):243–8. https://doi.org/10.1016/j.kjms.2018.01.009.
27. Gao S, Wang X, Xia Z, Zhang H, Yu J, Yang F. Artificial intelligence in dentistry: a narrative review of diagnostic and therapeutic applications. Med Sci Monit. 2025;31:e946676. https://doi.org/10.12659/MSM.946676.
28. Mallineni SK, Sethi M, Punugoti D, Kotha SB, Alkhayal Z, Mubaraki S, Almotawah FN, Kotha SL, Sajja R, Nettam V, Thakare AA, Sakhamuri S. Artificial intelligence in dentistry: a descriptive review. Bioengineering (Basel). 2024;11(12):1267. https://doi.org/10.3390/bioengineering11121267.

29. Schwendicke F, Samek W, Krois J. Artificial intelligence in dentistry: chances and challenges. J Dent Res. 2020;99(7):769–74. https://doi.org/10.1177/0022034520915714. Epub 2020.
30. Chen YW, Stanley K, Att W. Corrigendum: Artificial intelligence in dentistry: current applications and future perspectives. Quintessence Int. 2020;51(5):430. https://doi.org/10.3290/j.qi.a44465. Erratum for: Quintessence Int. 2020;51(3):248–57.
31. Ding H, Wu J, Zhao W, Matinlinna JP, Burrow MF, Tsoi JKH. Artificial intelligence in dentistry—a review. Front Dent Med. 2023;4:1085251. https://doi.org/10.3389/fdmed.2023.1085251.
32. Ossowska A, Kusiak A, Świetlik D. Artificial intelligence in dentistry-narrative review. Int J Environ Res Public Health. 2022;19(6):3449. https://doi.org/10.3390/ijerph19063449.
33. Rokaya D, Jaghsi AA, Jagtap R, Srimaneepong V. Artificial intelligence in dentistry and dental biomaterials. Front Dent Med. 2024;5:1525505. https://doi.org/10.3389/fdmed.2024.1525505.
34. Thurzo A, Urbanová W, Novák B, Czako L, Siebert T, Stano P, Mareková S, Fountoulaki G, Kosnáčová H, Varga I. Where is the artificial intelligence applied in dentistry? Systematic review and literature analysis. Healthcare (Basel). 2022;10(7):1269. https://doi.org/10.3390/healthcare10071269.
35. Mai HN, Ngo HC, Cho SH, Lee DH. Automated scoring and augmented reality visualization software program for evaluating tooth preparations. J Prosthet Dent. 2024;131(6):1104.e1–8. https://doi.org/10.1016/j.prosdent.2024.02.008. Epub 2024 Mar 14.
36. Zitzmann NU, Matthisson L, Ohla H, Joda T. Digital undergraduate education in dentistry: a systematic review. Int J Environ Res Public Health. 2020;17(9):3269. https://doi.org/10.3390/ijerph17093269.
37. Kihara T, Keller A, Ogawa T, Armand M, Martin-Gomez A. Evaluating the feasibility of using augmented reality for tooth preparation. J Dent. 2024;148:105217. https://doi.org/10.1016/j.jdent.2024.105217. Epub 2024 Jun 28.
38. Daud A, Matoug-Elwerfelli M, Khalid A, Ali K. The impact of virtual reality haptic simulators in pre-clinical restorative dentistry: a qualitative enquiry into dental students' perceptions. BMC Oral Health. 2024;24(1):988. https://doi.org/10.1186/s12903-024-04704-w.
39. Ayoub A, Pulijala Y. The application of virtual reality and augmented reality in Oral & Maxillofacial Surgery. BMC Oral Health. 2019;19(1):238. https://doi.org/10.1186/s12903-019-0937-8.
40. Joda T, Yeung AWK, Hung K, Zitzmann NU, Bornstein MM. Disruptive innovation in dentistry: what it is and what could be next. J Dent Res. 2021;100(5):448–53. https://doi.org/10.1177/0022034520978774. Epub 2020 Dec 16.
41. Song SJ, Tang M, Gwartzman B, Lee D, Romandini P, Salem M, Kwon P, Feiner SK, Sailer I. Augmented-reality-assisted intraoral scanning: a proof-of-concept study. J Prosthodont. 2024;33(6):550–7. https://doi.org/10.1111/jopr.13836. Epub 2024 Mar 20.
42. Alharbi NM, Osman RB. Augmented reality assisted intraoral scanning of mandibular arch: a proof-of-concept pilot clinical study. J Dent. 2024;150:105351. https://doi.org/10.1016/j.jdent.2024.105351. Epub 2024 Sep 10.
43. Marchand L, Touati R, Fehmer V, Ducret M, Sailer I. Latest advances in augmented reality technology and its integration into the digital workflow. Int J Comput Dent. 2020;23(4):397–408.
44. Touati R, Richert R, Millet C, Farges JC, Sailer I, Ducret M. Comparison of two innovative strategies using augmented reality for communication in aesthetic dentistry: a pilot study. J Healthc Eng. 2019;2019:7019046. https://doi.org/10.1155/2019/7019046.
45. Monterubbianesi R, Tosco V, Vitiello F, Orilisi G, Fraccastoro F, Putignano A, Orsini G. Augmented, virtual and mixed reality in dentistry: a narrative review on the existing platforms and future challenges. Appl Sci. 2022;12(2):877. https://doi.org/10.3390/app12020877.
46. Wang Q, Zhao Z, Li J, Zhao R, Zhou M, Tang K, Bai S, Ma C, Wang F. In vivo evaluation of T-Scan in quantifying occlusal contact. J Oral Rehabil. 2024;51(9):1675–83. https://doi.org/10.1111/joor.13732. Epub 2024 Jun 26.
47. Gözen M, Güntekin N. Comparison of occlusal force distribution and digital occlusal analysis methods of single posterior implant restorations: an in vivo study. BMC Oral Health. 2025;25(1):795. https://doi.org/10.1186/s12903-025-06205-w.

48. Biadsee A, Biadsee A, Khalifa A, Mtanis T, Ormianer Z. Clinical evaluation of the agreement between virtual and clinical occlusal registrations: A comparative clinical study. J Prosthet Dent. 2025;133(5):1250–9. https://doi.org/10.1016/j.prosdent.2023.07.018. Epub 2023 Aug 21.
49. Zheng Y, Zhang T, Liu Y, Pradíes G, Wang X, Ma D, Bai S. Evaluation methods and influencing factors on accuracy for static virtual articulation obtained by intraoral scanners: a critical review of the literature. J Esthet Restor Dent. 2025;37(2):378–99. https://doi.org/10.1111/jerd.13312. Epub 2024 Sep 27.
50. Al-Ani Z, Yar R. Evolution of dental occlusion: integrating digital innovations. Prim Dent J. 2025;14(1):53–65. https://doi.org/10.1177/20501684251320452. Epub 2025 May 13.
51. Wang F, Niu LN, Chen JH. [Digital occlusal analysis: solutions and efficacy]. Zhonghua Kou Qiang Yi Xue Za Zhi. 2025;60(8):822–8. Chinese. https://doi.org/10.3760/cma.j.cn112144-20250401-00113.
52. Mangano FG, Admakin O, Lerner H, Mangano C. Artificial intelligence and augmented reality for guided implant surgery planning: a proof of concept. J Dent. 2023;133:104485. https://doi.org/10.1016/j.jdent.2023.104485. Epub 2023 Mar 23.
53. Liu L, Wang X, Guan M, Fan Y, Yang Z, Li D, Bai Y, Li H. A mixed reality-based navigation method for dental implant navigation method: a pilot study. Comput Biol Med. 2023;154:106568. https://doi.org/10.1016/j.compbiomed.2023.106568. Epub 2023 Jan 24.
54. Mangano FG, Yang KR, Lerner H, Admakin O, Mangano C. Artificial intelligence and mixed reality for dental implant planning: a technical note. Clin Implant Dent Relat Res. 2024;26(5):942–53. https://doi.org/10.1111/cid.13357. Epub 2024 Jun 28.
55. Stadlinger B, Carvalho J, Menze B. AI in the field of oral surgery and implantology—an overview. ITI Forum Implantologicum. 2025; https://doi.org/10.63580/iti.fi.45752.
56. Shusterman A, Nashef R, Tecco S, Mangano C, Lerner H, Mangano FG. Accuracy of implant placement using a mixed reality-based dynamic navigation system versus static computer-assisted and freehand surgery: an in Vitro study. J Dent. 2024;146:105052. https://doi.org/10.1016/j.jdent.2024.105052. Epub 2024 May 9.
57. Pellegrino G, Mangano C, Mangano R, Ferri A, Taraschi V, Marchetti C. Augmented reality for dental implantology: a pilot clinical report of two cases. BMC Oral Health. 2019;19(1):158. https://doi.org/10.1186/s12903-019-0853-y.
58. Mai HN, Dam VV, Lee DH. Accuracy of augmented reality-assisted navigation in dental implant surgery: systematic review and meta-analysis. J Med Internet Res. 2023;25:e42040. https://doi.org/10.2196/42040.
59. Mosch R, Alevizakos V, Ströbele DA, Schiller M, von See C. Exploring augmented reality for dental implant surgery: feasibility of using smartphones as navigation tools. Clin Exp Dent Res. 2025;11(1):e70110. https://doi.org/10.1002/cre2.70110.
60. Engelschalk M, Al Hamad KQ, Mangano R, Smeets R, Molnar TF. Dental implant placement with immersive technologies: a preliminary clinical report of augmented and mixed reality applications. J Prosthet Dent. 2025;133(2):346–51. https://doi.org/10.1016/j.prosdent.2024.02.017. Epub 2024 Mar 12. Erratum in: J Prosthet Dent. 2024;132(3):656.
61. Kotler P, Kartajaya H, Setiawan I. Marketing 6.0: the future is immersive. New Jersey: Wiley; 2023.
62. Melnyk B. Research-innovation aspect of modern medical (dental) education in a mixed learning environment. Sci Bull Mukachevo State Univ Ser Pedag Psychol. 2023;9(2):28–37. https://doi.org/10.52534/msu-pp2.2023.28.
63. Kashwani R, Sawhney H. Dentistry and metaverse: a deep dive into potential of blockchain, NFTs, and crypto in healthcare [Internet]. Int Dent J Stud Res. 2023;11(3):94–8. https://doi.org/10.18231/j.idjsr.2023.021.
64. Roy S, Richert R, Tavares JMRS, Lahoud P. Editorial: Applications of digital twin technology in dentistry. Front Bioeng Biotechnol. 2025;13:1624734. https://doi.org/10.3389/fbioe.2025.1624734.

65. Durham M, Engel B, Ferrill T, Halford J, Singh TP, Gladwell M. Digitally augmented learning in implant dentistry. Oral Maxillofac Surg Clin North Am. 2019;31(3):387–98. https://doi.org/10.1016/j.coms.2019.03.003. Epub 2019 May 29.
66. Yan X, Yan Y, Cao M, Xie W, O'Connor S, Lee JJ, Ho MH. Effectiveness of virtual reality distraction interventions to reduce dental anxiety in paediatric patients: a systematic review and meta-analysis. J Dent. 2023;132:104455. https://doi.org/10.1016/j.jdent.2023.104455. Epub 2023 Feb 24.
67. Arroyo-Cruz G, Orozco-Varo A, Domínguez-Cardoso P, Árbol-Carrero AB, Jiménez-Castellanos E. FitJaw Mobile, a virtual reality device applied to dentistry: an analysis based on two patient treatments. J Prosthet Dent. 2025;133(3):805–10. https://doi.org/10.1016/j.prosdent.2023.04.018. Epub 2023 May 24.
68. Lepidi L, Galli M, Mastrangelo F, Venezia P, Joda T, Wang HL, Li J. Virtual articulators and virtual mounting procedures: where do we stand? J Prosthodont. 2021;30(1):24–35. https://doi.org/10.1111/jopr.13240.
69. Li J, Wang HL, Joda T. Digital dentistry and virtual patient integration: current applications and future directions. J Prosthet Dent. 2023;129(2):293–300. https://doi.org/10.1016/j.prosdent.2021.05.008.
70. Joda T, Gallucci GO. The virtual patient in dental medicine. Clin Oral Implants Res. 2015;26(6):725–6. https://doi.org/10.1111/clr.12379.
71. Revilla-León M, Gómez-Polo M, Vyas S, Barmak BA, Gallucci GO, Att W, Krishnamurthy VR. Artificial intelligence applications in implant dentistry: a systematic review. J Prosthet Dent. 2023;129(2):293–300. https://doi.org/10.1016/j.prosdent.2021.05.008.
72. Haku-Mizuhara K, Tanabe G, Kadempour A, Mirafzali S, Yotsuya M, Yamaguchi S. Development of a 4-dimensional virtual patient in motion: a digital concept. J Prosthet Dent. 2025; https://doi.org/10.1016/j.prosdent.2025.02.064.
73. Sohrabniya F, Hassanzadeh-Samani S, Ourang SA, Jafari B, Farzinnia G, Gorjinejad F, et al. Exploring a decade of deep learning in dentistry: a comprehensive mapping review. Clin Oral Investig. 2025;29(2):143. https://doi.org/10.1007/s00784-025-06216-5.
74. Revilla-León M, Zeitler JM, Fry E, Kois JC. Digital workflow to measure the mandibular range of motion using different jaw tracking technologies. J Prosthet Dent. 2025;134(4):1208–15. https://doi.org/10.1016/j.prosdent.2023.12.018.
75. Mangano FG, Veronesi G, Hauschild U, Mijiritsky E, Mangano C. Trueness and precision of four intraoral scanners in oral implantology: a comparative in vitro study. PLoS One. 2020;15(9):e0238266. https://doi.org/10.1371/journal.pone.0238266.
76. Marlière DAA, Demètrio MS, Picinini LS, Oliveira RG, Netto HDMC. Accuracy of computer-guided surgery for dental implant placement in fully edentulous patients: a systematic review. Eur J Dent. 2018;12(1):153–60. https://doi.org/10.4103/ejd.ejd_249_17.

Automated Tissue Segmentation

7

Mariana Balcewicz Pozza, Ji Yong Han,
Thi Ngoc Trang Tran, Rafik Akhmad, Malek Abu-Gharbieh,
Andreas Dominik Schwitalla, Florian Beuer,
and Arthur Rodriguez Gonzalez Cortes

The ability to generate precise 3D digital models from segmented imaging data is not merely a technical advancement but a clinical requirement for several techniques that directly impacts patient care and treatment outcomes. These models are indispensable for a wide range of diagnostic and therapeutic procedures, enabling a shift toward more predictable, patient-specific interventions. Among the main clinical applications in dentistry depending on accurate segmentations are implant dentistry, endodontics, orthodontics, and reconstructive surgery.

In implant guided surgery, accurate segmentations are critical to create virtual patients for 3D-guided implant surgery and the respective prosthetically driven treatment planning [1]. For this purpose, the final implant supported restoration is designed first to dictate the ideal implant position in relation to the bone structure available at the alveolar ridge, as further discussed in Chap. 9. Furthermore,

M. B. Pozza
GoBeyond Institute, Curitiba, Brazil

J. Y. Han
Seoul National University, Seoul, South Korea
e-mail: jiyong@snu.ac.kr

T. N. T. Tran · A. R. G. Cortes (✉)
Faculty of Dental Surgery, University of Malta, Msida, Malta
e-mail: thi-ngoc-trang.tran.22@um.edu.mt ; arthur.nogueira@um.edu.mt

R. Akhmad · A. D. Schwitalla · F. Beuer
Charité University, Berlin, Germany
e-mail: rafik.akhmad@charite.de; andreas.schwitalla@charite.de; florian.beuer@charite.de

M. Abu-Gharbieh
Institut für Werkzeugmaschinen und Fabrikbetrieb, Berlin, Germany
e-mail: abu-gharbieh@iwf.tu-berlin.de

A. R. G. Cortes (ed.), *Dental Clinical Procedures using Artificial Intelligence*,
https://doi.org/10.1007/978-3-032-24895-4_7

applications such as guided endodontics and apical surgeries depend on clear visualization of the root canal anatomy, which is made possible by means of precise tooth segmentation from CBCT data.

In the field of orthodontics, adequate segmentation technologies are integral to digital orthodontic workflows and virtual surgical planning for orthognathic surgery [2], allowing clinicians to simulate outcomes and plan complex skeletal movements with satisfactory accuracy, as further discussed in Chap. 8. This is also relevant for the surgical planning of reconstructive surgeries. Segmentation plays a vital role in planning procedures such as tooth autotransplantation and complex mandibular reconstruction following tumor ablation or trauma, where precise anatomical models guide the design of grafts and surgical guides.

7.1 Limitations of Traditional Segmentation Methods

In contrast to modern AI-driven approaches, traditional segmentation methods fall into two categories: manual and semiautomated. Manual segmentation, long considered the clinical standard, requires an expert clinician to meticulously outline anatomical structures slice-by-slice [3]. This process is exceptionally labor-intensive, time-consuming, and inherently susceptible to both interobserver (between different clinicians) and intra-observer (by the same clinician at different times) variability.

Semiautomated techniques, such as thresholding, were developed to improve efficiency. These methods attempt to distinguish structures based on their pixel intensity or gray values. However, they struggle significantly with the inherent limitations of CBCT imaging, which produces images with low contrast between tissues of similar density (e.g., dentin, cementum, and bone) and uncalibrated gray values that are not standardized such as Hounsfield units from conventional medical CT devices that present larger contrast scales. Consequently, these methods often fail to produce reliable results without substantial manual correction.

To overcome this limitation, a previous study validated a method of AI-driven image translation from CBCT to medical CT data, so that the pixel values from CBCT could be compatible with actual Hounsfield units for radiographic bone density and further imaging assessments [4]. The first stage of this proposed framework introduces explicit structural conditioning. Edge information derived from CBCT images is used as a surrogate representation of anatomical boundaries. These edge maps capture gradients corresponding to cortical bone, dental structures, and air-tissue interfaces, providing a geometry-preserving constraint during translation.

The next stage is the edge-guided unpaired learning, in which CBCT images are augmented with their corresponding edge representations and fed into an unpaired translation network. By jointly processing intensity and structural cues, the model learns to modify image contrast and texture while maintaining spatial consistency. A multi-scale discrimination strategy is employed to evaluate both global anatomical coherence and local textural realism. This allows the model to generate images that resemble CT in appearance while remaining faithful to the underlying CBCT

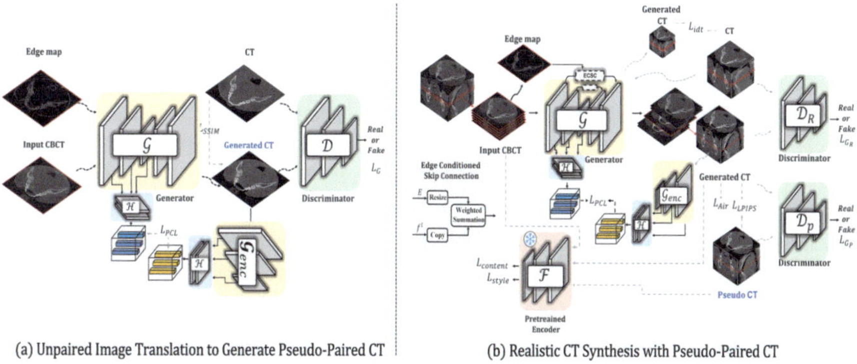

Fig. 7.1 Overview of the unpaired, edge-conditioned CBCT-to-pseudo-CT translation process. (**a**) Unpaired image translation to generate pseudo-paired CT. (**b**) Realistic CT synthesis with pseudo-paired CT

anatomy. The output of this stage is a set of pseudo-CT images. Although not identical to true CT scans, these images maintain voxel-level correspondence with their CBCT inputs and exhibit CT-like contrast characteristics (Fig. 7.1). These pseudo-CT images will be finally used for realistic CT synthesis in the next stage using a translation network based on a U-Net-like architecture.

7.2 Foundational Concepts of AI-Driven Segmentation

The transition from manual and semiautomated segmentation to automated AI algorithms represents a significant technological shift in medical image analysis and for dental professionals using CBCT devices. This evolution is driven by the clinical demand for greater efficiency, consistency, and the capacity to process the large, complex datasets generated by modern imaging technologies such as CBCT. AI models based on deep learning are trained to recognize intricate patterns and anatomical features from vast quantities of image data, enabling them to perform segmentation tasks with a level of speed and precision that is unattainable with traditional methods. Automated segmentation is now a recent feature of implant planning software programs [1, 5], due to the importance of creating the virtual patient from multiple combined imaging methods such as CBCT and intraoral scans.

The accuracy of a tissue segmentation is usually measured by quantifying the spatial overlap between the AI-generated model and the ground-truth model. The most common metrics are the Dice Similarity Coefficient (DSC) and Intersection over Union (IoU). A DSC score of 1.0 indicates perfect overlap, with scores above 0.7 considered a good overlap [6], while IoU scores above 0.9 are considered excellent [7]. Average distances and time efficiency can also be measured, as these are also clinically relevant aspects in dentistry.

7.3 Main AI Architectures in Dental Segmentation

The foundational technology behind modern AI-based medical image segmentation is a class of deep learning algorithms known as convolutional neural networks (CNNs) [2]. These networks are inspired by the human visual cortex and are exceptionally adept at recognizing visual patterns directly from pixelized images. Within the field of dentomaxillofacial imaging, the U-Net architecture and its variants (such as 3D U-Net and V-Net) have emerged as the most frequently employed and highly successful models, a finding consistently supported by multiple systematic reviews. The U-Net's unique encoder-decoder structure allows it to effectively capture both contextual and localized information, making it ideal for delineating complex anatomical boundaries. While U-Net is the dominant model, other advanced architectures, including the feature pyramid network (FPN) and generative adversarial networks (GANs), are also utilized to refine segmentation quality and enhance edge details.

7.4 Performance and Validation Metrics

To ensure that AI segmentation models are clinically reliable, their performance must be rigorously evaluated against a "ground-truth" standard, which is typically a meticulously prepared manual segmentation performed by an expert. This validation is conducted using a set of standardized quantitative metrics.

7.5 Applications of AI Segmentation by Anatomical Target

The technology being AI segmentation is best understood by examining the specific anatomical structures being targeted and the clinical decisions that hinge on their accurate delineation. The performance and clinical relevance of AI vary depending on the size, complexity, and imaging characteristics of the target anatomy. As mentioned in Chap. 1, it is important to understand the current state of AI segmentation for teeth, jawbones, and other critical structures, highlighting both its capabilities and its limitations in real-world clinical scenarios.

7.5.1 Tooth and Prosthetic Crown Segmentation

AI has demonstrated exceptional performance in segmenting individual teeth [6, 7], and prosthetic crowns [8], from CBCT data. This capability is useful for several applications, including prosthetically driven implant planning, designing guides for endodontic procedures, and virtual setups for orthodontic treatment. A meta-analysis of the existing literature reported a pooled Dice Similarity Coefficient (DSC) of 0.95 for AI-based tooth segmentation, indicating a very high degree of accuracy and overlap with expert manual segmentations [6]. Despite this strong overall performance, studies have identified a consistent pattern of lower accuracy in the apical region of the root. The complex anatomy and lower image contrast in this area make it more challenging for algorithms to precisely delineate the root tip, a critical consideration for endodontic and surgical planning.

7.5.2 Maxillofacial Bone Structure Segmentation

For larger and more distinct anatomical structures such as the maxilla and mandible, AI segmentation achieves even higher levels of accuracy [2], with reported DSC scores frequently exceeding 0.98. This high fidelity is essential for applications such as orthognathic surgery planning and trauma reconstruction. A particularly innovative application demonstrates AI's ability to "segment beyond the imaging data." Researchers have successfully trained AI models to generate anatomically valid edentulous (toothless) mandibular models from CT scans of dentate (tooth-bearing) patients [9]. This allows surgeons to create a virtual target geometry for reconstructive surgery using autologous bone grafts, such as those from the fibula or iliac crest. This capability highlights the potential of AI tools not just to replicate existing anatomy but to create clinically relevant predictive models for surgical planning.

7.5.3 Segmentation of Critical Anatomical Structures

Beyond teeth and jawbones, AI is increasingly being used to segment smaller but clinically critical structures, most notably the mandibular canal [10], which houses the inferior alveolar nerve. The primary clinical goal of segmenting this structure is to prevent iatrogenic nerve injury during procedures such as implant placement or third molar extractions. Accurately mapping the trajectory of the mandibular canal is therefore paramount for surgical safety. In this context, research in this area has underscored a critical factor for developing robust and reliable AI models, which is the dataset diversity. One multi-device study found that networks trained on varied datasets acquired from different CBCT machines consistently outperformed models trained on larger but more homogenous datasets from a single device [11]. This finding emphasizes that exposing an AI algorithm to a wide range of imaging characteristics is crucial for ensuring its generalizability and reliable performance in real-world clinical settings.

7.6 Analysis of Common Errors and Technical Challenges in AI Segmentation

Despite the high accuracy metrics reported in numerous studies, AI segmentation models are not infallible [12]. For AI to be implemented safely and effectively in clinical practice, it is crucial to understand the sources and patterns of its errors.

These challenges can compromise the reliability of the 3D models used for treatment planning and lead to adverse clinical outcomes if left uncorrected. This section systematically categorizes the most common challenges, ranging from inherent limitations in the source imaging data to the specific types of errors produced by algorithmic misinterpretations.

7.6.1 Imaging-Related Challenges

Many segmentation errors originate not from the AI algorithm itself, but from the quality and characteristics of the input CBCT data [11]. The following are the most significant imaging-related challenges:

7.6.1.1 Metal Artifacts

Beam-hardening artifacts from metal and hyperdense (radiopaque) structures are a primary cause of segmentation failure. High-density materials common in dentistry, such as metallic restorations, dental implants, and orthodontic brackets, may cause severe hypodense streaks and altered areas on the CBCT image. Furthermore, phenomena such as beam hardening and photon starvation also result in characteristic streak artifacts that obscure adjacent anatomical structures, making it difficult for AI algorithms to identify true anatomical boundaries.

7.6.1.2 Low Contrast and Noise

CBCT images inherently have lower contrast resolution compared to medical CT, making it challenging to distinguish between tissues with similar radiodensities (pixel values). The boundaries between cementum, dentin, and alveolar bone, for example, are often indistinct. This problem is further exacerbated by image noise, which can cause the algorithm to produce imprecise borders.

7.6.1.3 Patient Motion

Any patient movement during the scan, whether voluntary or involuntary (e.g., swallowing), introduces blurring and ghosting artifacts. These distortions create distorted or duplicated boundaries that may confuse AI algorithms, leading to grossly inaccurate segmentations.

7.6.2 Common AI Segmentation Error Types

Based on a review of AI performance in clinical settings, several common error patterns have been identified [12]. Understanding this taxonomy of failures is essential for clinicians tasked with verifying AI-generated models.

7.6.2.1 Boundary Errors

One of the most clinically relevant types of AI segmentation errors is the misinterpretation of anatomical borders. A common example is the failure to distinguish between a tooth root and surrounding bone or, in more extreme cases, misidentifying a normal radiolucent anatomical variation in the maxilla as the inferior alveolar nerve canal, which is located in the mandible.

7.6.2.2 Over-Segmentation

Excessive segmentations occur when the algorithm incorrectly includes adjacent structures as part of the target anatomy. A typical instance is the misclassification of dense mucosal tissue or bone graft material as part of the alveolar bone, resulting in a 3D model that overestimates the available bone volume.

7.6.2.3 Under-Segmentation

The omission of relevant anatomical structures from the final model is an important type of error. For instance, an AI model might fail to segment a reconstructed portion of a mandible because scattering artifacts from a metal fixation plate obscure the underlying bone, leading to an incomplete and clinically unusable model.

7.6.2.4 Misidentification

The most severe type of error occurs when one structure is misclassified as another, which is classified as "misidentification." In one documented case, an AI algorithm identified dense bone graft material as a tooth and even perceived an adjacent area of soft tissue integration as a "periapical lesion," a clear misinterpretation with significant clinical implications.

7.6.3 The Impact of Dataset and Device Heterogeneity

A critical challenge for the widespread adoption of AI segmentation is generalizability. An AI model trained on a limited, single-center dataset may perform exceptionally well on images from that specific institution but fail significantly when applied to data from different CBCT devices or diverse patient populations. Variations in scanning protocols, voxel sizes, and image processing across different manufacturers create subtle but important differences in image characteristics that can confound a narrowly trained algorithm. Systematic reviews consistently identify this lack of external validation as a key limitation in the current body of research. Studies that explicitly use multi-device datasets have confirmed that networks trained on more varied data are significantly more robust and perform better on unseen images. This underscores the necessity of moving beyond single-center studies to create AI tools that are reliable and effective across the entire spectrum of clinical practice.

7.7 Useful Tools and Techniques Involving AI-Driven Structural Segmentation

7.7.1 Image Thresholding for Oral and Maxillofacial Structures

Some of the modern AI and implant planning software programs present AI tools primarily dedicated for automating complex dental data preparation, such as the coDiagnostiX (Straumann; Fig. 7.2) and Diagnocat (Diagnocat Ltd.) software programs. Dedicated AI tools of these software programs can provide noise reduction of CBCT 3D reconstructed models. As per the discussion above based on the literature, these AI tools ultimately allow for faster and more accurate digital planning by automating segmentation of teeth and bone from CBCT scans, aligning 3D models, and enabling streamlined virtual tooth extractions and customized abutment designs. The intended benefit for clinicians is saving time and working load to focus on the treatment design rather than manual data processing.

7.7.2 Automated Superimposition or Alignment of CBCT and Intraoral Scans (IOS)

With advancements in digital dentistry, virtual surgical planning can be performed on virtual patients including bone and hard tissues from CBCT and crowns and soft tissues from IOS. These two different types of images are complementary to each other. On one hand, CBCT has limited spatial resolution to precisely define soft tissues and tooth crowns in occlusion. On the other hand, IOS provides no information on roots or the underlying alveolar bone structure.

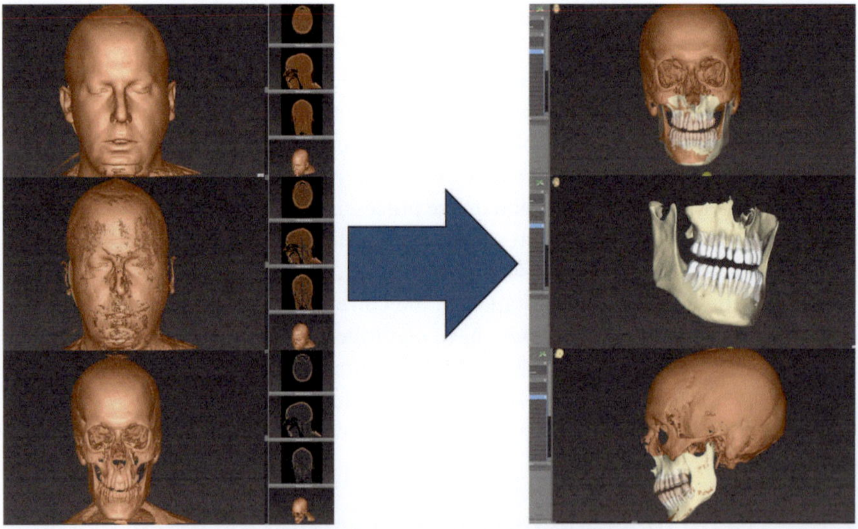

Fig. 7.2 AI-driven segmentation of teeth, maxilla, and mandible performed on coDiagnostiX software program to be used for dental implant planning. The left column shows the process of threshold optimization of the 3D CBCT reconstructed model to visualize bone structures. From this 3D model, every single tooth and the shapes of mandible and maxilla are automatically segmented by the AI tool of the software, which allows for exporting each tooth and structure as an independent STL file. (Software procedure performed by the Dr. Mariana Pozza and the planning center "Beyond Digital Solutions (BDS 3D)")

Therefore, these two types of scans are fundamentally different types of information. A CBCT scan is a collection of volumetric, cross-sectional images representing the density of various tissues (bone, skin, teeth), while an IOS scan is a high-resolution surface point cloud.

Both scans capture more than just the teeth. CBCT includes the entire craniofacial skeleton, skin, and muscle, while IOS captures both teeth and contours of the gingival tissue. The essential first step is to digitally isolate the teeth as a "region of interest" from all the surrounding data. Traditionally, this registration has been done manually using commercial software. However, this method is time-consuming, labor-intensive, and highly dependent on the skill of the operator, which can lead to inconsistent and unreliable results. To overcome these obstacles, a novel automated workflow has been developed by AI software manufacturers to prepare and align these data with high precision (Fig. 7.3).

Every STL file exported from AI or implant planning software programs can be imported into computer-aided design (CAD) software programs such as the Modellier (Zirkonzahn) (Fig. 7.4), to take part in the prosthetically driven treatment plan of the patient [3]. These STL files and the corresponding structures will generally be imported automatically in the same 3D coordinates of the CAD project, which is a very important advantage for an adequate and less time-consuming treatment plan involving digital prosthetic designs and occlusal devices.

Another useful CAD software program with advanced supporting AI tools for segmentations of virtually articulated images is the Modifier software (Zirkonzahn, Gais, Italy). The software offers useful types of automatisms that support the user during the workflow for designing restorations, which may leverage some basic AI principles (e.g., machine learning algorithms for pattern recognition) but is primarily algorithm-based. One feature useful for cases with overlapping scan areas between maxilla and mandible in occlusion (Figs. 7.5, 7.6, and 7.7) is the "Optimize occlusion" tool (under the menu "Extras" within option "Maximum occlusion") to correct the overlapping areas and refine the accuracy of the occlusal relationship.

After this AI-driven optimization of the digital occlusion of the patient, it is possible to perform an automated segmentation of individual teeth and anatomical structures as well as the alignment between CBCT DICOM data and the upper and lower intraoral scans mounted on the virtual articulator (Figs. 7.8, 7.9, and 7.10), enabling proper treatment planning and digital designs considering all tissues of the patient, along with simulation of occlusal movements such as protrusion and lateral excursion.

Dental clinicians and professionals who are busy could also visualize all the STL files exported from AI software programs in CAD/CAM viewers (Fig. 7.11), which are applications available for mobile devices to open STL files in a 3D space considering their original coordinates.

The accuracy of a tooth segmentation from CBCT data will depend on the quality and resolution of the scan. Factors such as noise, artifacts, and scanning parameters such as greater voxel sizes and field-of-views may significantly affect the outcomes of tissue segmentations.

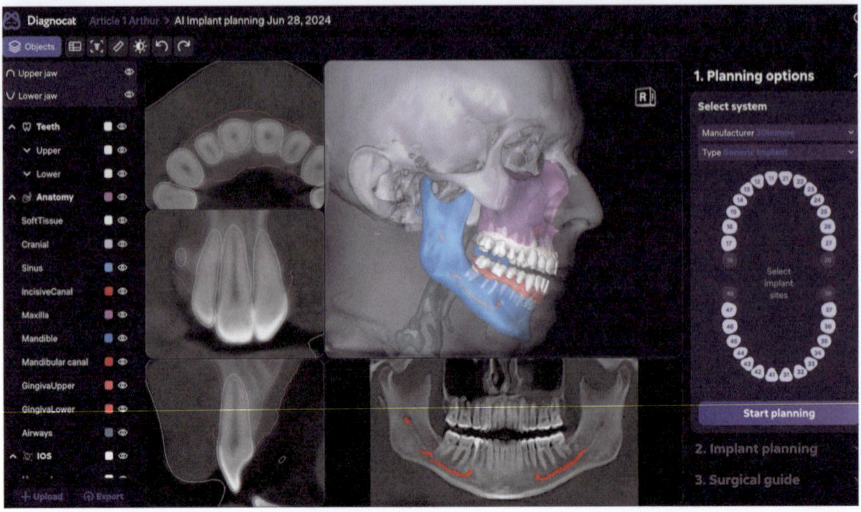

Fig. 7.3 AI automated alignment of CBCT and IOS images performed by the implant planning tool of the Diagnocat software. Note that the outlined structures can also be visualized in the 2D multiplanar reconstruction, to ensure quality of contours of the AI segmentation. All the anatomical structures mentioned in Chap. 1 are also automatically segmented and displayed in different colors to be considered during the dental implant planning. With this software, each tooth or structured segmented, as well as virtual implants and surgical guides, can also be exported as independent STL files

A software such as Geomagic Control X (Oqton) can be used to assess the alignment of meshes from two different scans of the same objects (Fig. 7.12). In this context, Geomagic software compares 3D images by aligning a measured scan (point cloud or mesh) to a reference mesh (often CAD file or a master scan). For this purpose, the software uses best-fit algorithms and color maps to show deviations (Fig. 7.13), enabling the assessment of 2D cross sections, dimensioning, and automated quality reports to find fit, form, and function issues, as part of an intuitive 3D inspection process.

7.7.2.1 Acknowledgments

The editor would like to thank the dental technician, Mr. Jürgen Feierabend, for his support and encouragement in the preparation of this section of the chapter.

7.7.3 Optimization of AI Segmented Areas

Several modern imaging devices use AI tools to optimize outcomes from automated segmentations. One of the examples is the SIRIOS intraoral scanner (Straumann), which uses AI primarily for automated scan cleanup and optimization, with an AI Smart Filtering Tool that intelligently removes soft tissue, cheeks, or other unwanted

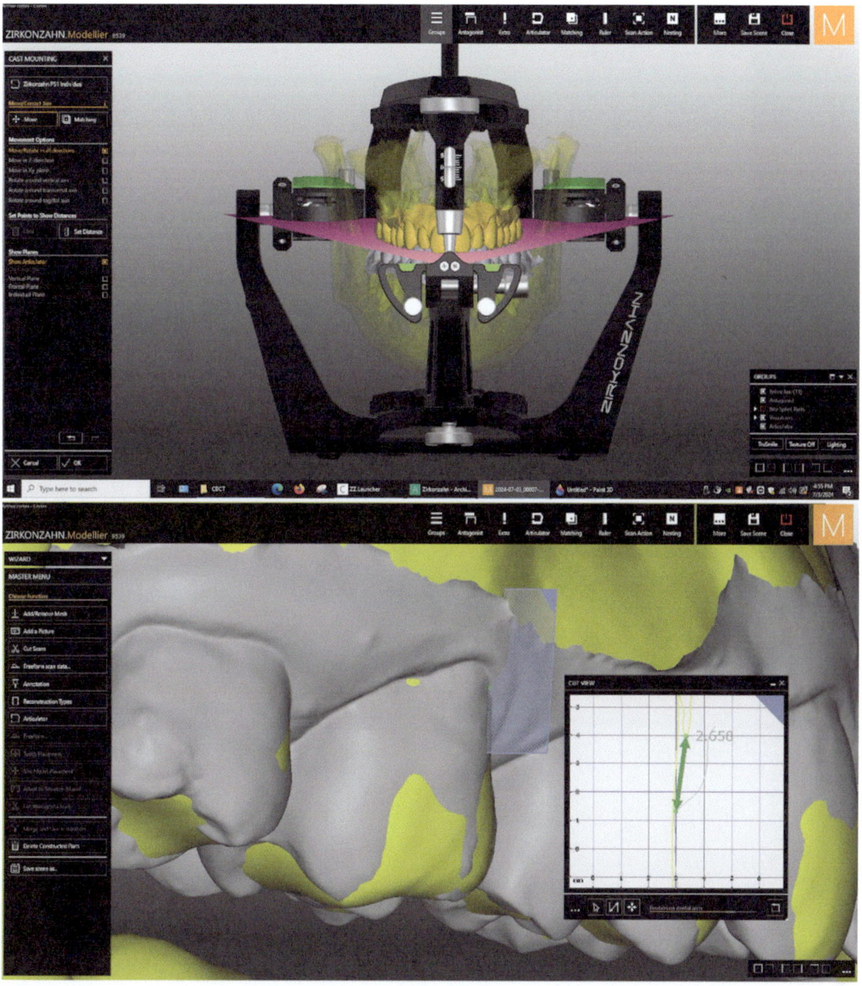

Fig. 7.4 Computer-aided design project created in a CAD software (Modellier, Zirkonzahn) with the virtual patient generated from the STL files of the AI segmentation of Fig. 7.2. The case was mounted on a virtual articulator (top) for digital prosthetic planning. Once in a CAD software, it is possible to design veneers, crowns, fixed partial dentures, occlusal splints, snoring, and other devices to be 3D-printed or milled. Since the virtual patient data includes well-aligned CBCT and intraoral scans, it is possible to measure the distance between the marginal gingiva and the alveolar crest (bottom), which includes the biological width plus the depth of the gingival sulcus. These two components should ideally have sufficient space to prevent inflammation, which is the reason why the distance between the margins of a restoration and the alveolar crest should generally be at least 3 mm

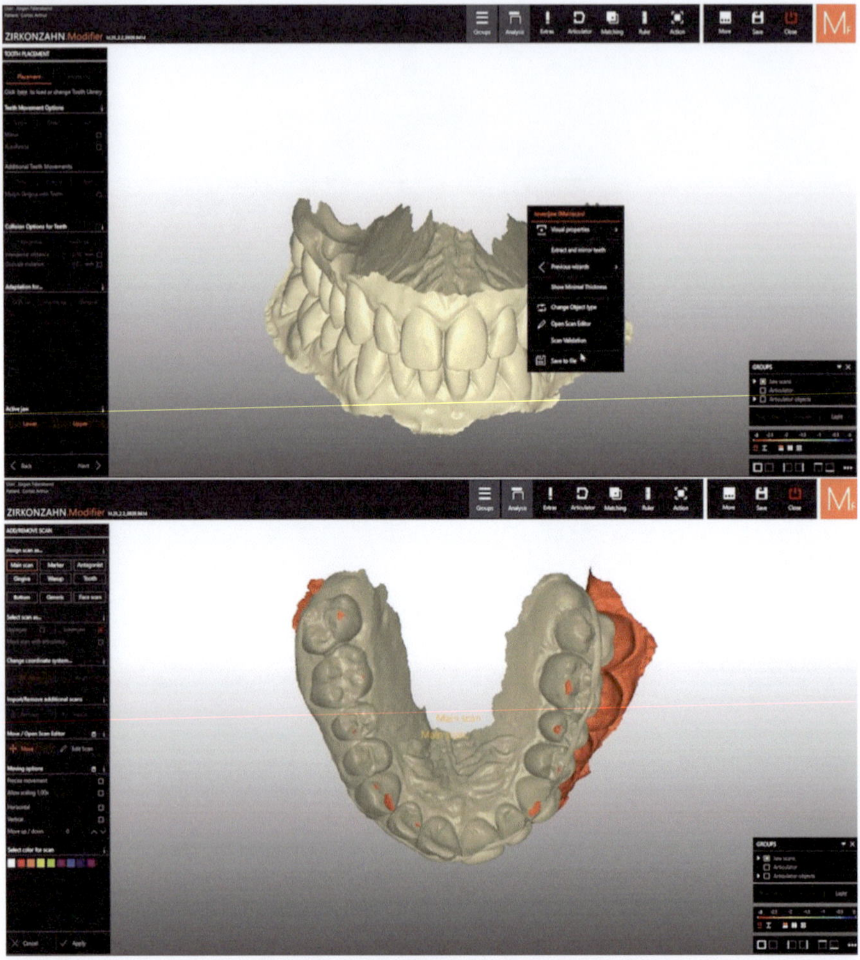

Fig. 7.5 Screenshot of the Zirkonzahn Modifier software visualizing the articulated intraoral scans from the top. Note the overlapping cusps of teeth from the lower intraoral scan (orange) trespassing the mesh of the upper intraoral scan (brown)

items, preserving crucial gingiva around implants or teeth (Fig. 7.14). This scanner also features an AI model trained on extensive dental data to improve image realism (tool explained on the previous chapter), provide margin line detection, and enable automated scan body recognition with alignment of different intraoral scans and their components for the same patient.

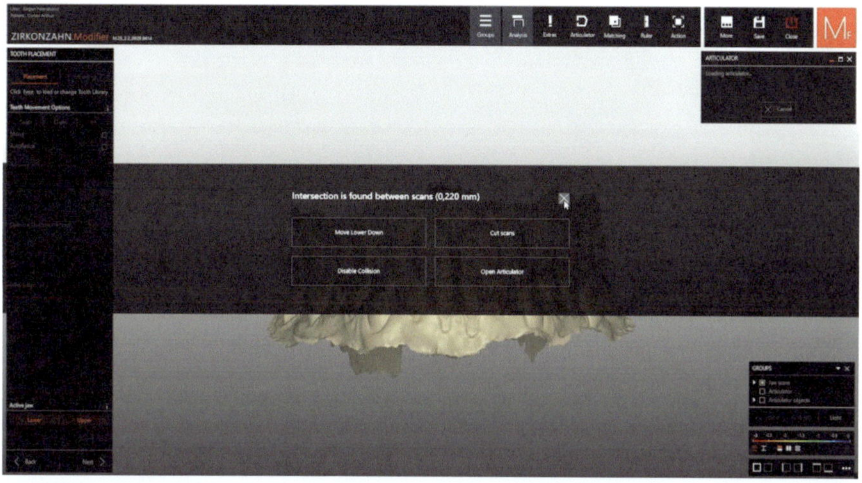

Fig. 7.6 Screenshot of the Zirkonzahn Modifier software after an attempt to simulate occlusal movements. The software warned the user about the overlapping areas between mandibular and maxillary intraoral scans, which affects the occlusal registration

7.7.4 Root-Analogue Dental Implants (Technique Presented by Dr. Rafik Akhmad, Dr. Malek Abu-Gharbieh, and Prof. Andreas D. Schwitalla)

AI-based segmentation and planning tools facilitate patient-specific treatment planning and therapies. In this context, nature serves as a central blueprint, e.g., natural tooth anatomy becomes the morphological and biomechanical reference for the design of future implants.

The convergence of AI and additive manufacturing allows patient-specific implants with complex, nature-inspired geometries, including root-analogue implant bodies and biomimetic crown morphologies tailored to individual anatomical and biomechanical conditions. Longitudinal digital data, such as intraoral scans and CBCT datasets, can be reused to manufacture "spare parts" when needed, for example, after tooth loss or implant failure.

Biomimetic design concepts, such as gyroid structures, provide highly organized porous architectures with high strength, low weight, and large internal surface areas that support biological integration. This chapter outlines the biomechanical rationale, concept, and workflow of patient-specific individualized implants, from data acquisition and AI-assisted segmentation to semiautomated design, hybrid (additive and subtractive) manufacturing, and post-processing, and highlights the potential of biomimetic structures to bridge the gap between natural tooth anatomy and future implant design in order to optimize the integration of the alloplastic implant into the human organism.

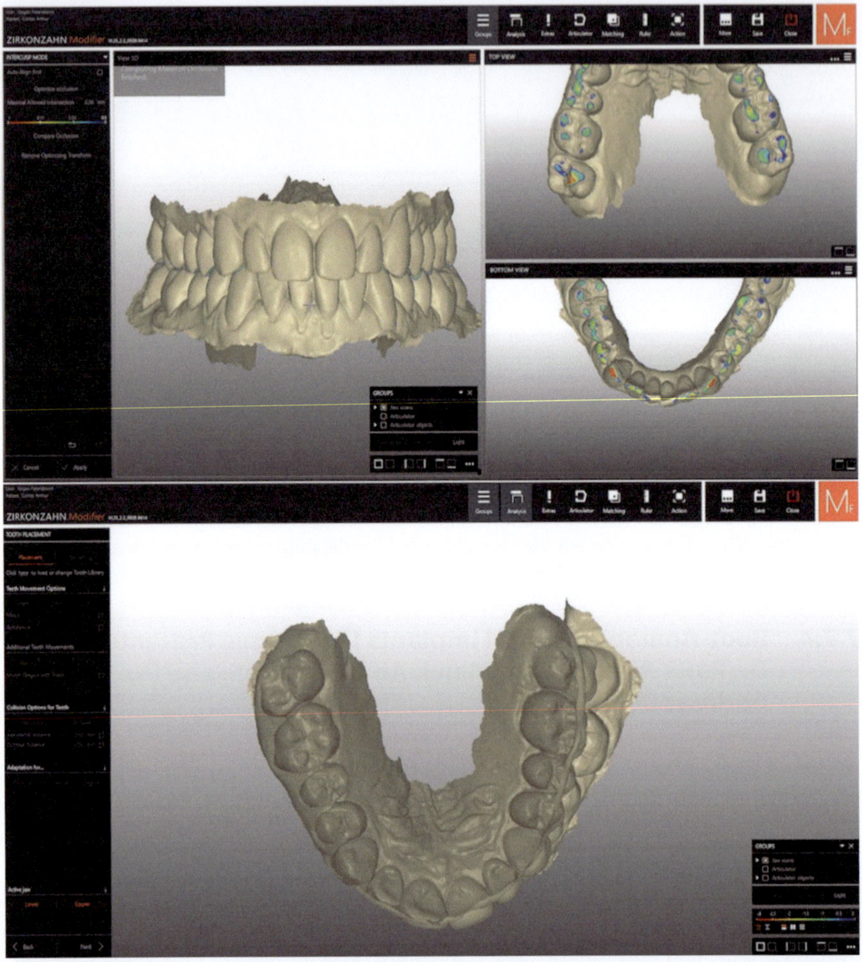

Fig. 7.7 Screenshot of the Zirkonzahn Modifier software visualizing the articulated intraoral scans from the top after the use of the "Optimize occlusion" tool. Note the confirming of the absence of overlapping areas and an adequate occlusal registration

7.7.4.1 Biomechanical and Anatomical Rationale

The design of patient-specific individualized implants is fundamentally grounded in the anatomy and biomechanics of the natural teeth. The tooth-periodontium complex represents a highly optimized biological structure in which form and function are tightly interrelated [13]. Tooth morphology, root geometry, and the properties of the surrounding tissues have evolved to transmit masticatory forces efficiently while minimizing local stress peaks and preserving tissue vitality over decades [14–16].

From this perspective, tooth shape is not arbitrary. Parameters such as root taper, length, curvature, cross-sectional form, number of roots, and surface texture can all be related to specific biomechanical tasks [17–19]. Slender and tapered roots enable

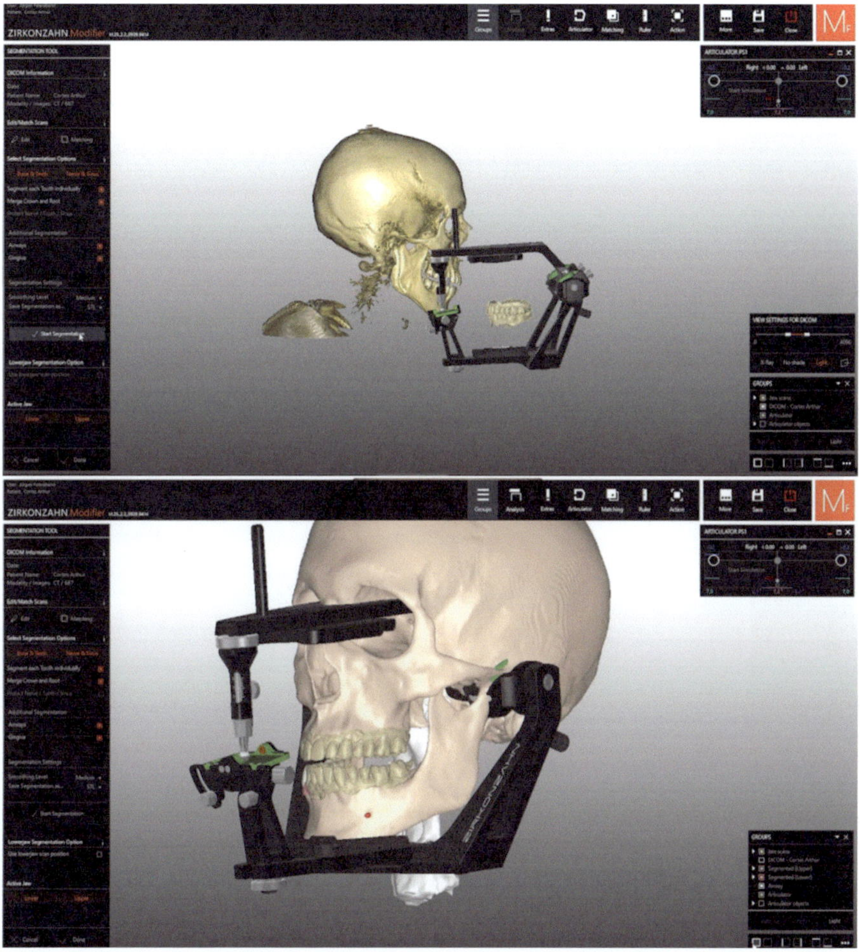

Fig. 7.8 Screenshot of the Zirkonzahn Modifier software before (top) and after (bottom) activation of the automated segmentation tool, aligning CBCT and articulated intraoral scans

gradual load transfer from the crown to the apex, improving the resistance to shear [14].

Finite element analysis and experimental studies consistently show that changes in these morphological parameters alter the stress distribution within dentin, periodontal ligament, and alveolar bone [20, 21]. Even subtle variations in root form or crown morphology can influence how forces are guided through periodontium complex, affecting micromobility, load sharing, and the risk of mechanical and biological failure [22–25].

Experimental in vivo data further underlines that natural teeth behave in a fundamentally different way from conventional osseointegrated implants. Because of the periodontal ligament, natural teeth exhibit pronounced creep, stress relaxation, and

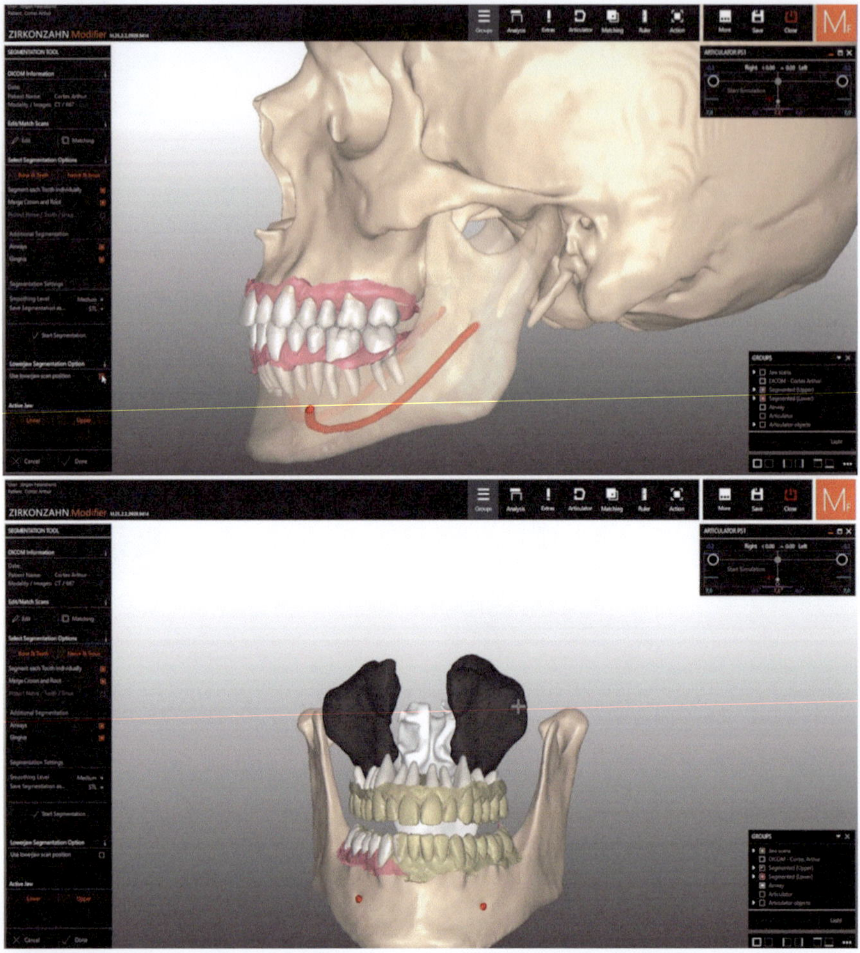

Fig. 7.9 Screenshot of the Zirkonzahn Modifier software showing segmented teeth and anatomical structures including the mandibular canal (red) and the maxillary sinuses (black). Every single tooth and structure can be exported as an individual STL file

hysteresis, dissipating approximately 50-fold more energy under axial loading than implants. This viscoelastic behavior contributes to shock absorption and controlled micromobility [26]. For individualized implant concepts, the goal is therefore not only to copy the outer form of the tooth but also to recreate a load transfer pattern and strain environment that are as physiological as possible.

Root-analogue dental implants represent one approach to restore the function and esthetics of missing teeth by mimicking the original root morphology as closely as possible. As individualized treatment solutions, they are designed to reproduce the patient's anatomy and thus approximate the biomechanical behavior of the natural tooth more closely than conventional standardized implants [27].

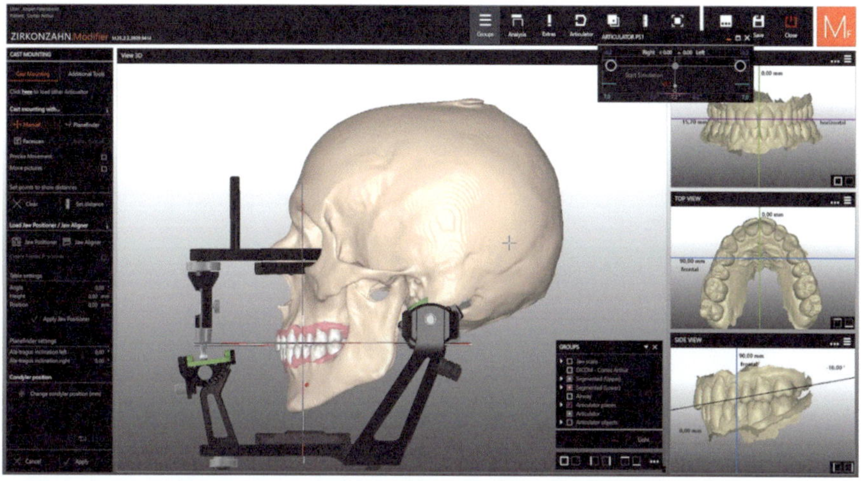

Fig. 7.10 Screenshot of the Zirkonzahn Modifier software using the virtual patient for adjustments and occlusal movement simulation. Note that the virtual articulator of Zirkonzahn uses the mastoid process as the fixed center of rotation, rather than the condyle head, along with other anatomical landmarks as reference points. The rationale for this choice is based on the fact that the mastoid process is always in a fixed position in all the patients

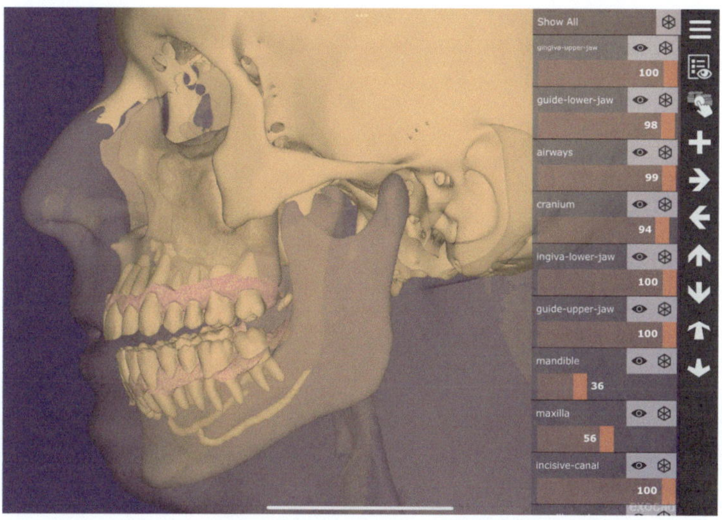

Fig. 7.11 STL files from the AI segmentation of the previous figures, imported into the Exocad viewer for iPad (Apple), providing general visualization of the virtual patient. Note the list of STL files and their respective visualization contrast on the column at the right side

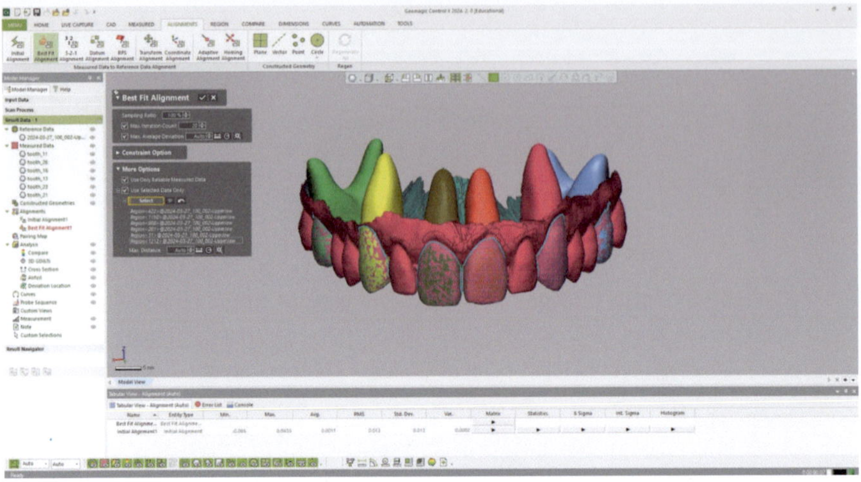

Fig. 7.12 Comparison between STL meshes from the AI segmentation of several teeth and the respective intraoral scan with the Geomagic Control X software. Note the outcome columns below. One of the variables displayed is the RMS (root mean square), which is a statistical measure used to quantify the average magnitude of the geometric deviation or distance between two meshes or a mesh and a desired reference surface

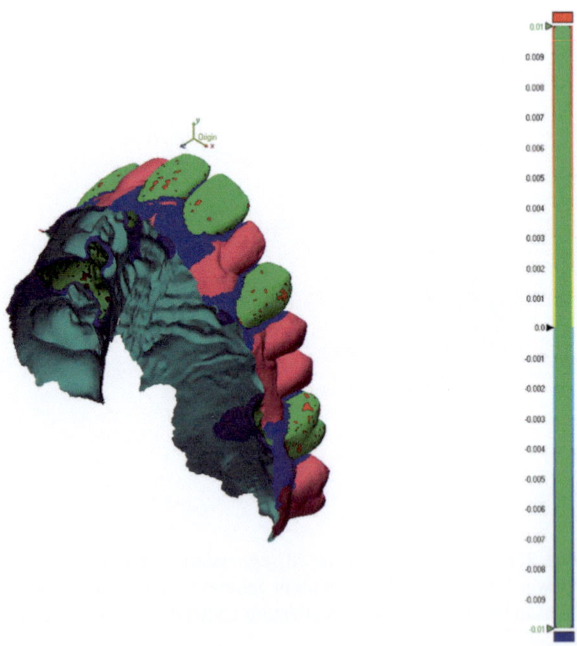

Fig. 7.13 Color map of the comparison between STL meshes from the AI segmentation of maxillary central incisors, canines and first molars, and the respective intraoral scan with the best-fit algorithm of the Geomagic Control X software. Note that green color depicts deviations close to zero, which generally indicates satisfactory accuracy of the scans

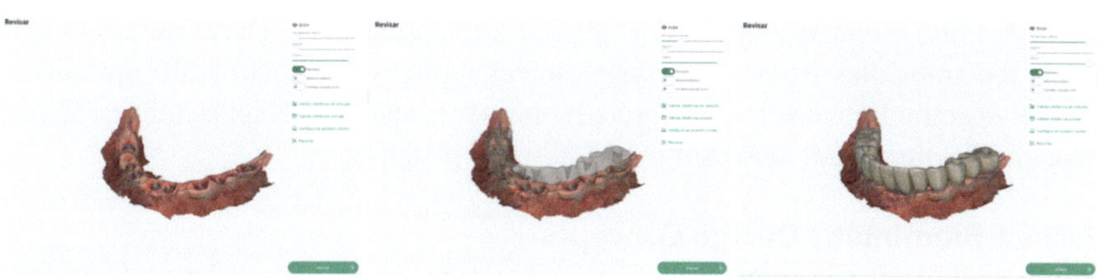

Fig. 7.14 Intraoral scans automatically optimized and aligned with teeth shapes on the software of the SIRIOS intraoral scanner (Straumann). (Courtesy of Dr. Alan Costa)

Historically, the idea of replacing teeth with root-shaped structures is not new. Archaeological findings, such as mandibular fragments with mussel shells shaped like a tooth, demonstrate early attempts to restore lost teeth by inserting artificial (xenogenic) teeth into the jawbone [28]. Although these treatments were far from today's concepts of osseointegration, they illustrate the intention to copy tooth morphology rather than the use of generic shapes.

The modern scientific history of RAIs starts in 1969, when Hodosh and coworkers introduced the dental polymer implant concept. Custom-made polymethylmethacrylate (PMMA) with or without particles of freeze-dried bovine bone were fabricated after extraction using a transfer technique that copied the anatomical shape. Because healing resulted mainly in connective tissue encapsulation instead of bone contact, the concept was abandoned [29].

In the early 1990s, the concept was revived with titanium as a more suitable implant material. Lundgren and collaborators placed machined root-analogue titanium implants in extraction sockets of beagle dogs and reported high rates of osseointegration [30]. Shortly afterward, Kohal and colleagues developed CAD/CAM fabricated root-analogue titanium implants for monkeys [31], and Strub and collaborators introduced the Re-Implant System [32]. Despite excellent primary stability, a considerable number of implants failed early, mainly due to limitations in imaging accuracy, manufacturing precision, and surface design [33].

With the help of high-resolution CBCT, digital workflows, and improved ceramic and titanium processing, a second wave of RAI concepts emerged in the 2000s and 2010s. These include custom-made zirconia RAIs with differentiated surface design, direct laser metal sintering (DLMS) of titanium RAIs, and fully digital CAD/CAM systems such as the Replicate System and other commercial solutions [34–38]. All of these designs are one-piece implants fabricated either after extraction from the tooth or socket replica or pre-extraction from CBCT data and inserted with a tapping technique [39]. A small number of two-piece or two-stage systems have been proposed to combine anatomic root fit with prosthetic flexibility, continuing the development from the early titanium systems to current concepts [40].

More recently, additive manufacturing has enabled RAIs with porous and biomimetic macro- and microgeometries, including triply periodic minimal surface structures and graded lattices. Examples include porous one-piece mandibular molar RAIs and additively manufactured root-analogue designs specifically optimized through finite element analysis and digital simulation [41]. These developments mark the transition from simple anatomical replicas to functionally optimized, patient-specific implants that integrate biomimetic design principles, advanced surface architectures and, increasingly, AI-assisted planning.

7.7.4.2 Biomimetic Design Concepts

Biomimetic design in implant dentistry aims to translate the mechanical and biological logic of the natural tooth-periodontium complex into artificial structures. This involves not only copying overall root and crown shape but engineering the internal architecture and surface morphology across multiple length scales. On the macro level, root and crown geometry define load paths and occlusal function; on the micro level, porous architectures and graded materials modulate stiffness and tissue ingrowth; on the nano level, surface chemistry and topography influence protein adsorption, cell adhesion, and early bone formation. At the same time, biomimetics are not restricted to dental anatomy alone: principles derived from other biological systems such as bone, shells, wood, or plant stems can be similarly applied to the macro-, micro-, and nano-design of individualized implants [42, 43].

For patient-specific individualized implants, the root surface is not only a mechanical interface but also a biological and informational interface. Its macro-, micro-, and nano-geometry determines how forces are transmitted into the surrounding bone and how cells attach, migrate, and differentiate at the implant-tissue interface [44].

Organized porous architectures such as gyroid lattices and other triply periodic minimal surface (TPMS) structures offer a highly interconnected pore network with a large internal surface area. Their continuous curvature avoids sharp edges and local stress peaks, while the pore size and porosity can be tuned to fall within ranges known to support osteoconduction and vascularization [45]. On the cellular level, such curved, interconnected geometries guide osteoblast and osteocyte orientation, facilitate nutrient and oxygen diffusion, and provide protected niches for new bone formation [46].

Experimental and finite element analysis studies on porous custom-made root-analogue implants underline this biological potential. In Ti6Al4V RAIs with an interconnected porous surface (porosity $\approx$ 80%, pore size $\approx$ 550 μm), the elastic modulus of the implant is substantially reduced compared with dense titanium, while compressive strength remains sufficient for clinical loading. The surrounding bone experiences a more homogeneous stress distribution with higher median but lower peak von Mises stresses than around conventional implants, and the resulting strain values fall within a range considered conducive to bone formation and remodeling. In vivo, these porous RAIs show faster and deeper bone ingrowth into the interconnected pore system and higher fixation strength than bulk implants, indicating a biologically more favorable and mechanically more stable anchorage [47–49].

From a biomimetic perspective, these findings suggest that an anatomically inspired root macro-shape, combined with gyroid-based or similar porous micro-architectures, appears to result in physiological load transfer to the bone, whereas stresses are sufficiently high to stimulate bone apposition and prevent disuse atrophy on the one hand but low enough to avoid overload and resorption on the other hand. At the same time, the 3D pore geometry actively shapes cell behavior by providing specific curvature, confinement, and connectivity conditions at the micro- and nanoscale.

Thus, root surface modification with organized porous structures is not merely a mechanical design feature, but a biological design tool. By tailoring cell-geometry interaction on the root surface, patient-specific individualized implants can approach a more physiological coupling between mechanical loading, cellular response, and long-term bone stability. Such complex geometries can be implemented using additive processes, whereas subtractive processes reach their limits.

7.7.4.3 Digital Workflow for Patient-Specific Individualized Implants

To design a two-piece root-analogue implant, a cloud-based configurator software was developed by the 3D-design software company trinckle 3D GmbH in cooperation with Charité-University Medicine Berlin and Technische Universität Berlin to embed medical and manufacturing expertise.

Similarly to conventional digital implant planning, planning a two-piece root-analogue implant requires a surface scan (STL file, e.g., from an intraoral scan, IOS) of the dental arch containing the tooth to be replaced by a root-analogue implant, as well as a DICOM file from a 3D radiographic image (CBCT or CT). These are required to perform segmentation of the anatomical structures (teeth, gingiva, and jawbone) in a first step. This can be done by activating the main button (1) on the left side of the homepage of the cloud-based planning software (Fig. 7.15a).

The user will then be directed to the menu shown in Fig. 7.15b where you can upload the DICOM dataset and the STL file of the respective jaw. The software is designed so that no patient data are stored in the cloud in order to comply with data protection regulations.

When the lower "SUBMIT" button is clicked, AI-based segmentation (Relu® Engine, Relu BV, Leuven Belgium) of the anatomical structures is performed automatically. A folder is then downloaded containing the STL files of the teeth, jawbone, and gingiva. These can then be uploaded in the corresponding menu shown in Fig. 7.15c by clicking the main button (2) on the right side of the homepage in Fig. 1a, namely, the tooth to be replaced and the surrounding jawbone ("mandible/maxilla") with gingiva. After clicking the "SUBMIT" button below, you are taken to the implant planning menu (Fig. 7.15d).

Using the buttons along the left side of the interface ((1)–(9)), the two-piece root-analogue (bone-level) implant can then be planned as described below.

First, two split planes must be defined—one to define the implant shoulder and a second to define the crown base. To do this, click on button (4) ("Split model")—Ih opens the "Split Model" menu and hides the gingiva model. The jawbone model is now visible to help orient the implant shoulder at the level of the alveolar ridge. This is done by clicking the "Define Split Plane" button under "JAW-LEVEL SPLIT." A point can then be placed on the root surface at the desired level (arrow, Fig. 7.15e). The "Define Split Plane" button now becomes "Split Model" and must be clicked again. The gingiva model then reappears, enabling orientation for the crown base.

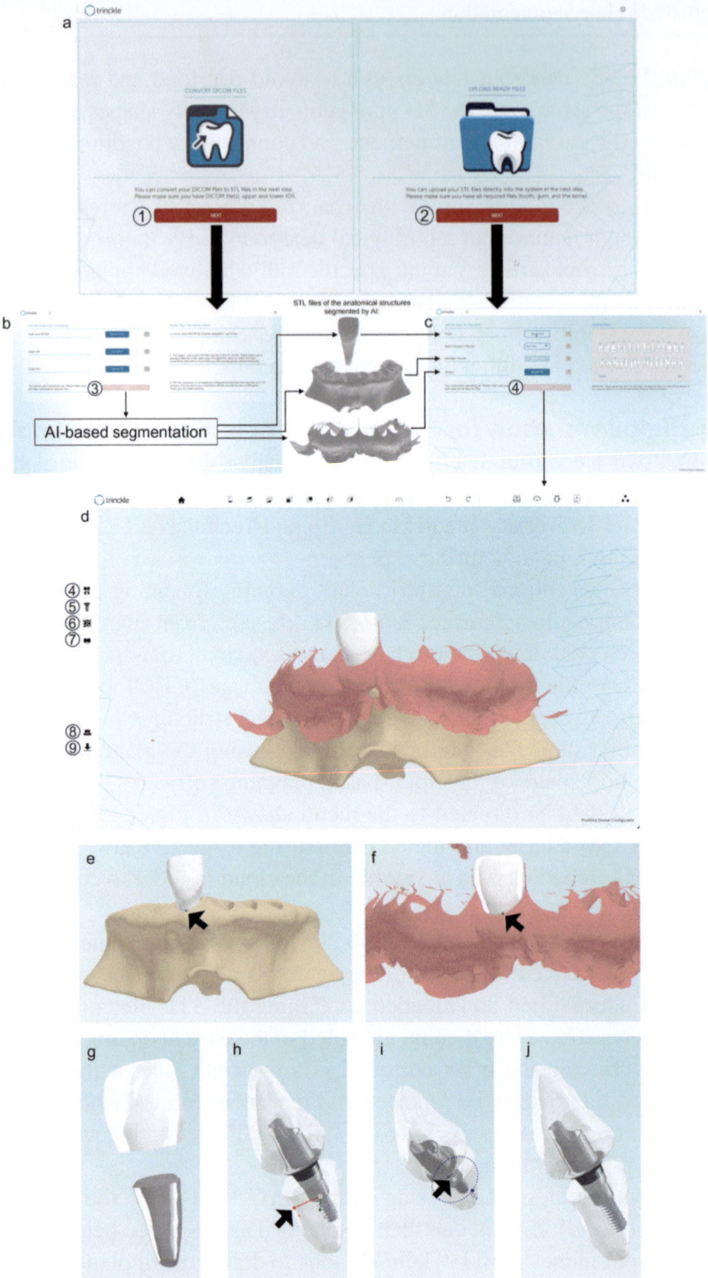

Fig. 7.15 Step-by-step workflow in the cloud-based planning software for generating a two-piece root-analogue implant, beginning with the homepage, where the menu on the left performs AI-based automatic segmentation of anatomical structures based on the uploaded patient files (DICOM from CBCT/CT scan and STL from IOS). The resulting STL datasets of teeth, bone, and gingiva are automatically downloaded into a folder called "outputs." These can then be uploaded in menu I, opened by clicking button (2) on the right side of the homepage, to design the root-analogue implant from a selected tooth. Figure 7.15j shows the final positioning of a commercial abutment (iSy Titanium Base CAD/CAM free, Crown (item number: P2247.4510), CAMLOG Biotechnologies GmbH, Basel, Switzerland)

Under "GUM-LEVEL SPLIT," a second "Define Split Plane" button must be clicked. Ir point can then be placed on the crown surface at the desired section level (arrow, Fig. 7.15f). The section planes are automatically aligned perpendicular to the long-axis of the tooth defined by the software (Fig. 7.15g). A bevel in the form of a slight "reverse taper" is automatically added to the implant shoulder—Ih is intended to be overgrown by peri-implant bone. By clicking button (5) ("Insert abutment") in Fig. 7.15d, the menu for integrating a commercial abutment opens. Clicking the button "Select Abutment Type" opens an integrated library containing commercial abutments.

On the one hand, this offers the possibility of selecting an abutment that is better suited to the implant. On the other hand, the openness of the system ensures that users can continue to use their standard system-dependent instruments. After selecting the desired abutment, it is inserted into the implant together with the abutment screw (Fig. 7.15h). If the abutment intersects the outer surface of the root-analogue implant and the crown, an error message appears. The abutment can be optimally positioned (arrow, Fig. 7.15h) and rotated (arrow, Fig. 7.15i), until the abutment is ideally aligned with both the root-analogue implant and the crown (Fig. 7.15j). Figure 7.16 shows examples of implant designs using two other commercial abutment types.

After positioning the abutment, the "Cutout" button must be clicked, causing the abutment to disappear and the crown and implant to receive its negative form.

Next, button (6) ("Adjust surface layer") in Fig. 7.15d is activated to introduce pores into the implant surface to increase surface area. These pores can be adjusted with respect to their radius, depth, and density.

Clicking the lower "Add Pores" button adds them to the implant surface (Fig. 7.17a). Clicking button (7) ("Process crown") in Fig. 7.15d opens the menu for modifying the screw channel. The user can select between a straight ("Straight") or angled ("Angled") screw channel under "Add screw axis insertion type" (Fig. 7.17b, c).

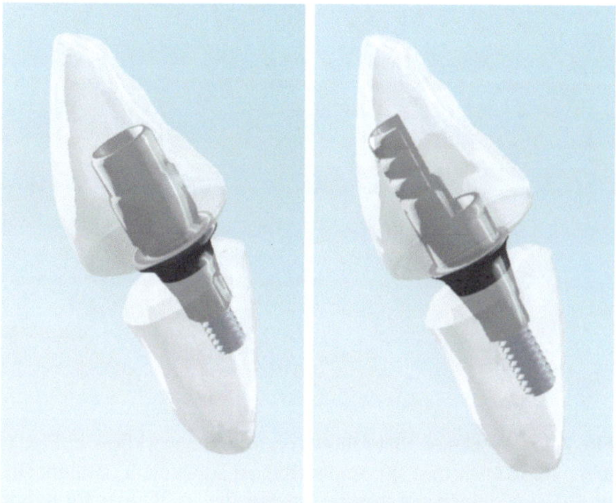

Fig. 7.16 Examples of root-analogue implant designs combined with two different commercial abutments (copaSKY uni. fit titanium base (item number: COPAUTB2), bredent medical GmbH & Co. KG, Senden, Germany, left; Medentika ASC Flex 2-09-19-SF 3.5 RI GH1.2, Medentika GmbH, Hügelsheim, Germany, right)

The lower "Cutout" button must be clicked to finalize the 3D files of the crown and the root-analogue implant.

In the menu opened with button (8) ("Add support") in Fig. 7.15d, clicking "Add marker" allows placement of an orientation marker, e.g., on the buccal side of the implant shoulder, so that the user can recognize the orientation of the implant during implant insertion.

To prepare for subtractive post-processing, which is necessary for optimal fit between the commercial abutment and implant after additive manufacturing, a fixation support must be added by clicking "Add support."

Finally, under the menu opened with button (9) ("Download models") in Fig. 7.15d, all STL and STEP files required for both additive and subtractive manufacturing can be downloaded. Data is provided for three models that differ slightly in size. This allows the users to have all three implant models manufactured so that, if necessary, they can switch to an alternative size during surgery. The 3D data is coordinated in such a way that the additive and subtractive processes are aligned for the simplest possible production.

Figure 7.18 shows a complete assembly of a two-piece RAI with a screw-retained crown of hybrid ceramic (VarseoSmile Crown plus, BEGO GmbH & Co. KG, Bremen, Germany) on a titanium base abutment (iSy Titanium Base CAD/CAM free, Crown (item number: P2247.4510), CAMLOG Biotechnologies GmbH, Basel, Switzerland) after hybrid manufacturing of the implant, which was first manufactured additively via powder bed fusion of metals using a laser beam (PBF-LB/M) from titanium grade II and subsequently subtractively finished to create the implant-abutment interface.

The surface pores of the implant shown are only slightly pronounced and therefore almost invisible. In any case, as mentioned above, this manufacturing technique offers the possibility of designing the surface layers of the implant from complex (lattice) structures, which will be further investigated in the future.

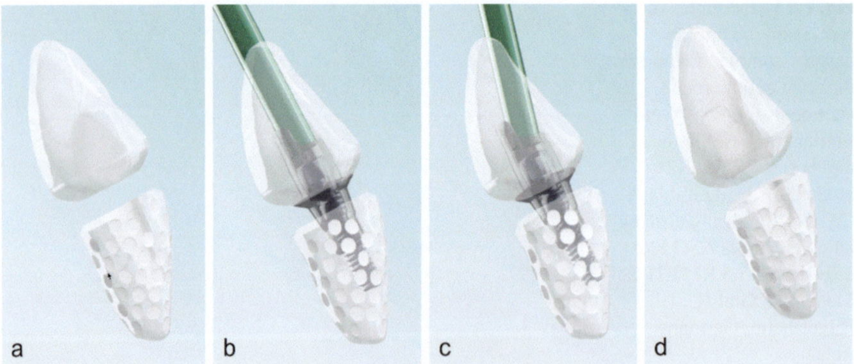

Fig. 7.17 Workflow that follows on from the workflow in Fig. 1 showing the application of pores to the implant surface (**a**); screw channel adjustment (straight (**b**) vs. angled (**c**)); and the resulting final design, which can then be downloaded as 3D files for hybrid manufacturing (**d**)

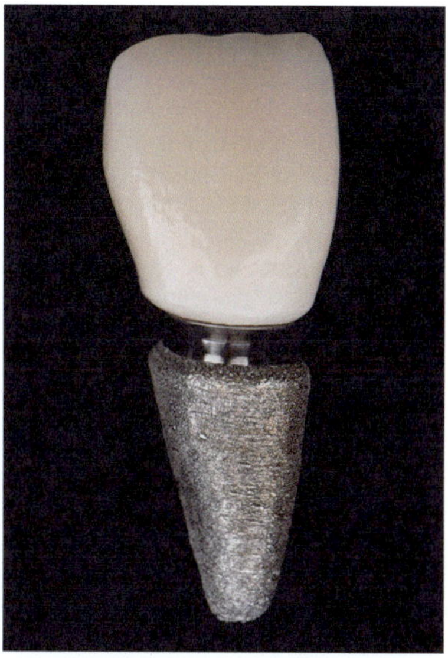

Fig. 7.18 Final implant-abutment-crown complex

7.7.4.4 Acknowledgments

The publication of this technique is based on results obtained within a project funded by the Program for the Promotion of Research, Innovation, and Technology (Pro FIT) by the State of Berlin and by the European Union (ERDF).

References

1. Ayres AP, Correa DS, de Moura e Costa AJ, Pradíes G, Cortes ARG. The use of artificial intelligence to create a virtual patient for oral and maxillofacial surgical planning. SciLet. 2024;1(1):6. https://doi.org/10.48797/sl.2024.124.
2. Iacob AM, Verdecchia A, García-Mesa Y, Spinas E, Cobo T. Effectiveness of automated segmentation of maxillofacial structures in cone-beam computed tomography images using artificial intelligence: a systematic review. Int Orthod. 2026;24:101081.
3. Cortes ARG. Digital dentistry: a step-by-step guide and case atlas. Hoboken, NJ: Wiley; 2022. https://doi.org/10.1002/9781119852025.
4. Han JY, Yang S, Kim S, Kim S, Lim SH, Yun H, Kim D. Semi-supervised deformation-free image-to-image translation for realistic CT synthesis from CBCT. In: Gee JC, et al., editors. Medical image computing and computer assisted intervention—MICCAI 2025. MICCAI 2025, Lecture notes in computer science, vol. 15962. Cham: Springer; 2026. https://doi.org/10.1007/978-3-032-04947-6_55.
5. Ntovas P, Sirirattanagool P, Asavanamuang P, Jain S, Tavelli L, Revilla-León M, Galarraga-Vinueza ME. Accuracy and time efficiency of artificial intelligence-driven tooth segmentation on CBCT images: a validation study using two implant planning software programs. Clin Oral Implants Res. 2025;36(10):1312–23. https://doi.org/10.1111/clr.70003.
6. Xiang B, Lu J, Yu J. Evaluating tooth segmentation accuracy and time efficiency in CBCT images using artificial intelligence: a systematic review and Meta-analysis. J Dent. 2024;146:105064.
7. Lahoud P, EzEldeen M, Beznik T, et al. Artificial intelligence for fast and accurate 3-dimensional tooth segmentation on cone-beam computed tomography. J Endodont. 2021;47(5):827–35.

8. Elgarba BM, Ali S, Fontenele RC, Meeus J, Jacobs R. An AI-based tool for prosthetic crown segmentation serving automated intraoral scan-to-CBCT registration in challenging high artifact scenarios. J Prosthet Dent. 2025;134:191–8.
9. Raith S, Pankert T, Jaganathan S, et al. Segmenting beyond the imaging data: creation of anatomically valid edentulous mandibular geometries for surgical planning using artificial intelligence. Clin Oral Investig. 2025;29:501.
10. Aung MTZ, Lim SH, Han J, et al. Deep learning-based automatic segmentation of the mandibular canal on panoramic radiographs: a multi-device study. Imaging Sci Dent. 2024;54(1):81–91.
11. Shaheen E, Khalil W, Ezeldeen M, et al. Accuracy of segmentation of tooth structures using 3 different CBCT machines. Oral Surg Oral Med Oral Pathol Oral Radiol. 2017;123(1):123–8.
12. Lawand G, Gonzaga L, Issa J, Revilla-Leon M, Tohme H, Saleh A, Martin W. Artificial intelligence segmentation errors in implant planning software programs: an overview. Clin Implant Dent Relat Res. 2025;27(5):e70095. https://doi.org/10.1111/cid.70095.
13. Santos MS, Silva JC, Carvalho MS. Hierarchical biomaterial scaffolds for periodontal tissue engineering: recent progress and current challenges. Int J Mol Sci. 2024;25(16):8562. https://www.mdpi.com/1422-0067/25/16/8562.
14. Abdelfattah RA, Nawar NN, Kataia EM, Saber SM. How loss of tooth structure impacts the biomechanical behavior of a single-rooted maxillary premolar: FEA. Odontology. 2024;112(1):279–86. https://doi.org/10.1007/s10266-023-00829-6.
15. Dorado S, Arias A, Jimenez-Octavio JR. Biomechanical modelling for tooth survival studies: mechanical properties, loads and boundary conditions—a narrative review. Materials (Basel). 2022;15(21). https://doi.org/10.3390/ma15217852.
16. Nikolaus A, Currey JD, Lindtner T, Fleck C, Zaslansky P. Importance of the variable periodontal ligament geometry for whole tooth mechanical function: a validated numerical study. J Mech Behav Biomed Mater. 2017;67:61–73. https://doi.org/10.1016/j.jmbbm.2016.11.020.
17. Flatten J, Gedrange T, Bourauel C, Keilig L, Konermann A. The role of bone and root resorption on the biomechanical behavior of mandibular anterior teeth subjected to orthodontic forces: a finite element approach. Biomedicine. 2024;12(9):1959. https://www.mdpi.com/2227-9059/12/9/1959.
18. Kırmalı Ö, Türker N, Akar T, Yılmaz B. Finite element analysis of stress distribution in autotransplanted molars. J Dent. 2022;119:104082. https://doi.org/10.1016/j.jdent.2022.104082.
19. Soares PV, Souza LV, Veríssimo C, Zeola LF, Pereira AG, Santos-Filho PCF, Fernandes-Neto AJ. Effect of root morphology on biomechanical behaviour of premolars associated with abfraction lesions and different loading types. J Oral Rehabil. 2014;41(2):108–14. https://doi.org/10.1111/joor.12113.
20. Baghani Z, Soheilifard R, Baghani Z. How does the first molar root location affect the critical stress pattern in the periodontium? A finite element analysis. J Dent. 2023;24(2):182–93. https://doi.org/10.30476/dentjods.2022.93271.1704.
21. Magne P, Versluis A, Douglas WH. Rationalization of incisor shape: experimental-numerical analysis. J Prosthet Dent. 1999;81(3):345–55. https://doi.org/10.1016/s0022-3913(99)70279-9.
22. Agrawal R, Narang S, Ahmed H, Prasad S, Reddy S, Aila S. Influence of occlusal bite forces on teeth with altered periodontal support: a three-dimensional finite element stress analysis. J Pharm Bioallied Sci. 2021;13(Suppl 1):S688–91. https://doi.org/10.4103/jpbs.JPBS_785_20.
23. Choy K, Pae E-K, Park Y, Kim K-H, Burstone CJ. Effect of root and bone morphology on the stress distribution in the periodontal ligament. Am J Orthod Dentofacial Orthop. 2000;117(1):98–105. https://doi.org/10.1016/S0889-5406(00)70254-X.
24. Heravi F, Salari S, Tanbakuchi B, Loh S, Amiri M. Effects of crown-root angle on stress distribution in the maxillary central incisors' PDL during application of intrusive and retraction forces: a three-dimensional finite element analysis. Prog Orthod. 2013;14(1):26. https://doi.org/10.1186/2196-1042-14-26.
25. Oyama K, Motoyoshi M, Hirabayashi M, Hosoi K, Shimizu N. Effects of root morphology on stress distribution at the root apex. Eur J Orthod. 2007;29(2):113–7. https://doi.org/10.1093/ejo/cjl043.

26. Chang HH, Yeh CL, Wang YL, Huang YC, Tsai SJ, Li YT, Yang JH, Lin CP. Differences in the biomechanical behaviors of natural teeth and dental implants. Dent Mater. 2021;37(4):682–9. https://doi.org/10.1016/j.dental.2021.01.003.
27. Wood-Bailey AP, Smith C, Fitton LC, Sharp AC. Biomechanical impact of tooth root morphology to inform dental implant design. Arch Oral Biol. 2026;181:106455. https://doi.org/10.1016/j.archoralbio.2025.106455.
28. Pasqualini U, Pasqualini ME. In treatise of implant dentistry: the Italian tribute to modern implantology. Ariesdue © copyright 2009 Azienda Pubblica di Servizi alla Persona "Suor Agnese"; 2009.
29. Hodosh M, Povar M, Shklar G. The dental polymer implant concept. J Prosthet Dent. 1969;22(3):371–80. https://doi.org/10.1016/0022-3913(69)90200-5.
30. Lundgren D, Rylander H, Anderssong M, Johansson C, Albrektsson T. Healing-in of root analogue titanium implants placed in extraction sockets. An experimental study in the beagle dog. Clin Oral Implants Res. 1992;3(3):136–44. https://doi.org/10.1034/j.1600-0501.1992.030306.x.
31. Kohal R-J, Hürzeler MB, Mota LF, Klaus G, Caffesse RG, Strub JR. Custom-made root analogue titanium implants placed into extraction sockets. An experimental study in monkeys. Clin Oral Implants Res. 1997;8(5):386–92. https://doi.org/10.1034/j.1600-0501.1997.080505.x.
32. Strub JR, Kohal RJ, Klaus G, Ferraresso F. The Re implant system for immediate implant placement. J Esthet Dent. 1997;9(4):187–96. https://doi.org/10.1111/j.1708-8240.1997.tb00940.x.
33. Dantas T, Rodrigues F, Araujo J, Vaz P, Silva F. Customized root-analogue dental implants—procedure and errors associated with image acquisition, treatment, and manufacturing technology in an experimental study on a cadaver dog mandible. J Mech Behav Biomed Mater. 2022;133:105350. https://doi.org/10.1016/j.jmbbm.2022.105350.
34. Anssari Moin D, Hassan B, Wismeijer D. A novel approach for custom three-dimensional printing of a zirconia root analogue implant by digital light processing. Clin Oral Implants Res. 2017;28(6):668–70. https://doi.org/10.1111/clr.12859.
35. Bose MWH, Hildebrand D, Beuer F, Wesemann C, Schwerdtner P, Pieralli S, Spies BC. Clinical outcomes of root-analogue implants restored with single crowns or fixed dental prostheses: a retrospective case series. J Clin Med. 2020;9(8). https://doi.org/10.3390/jcm9082346.
36. Figliuzzi M, Giudice A, Rengo C, Fortunato L. A direct metal laser sintering (DMLS) root analogue implant placed in the anterior maxilla. Case report. Ann Ital Chir. 8:2019.
37. Moin DA, Hassan B, Mercelis P, Wismeijer D. Designing a novel dental root analogue implant using cone beam computed tomography and CAD/CAM technology. Clin Oral Implants Res. 2013;24:25–7. https://doi.org/10.1111/j.1600-0501.2011.02359.x.
38. Sokolowski AA, Sokolowski AA, Kammerhofer J, Madreiter-Sokolowski CT, Payer M, Koller M, Jakse N, Wegscheider WA. Accuracy assessment of 3D-printed tooth replicas. Int J Comput Dent. 2019;22(4):321–9.
39. Saeidi Pour R, Freitas Rafael C, Engler M, Edelhoff D, Klaus G, Prandtner O, Berthold M, Liebermann A. Historical development of root analogue implants: a review of published papers. Br J Oral Maxillofac Surg. 2019;57(6):496–504. https://doi.org/10.1016/j.bjoms.2019.01.021.
40. Yu X, Feng B, Lan Y, Li J, Ye G, Li Q, Zhao F, Gu Y, You D, Zhu Y, Yu M, Wang H, Yang H. A 2-stage root analog implant with compact structure, uniform roughness, and high accuracy. J Dent Res. 2023;102(6):636–44. https://doi.org/10.1177/00220345231160670.
41. Liu T, Chen Y, Apicella A, Mu Z, Yu T, Huang Y, Wang C. Effect of porous microstructures on the biomechanical characteristics of a root analogue implant: an animal study and a finite element analysis. ACS Biomater Sci Eng. 2020;6(11):6356–67. https://doi.org/10.1021/acsbiomaterials.0c01096.
42. Jaggessar A, Shahali H, Mathew A, Yarlagadda PKDV. Bio-mimicking nano and micro-structured surface fabrication for antibacterial properties in medical implants. J Nanobiotechnol. 2017;15(1):64. https://doi.org/10.1186/s12951-017-0306-1.

43. Lackington WA, Bellon B, Guimond S, Schweizer P, Cancellieri C, Ambeza A, Chopard-Lallier A-L, Pippenger B, Armutlulu A, Maeder X, Schmutz P, Rottmar M. Bio-inspired micro- and nano-scale surface features produced by Femtosecond Laser-Texturing Enhance TiZr-Implant Osseointegration. Adv Healthc Mater. 2024;13(23):2400810. https://doi.org/10.1002/adhm.202400810.
44. Zhang Y, Li S, Lin Y, Di P, Liu Y. Macro to micro: surface modification of titanium dental implants. In: Gulati K, editor. Surface modification of titanium dental implants. Springer International Publishing; 2023. p. 61–82. https://doi.org/10.1007/978-3-031-21565-0_3.
45. Alemayehu DB, Todoh M, Huang S-J. Hybrid biomechanical design of dental implants: integrating solid and gyroid triply periodic minimal surface lattice architectures for optimized stress distribution. J Funct Biomater. 2025;16(2):54. https://www.mdpi.com/2079-4983/16/2/54.
46. Jíra A, Šejnoha M, Krejčí T, Vorel J, Řehounek L, Marseglia G. Mechanical properties of porous structures for dental implants: experimental study and computational homogenization. Materials. 2021;14(16):4592. https://doi.org/10.3390/ma14164592.
47. Li L, Lee J, Amara HB, Lee JB, Lee KS, Shin SW, Lee YM, Kim B, Kim P, Koo KT. Comparison of 3D-printed dental implants with threaded implants for osseointegration: an experimental pilot study. Materials (Basel). 2020;13(21). https://doi.org/10.3390/ma13214815.
48. Liu C, Huang S, Guo F, Li Y, Zhao B, Luo A, Liu H, Wang C, Hu M, Zhou H. Immediate, non-submerged, three-dimensionally printed, one-piece mandibular molar porous root-analogue titanium implants: a 2-year prospective study involving 18 patients. J Stomatol Oral Maxillofac Surg. 2022;123(6):e770–6. https://doi.org/10.1016/j.jormas.2022.05.019.
49. Yang E, Leary M, Lozanovski B, Downing D, Mazur M, Sarker A, Khorasani A, Jones A, Maconachie T, Bateman S, Easton M, Qian M, Choong P, Brandt M. Effect of geometry on the mechanical properties of Ti-6Al-4V Gyroid structures fabricated via SLM: a numerical study. Mater Des. 2019;184:108165. https://doi.org/10.1016/j.matdes.2019.108165.

Artificial Intelligence in Orthodontics

8

Adriana Bartolo, Juliana No-Cortes, Adam Bartolo, and Arthur Rodriguez Gonzalez Cortes

8.1 AI in Class II Malocclusion Treatment Planning

The treatment of Class II malocclusion represents a significant strategic challenge in orthodontics, involving complex decisions that weigh the benefits of growth modulation in younger patients against camouflage or surgical interventions in adults. The selection of the optimal pathway is critical for achieving functional and aesthetic success. The application of AI in this domain aims to bring data-driven consistency and objective support to these pivotal decisions, reducing practitioner-dependent variability.

A comparative study has evaluated four distinct machine learning (ML) models to predict the most appropriate treatment pathway for Class II malocclusion [1]. The random forest (RF) and support vector machine (SVM) models demonstrated superior and identical performance, significantly outperforming the logistic regression (LR) and decision tree (DT) models. The performance of these models, measured by the area under the precision-recall curve (AUC-PR), reveals significant differences in their predictive capabilities.

Analysis of the highest-performing models (RF and SVM) identified a consistent set of clinical and demographic features that were most influential in predicting treatment pathways. These features underscore the importance of specific skeletal, soft tissue, and patient-specific indicators in expert decision-making.

A. Bartolo
BroadStreet Dental Centre, Hamrun, Malta
e-mail: adriana@broadstreet.com.mt

J. No-Cortes · A. Bartolo · A. R. G. Cortes (✉)
Faculty of Dental Surgery, University of Malta, Msida, Malta
e-mail: adam.bartolo@um.edu.mt; arthur.nogueira@um.edu.mt

A. R. G. Cortes (ed.), *Dental Clinical Procedures using Artificial Intelligence*,
https://doi.org/10.1007/978-3-032-24895-4_8

- ANB angle: This skeletal measurement, which indicates the anteroposterior relationship of the maxilla and mandible, was a consistently strong predictor across models.
- SNA angle: Reflecting the position of the maxilla relative to the cranial base, this feature was crucial for distinguishing between skeletal discrepancies.
- Nasolabial angle: As a key soft tissue metric, this angle helps assess the harmony of the upper lip and nose, influencing aesthetic considerations in treatment planning.
- H angle (holdaway): This soft tissue feature, which assesses lip-to-face harmony, proved to be a decisive/important factor in predicting treatment pathways.
- Age: This demographic feature was highly predictive, particularly for identifying candidates for growth modulation, which is most effective in growing patients.

The high accuracy of the RF and SVM models suggests significant clinical utility as decision-support systems. By training on a dataset of treatment plans established by the consensus of a panel of orthodontists with over two decades of experience, these AI systems can function as a reliable "second opinion." This capability helps to guide practitioners—particularly those with less experience—toward decisions that reflect an expert-level standard of care, thereby enhancing diagnostic consistency and standardizing treatment approaches for complex Class II cases. Building upon the classification of malocclusion, another fundamental decision point in orthodontics is whether to proceed with tooth extraction, a domain where AI is also being actively investigated.

8.2 AI in Orthodontic Extraction Decision-Making

The decision to extract teeth is one of the most consequential in orthodontic treatment planning, fundamentally influencing the patient's facial profile, occlusal stability, and overall treatment outcome. This choice involves a complex interplay of skeletal, dental, and soft tissue factors, and AI offers a promising avenue to standardize this process by learning from vast datasets of expert clinical judgments. A systematic review and meta-analysis evaluated the overall diagnostic accuracy of AI models in predicting the need for orthodontic extractions [2]. The analysis revealed promising, albeit variable, performance. The pooled results indicated a sensitivity of 70% (95% CI: 61–78) and a specificity of 90% (95% CI: 87–92).

This marked difference suggests that current AI models are more reliable at correctly identifying non-extraction cases (ruling out the need for extraction) than they are at consistently identifying cases that genuinely require extraction. The meta-analysis mentioned above found an extremely high level of statistical heterogeneity for both sensitivity (I^2 = 96.7%) and specificity (I^2 = 93.7%) [2]. This indicates significant variability in AI performance across the included studies, warranting a deeper analysis of the underlying model architectures and study designs.

To explore the sources of this heterogeneity, a subgroup analysis was performed based on the type of AI model used [2]. This analysis revealed that convolutional neural network (CNN)-based models demonstrated significantly superior and more consistent performance compared to other architectures. This highlights the strength of modern deep learning architectures. The CNN-based models (ResNet and VGG) not only achieved high sensitivity and specificity but also showed no statistical heterogeneity ($I^2 = 0.0\%$). This consistency suggests that these models are more robust and reliable for this specific diagnostic task. In contrast, random forest and neural network (MLP) models exhibited substantial heterogeneity, indicating that their performance is less predictable across different datasets and clinical scenarios.

The high heterogeneity observed in the overall meta-analysis can be attributed to several important factors that influence AI model performance, including the AI model type, training datasets, and population characteristics [2]. Understanding these variables is essential for the development and validation of future clinical AI tools. As demonstrated in the subgroup analysis, the choice of model architecture is suggested to be a primary driver of performance consistency. Advanced architectures such as CNNs, which excel at feature extraction from images, appear better suited for orthodontic diagnostic tasks than traditional machine learning models. Moreover, the composition of the training data significantly impacts model behavior. Imbalances in datasets, such as a higher prevalence of extraction cases, can bias a model's predictions, leading to higher reported sensitivity but potentially lower generalizability to populations with different case distributions. Finally, variations in patient demographics across studies, including different age ranges, can influence model accuracy. An AI model trained on an adolescent population may not perform as well when applied to adult patients, and vice versa.

8.3 AI in Orthodontic Aligner (Invisalign) Treatment Planning

Orthodontic aligner therapy, exemplified by Invisalign, presents a unique set of challenges for treatment planning. The complexity of this modality is compounded by factors such as the biological response of teeth to aligning forces, the properties of aligner materials, slipping motions, and variability in patient compliance. Inaccuracies in planning can lead to extended treatment times, increased costs, and compromised results. AI and machine learning offer a powerful approach to enhance the predictability and personalization of these treatments by analyzing complex patient data to forecast outcomes.

A previous study evaluated four machine learning models for their ability to predict the success or failure of Invisalign treatment based on a comprehensive dataset of patient records [3]. The four AI models assessed were decision tree, random forest, artificial neural network (ANN), and the XGBoost model, which presented the best diagnostic performance (accuracy of 94.34%, sensitivity of 97.12%, and specificity of 90.36%), demonstrating superior accuracy in classifying treatment outcomes.

A significant barrier to the adoption of advanced AI models such as XGBoost and ANNs in clinical practice is their "black box" nature, in which the reasoning behind a prediction is not transparent. Explainable AI (XAI) is a field dedicated to addressing this challenge. Interpretability refers to the extent to which a human can understand the rationale behind a model's decision, while explainability concerns the transparency of the internal operations of a model.

A previous study has described the use of SHapley Additive exPlanations (SHAP) in orthodontics [3]. SHAP is a novel XAI method that deconstructs the output of a complex model, allowing clinicians to visualize the precise impact of each individual feature on a prediction. For example, a SHAP analysis can show exactly how much the "treatment time" or "number of aligners" contributed to a model's forecast of success or failure. This transparency is crucial for building clinical trust, supporting informed consent, and ensuring the ethical application of AI in patient care.

8.3.1 Important Predictors of Invisalign Outcomes

The SHAP analysis identified several important factors that significantly influence the success or failure of Invisalign treatment, such as treatment time, number of aligners and submission option. These data-driven insights can help clinicians optimize treatment plans and manage patient expectations.

Longer treatment times were negatively correlated with success, which the study suggests is reflective of more comprehensive cases and potential patient compliance issues. Furthermore, a higher number of aligners was positively associated with success, which may indicate well-planned and comprehensive treatment protocols. It is noteworthy that the "Teen" submission option had a positive impact on outcomes, an effect attributed to higher biological responsiveness and that accelerated tooth movement in younger patients. Finally, the "Scan" submission process showed a negative impact, a finding potentially linked to variability in operator training and quality control of digital scanning techniques.

While these specialized models provide deep, interpretable insights for specific clinical tasks, the field is also exploring the capabilities of general-purpose generative AI for broader diagnostic applications.

8.3.2 Clinical Case Study: Invisalign (Case by Dr. Juliana No-Cortes)

A 13-year-old male patient with no relevant medical conditions presented for orthodontic treatment. At the clinical examination, an asymmetric overbite with longer vertical overlapping distances at the left side was noted. A conventional impression with PVS (Aquasil, Dentsply-Sirona) was taken and sent to be digitalized. The resulting STL files were used in the ClinCheck Pro 6 cloud-based software (Align Technology) to plan the orthodontic treatment with Invisalign (Align technology). A 3D digital plan was performed mapping out how the resulting custom aligners would apply gentle and consistent orthodontic forces. The orthodontic strategy was generally to slightly intrude the maxillary central incisors and mandibular anterior teeth, with further small adjustments on the dental arches to correct asymmetry. Based on this plan, a series of clear orthodontic aligners (Invisalign) were fabricated to execute the treatment.

It is noteworthy that the dentist can always edit the treatment plan to modify tooth movements, add attachments, or adjust treatment approaches before confirming final approval. An AI tool of the software (ClinCheck In-Face Visualization) merges a 2D photograph of the face of the patient with the corresponding 3D Invisalign treatment plan to create a realistic simulation of their potential posttreatment smile (Fig. 8.1). The software interface also enables streamlining communication with dental technicians to ensure success of the treatment plan.

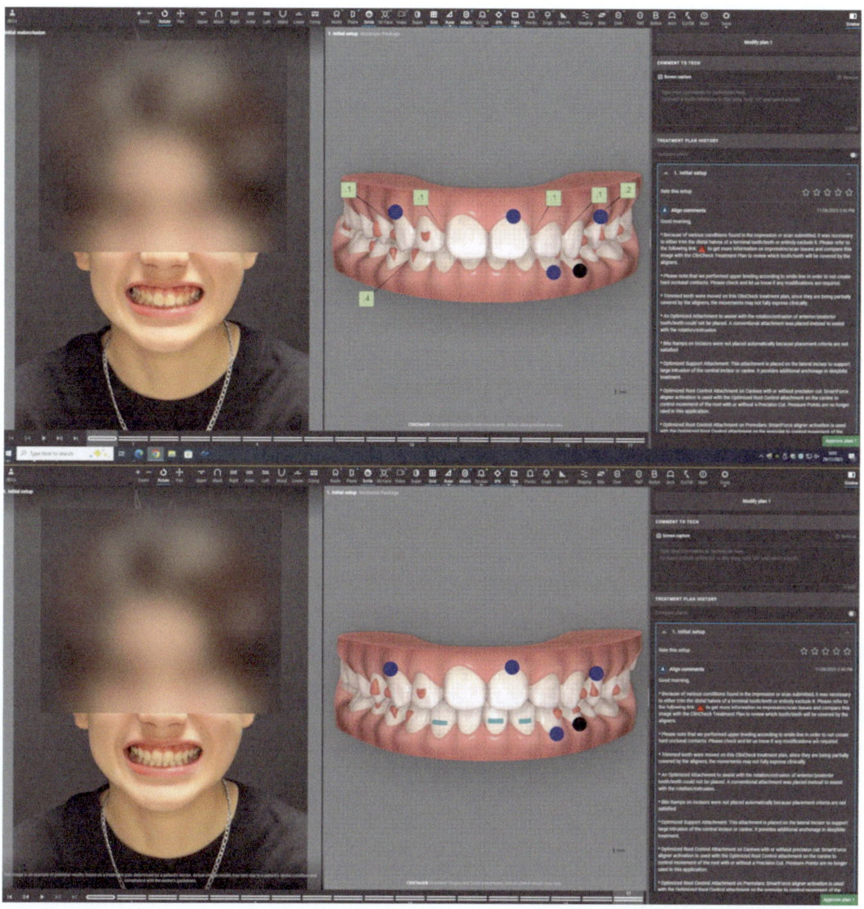

Fig. 8.1 AI-driven treatment plan designed with the ClinCheck software (Align Technology). Note the differences between the initial situation (top) and the predicted orthodontic outcome (bottom)

8.4 Generative AI for Dental Crowding Assessment

As discussed previously in this book, a new frontier in medical AI involves the application of generative multimodal large language models (MLLMs), such as ChatGPT and Microsoft Copilot. Unlike the specialized, task-specific models previously discussed, these are general-purpose AIs designed to process and generate humanlike text and interpret various data inputs, including images. Recent studies have begun to test their capabilities for visual diagnostic tasks in orthodontics, such as assessing the severity of dental crowding from intraoral photographs.

A study evaluated the performance of three commercial MLLMs in classifying dental crowding severity (mild, moderate, or severe) and identifying the dental arch (maxillary or mandibular) from 120 occlusal images [4]. The results revealed limited and inconsistent accuracy. The performance of these MLLMs was suboptimal when compared to the substantial agreement achieved by experienced human orthodontists, who reached a Cohen's kappa of 0.87 on the same task. This disparity underscores a critical paradox in the current state of generative AI for clinical use: Claude 3.5 Sonnet, the model with the best initial performance in crowding classification (50% accuracy), was also the most erratic upon reevaluation, demonstrating the lowest consistency (43% repeatability). This contradiction—where the most accurate model is also the least reliable—decisively proves that these general-purpose tools are not yet ready for clinical deployment in specific visual diagnostic tasks. The lack of specialized training and inherent variability in their outputs makes them unsuitable for applications where precision and consistency are paramount. The variable performance of these MLLMs transitions the discussion into a broader overview of the current status and future direction of AI in the field.

8.5 AI Orthodontic Reports by Dental Commercial Software Programs

AI algorithms have been applied to automate several diagnostic tasks related to orthodontic treatment planning and the respective reports, enhancing both speed and consistency. The primary areas of application include image indexing and archiving, maturation determination, diagnosis of occlusal traits, and upper airway assessment.

CNNs are used to automatically classify and sort shuffled clinical and radiological images (e.g., facial photos, intraoral photos, cephalograms) into their respective categories. One study demonstrated that this task could be completed with 99% accuracy in only 0.08 min, dramatically reducing the administrative burden on clinicians [5].

Furthermore, AI offers a highly efficient method for assessing cervical vertebrae maturation (CVM) from lateral cephalograms, a crucial step for determining the optimal timing for treatment. One AI model was able to produce a CVM staging assessment in under 0.1 s [6]. While the performance of these systems is nearly comparable to that of expert manual assessments, their reliability is not yet sufficient to be fully trusted without ongoing human validation [7].

It is also noteworthy that AI algorithms can provide a one-step diagnosis of dentoskeletal classifications directly from images such as lateral cephalometry, eliminating the need for time-consuming manual landmark detection and its associated errors. Studies have reported high accuracy rates, with one model achieving over 90% accuracy for diagnosing sagittal and vertical malocclusions [8].

Finally, the evaluation of the upper airway is critical in orthodontics, as conditions such as adenoid hypertrophy can influence craniofacial development and lead to malocclusion [9]. AI provides a rapid method for segmenting and evaluating these structures from CBCT images. A CNN-based model achieved a Dice similarity coefficient (DSC) of 97% for automatically segmenting the pharyngeal airway space, demonstrating high precision [10].

AI orthodontic reports from dental commercial AI software programs are an example of clinical application of the AI technologies described and discussed in the scientific literature. For this purpose, the AI software can automatically detect the patient's head orientation, reconstruct a synthetic lateral cephalogram, identify cephalometric landmarks, and produce automated tracings and measurements.

A CBCT-generated lateral cephalogram will normally show the teeth in the same occlusal relationship as they were during the CBCT scan, but this depends entirely on how the patient was positioned when the CBCT was taken. However, CBCT scans are often taken with the patient biting on a bite block or in a slightly open position. If the jaws are not fully intercuspated, the AI-generated cephalogram will not match a conventional lateral one taken in centric occlusion (Fig. 8.2). For orthodontic analysis, this can affect measurements involving overbite, overjet, and

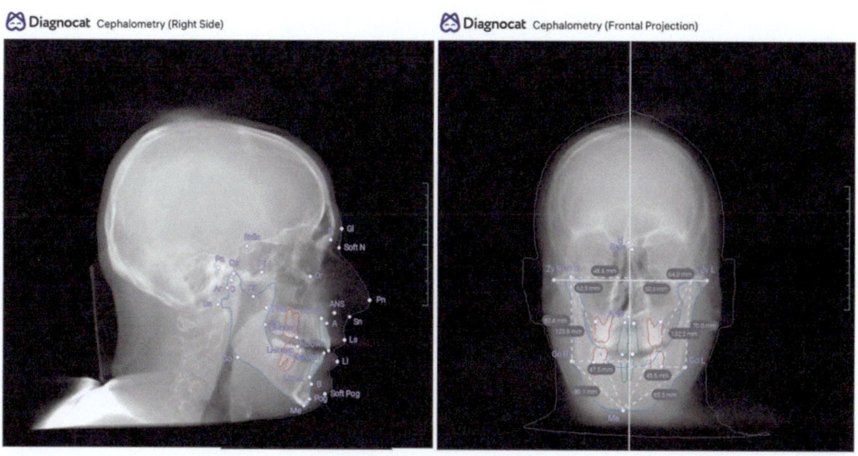

Fig. 8.2 Examples of AI-driven cephalograms generated with the Diagnocat software. These images do not meet requirements for proper orthodontic assessment, as teeth should be in centric occlusion and Frankfort plane should be parallel to the ground. Lips should be in a natural position and touching if the patient has competent lips

incisor inclination. For this reason, ensuring the patient is in centric occlusion at the time of CBCT acquisition is essential if occlusal measurements are required.

One of the related examples of AI platform is the Diagnocat software (Diagnocat Ltd.). For cephalometric analysis, the AI tool of the Diagnocat software creates posterior-anterior and lateral projections from the CBCT scans, for both the left and right sides. A fully automated cephalometric analysis is then performed with an interpretation of all measured values (Figs. 8.3 and 8.4). This includes a symmetry analysis on frontal projections and Penn analysis to compare maxillary and mandibular widths in the molar region. The report also offers organized cross-sectional images of teeth, jaws, and TMJ (Fig. 8.5). An analysis of the airways with related measurements can also be provided (Fig. 8.6). The Final Output is a patient-friendly report that can be exported as a PDF file, printed or downloaded for inclusion in patient records or for educational purposes. One of the drawbacks, however, is that some analyses such as TMD and airways require large CBCT scanning field-of-views (Fig. 8.7), which increases the ionizing radiation doses for the patient. Despite studies describing an increased reliability of 3D cephalometric analysis as compared with the 2D conventional one [11], all important radiation guidelines such as the ALARA principle should be followed by the dental professionals by using the radiographic methods only when there is a clear diagnostic benefit for the patient.

AI orthodontic reports have potential to address two important challenges of manual orthodontic workflows identified in the literature, which are excessive time

Diagnocat Cephalometry (Right Side)

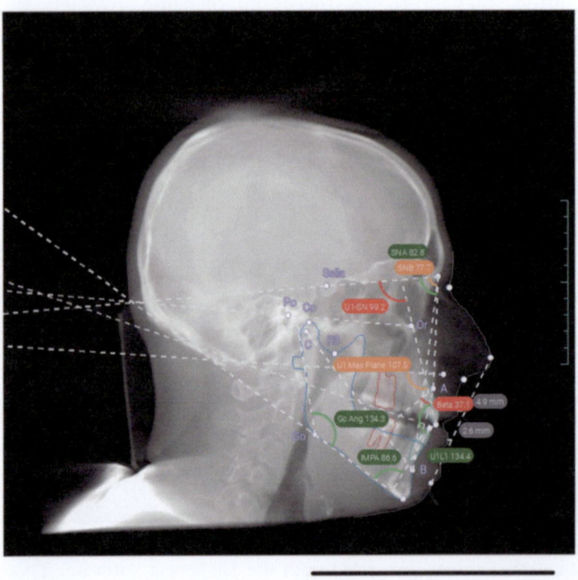

	Name	Value R	Norm	Dev R
Vertical Relationship	SN-MP	39.8	32 ± 2	5.8
	FH-OP	13.4	9 ± 4	0.4
	Go Ang	134.3	130 ± 7	-
	Mid Height	44.2	49 ± 4	0.8
	Low Height	55.8	50 ± 5	0.8
A-Po Relationship	Beta	37.1	31 ± 2	4.1
	Wits	-3.2	0 ± 1	2.2
	NSeAr	120.3	124 ± 5	-
	SNA	82.8	82 ± 2	-
	SNB	77.7	80 ± 2	0.3
	ANB	5.2	2 ± 2	1.2
	MP	67.8	71 ± 2	1.2
	S-N	70.2	70 ± 3	-
Soft	ULip to Eline	-4.9	-4 ± 2	-
	LLip to Eline	-2.6	-2 ± 2	-
Incisor Relationship	Overjet	3.0	3 ± 1	-
	Overbite	2.2	3 ± 1	-
	U1-SN	99.2	105 ± 2	3.8
	U1-PP	107.5	110 ± 2	0.5
	U1-TVL (ANS)	-4.8	0 ± 1	3.8
	Interincisal	134.4	130 ± 6	-
	Li-MP	86.6	90 ± 5	-
	Shimbashi	22.7	18 ± 1	3.7

Moderate 1-2 deviations Severe >2 deviations

Fig. 8.3 Examples of AI-driven cephalometric measurements with the Diagnocat software. Note that this example would not be clinically valid, as molars are not in occlusion on the CBCT

Diagnocat Cephalometry (Comments) — Moderate 1-2 deviations; Severe >2 deviations

	Comments L	Deviation L	Value L	Name	Norm	Value R	Deviation R	Comments R	
Vertical Relationship	high angle	0.8	34.8	SN-MP	32 ± 2	39.8	5.8	high angle	Vertical Relationship
	normal growth pattern	-	9.8	FH-OP	9 ± 4	13.4	0.4	hyperdivergent growth pattern	
	normal growth pattern	-	124.6	Go Ang	130 ± 7	134.3	-	normal growth pattern	
	short mid height	0.8	44.2	Mid Height	49 ± 4	44.2	0.8	short mid height	
	long lower height	0.8	55.8	Low Height	50 ± 5	55.8	0.8	long lower height	
A-Po Relationship	skeletal class III	3.6	36.6	Beta	31 ± 2	37.1	4.1	skeletal class III	A-Po Relationship
	skeletal class II	1.2	2.2	Wits	0 ± 1	-3.2	2.2	skeletal class III	
	skeletal class II	5.0	114.0	NSeAr	124 ± 5	120.3	-	skeletal class I	
	normal maxillary position	-	82.8	SNA	82 ± 2	82.8	-	normal maxillary position	
	mandibular retroposition	0.3	77.7	SNB	80 ± 2	77.7	0.3	mandibular retroposition	
	skeletal class II	1.2	5.2	ANB	2 ± 2	5.2	1.2	skeletal class II	
	mandibular micrognathia	1.2	67.8	MP	71 ± 2	67.8	1.2	mandibular micrognathia	
	skull base length	-	70.2	S-N	70 ± 3	70.2	-	skull base length	
Soft	normal upper lip	-	-4.9	ULip to Eline	-4 ± 2	-4.9	-	normal upper lip	Soft
	normal lower lip	-	-2.6	LLip to Eline	-2 ± 2	-2.6	-	normal lower lip	
Incisor Relationship	normal overjet	-	2.8	Overjet	3 ± 1	3.0	-	normal overjet	Incisor Relationship
	normal overbite	-	3.5	Overbite	3 ± 1	2.2	-	normal overbite	
	upper incisor retrusion	1.8	101.2	U1-SN	105 ± 2	99.2	3.8	upper incisor retrusion	
	normal inclination of the upper incisors	-	109.5	U1-PP	110 ± 2	107.5	0.5	upper incisor retrusion	
	upper incisor retrusion	3.3	-4.3	U1-TVL (ANS)	0 ± 1	-4.8	3.8	upper incisor retrusion	
	normal incisors inclination	-	132.1	Interincisal	130 ± 6	134.4	-	normal incisors inclination	
	normal inclination of the upper incisors	-	91.8	Li-MP	90 ± 5	86.6	-	normal inclination of the upper incisors	
		4.9	23.9	Shimbashi	18 ± 1	22.7	3.7		

Fig. 8.4 AI-driven cephalometric analyses with the Diagnocat software. Note that this example would not be clinically valid, as molars are not in occlusion on the CBCT

consumption and high observer variability. However, the current scientific evidence indicates that AI orthodontic reports should act as decision-support systems, and not a replacement for the orthodontist. The presence of patient-friendly reports with potential to motivate patients suggests that commercial tools are engineered not only for clinical efficiency but also for improving treatment acceptance from patients. Therefore, despite profound technological advances for AI-driven orthodontic reports, the clinical judgment, ethical responsibility, and expert supervision of the orthodontist remain indispensable for ensuring optimal and patient-specific care.

8.5.1 Clinical Case Analysis: AI-Driven Orthodontic Report (Case by Dr. Adriana Bartolo)

The management of impacted maxillary canines is a significant and relatively frequent challenge in orthodontics. This clinical scenario often necessitates a multidisciplinary approach involving both surgical and orthodontic expertise. The complex mechanics required to guide an impacted tooth into the dental arch can lead to prolonged treatment times, increased costs, and potential complications involving the supporting periodontal tissues. Consequently, the importance of an early and accurate diagnosis cannot be overstated, as it is paramount to intervening efficiently and mitigating associated risks [12].

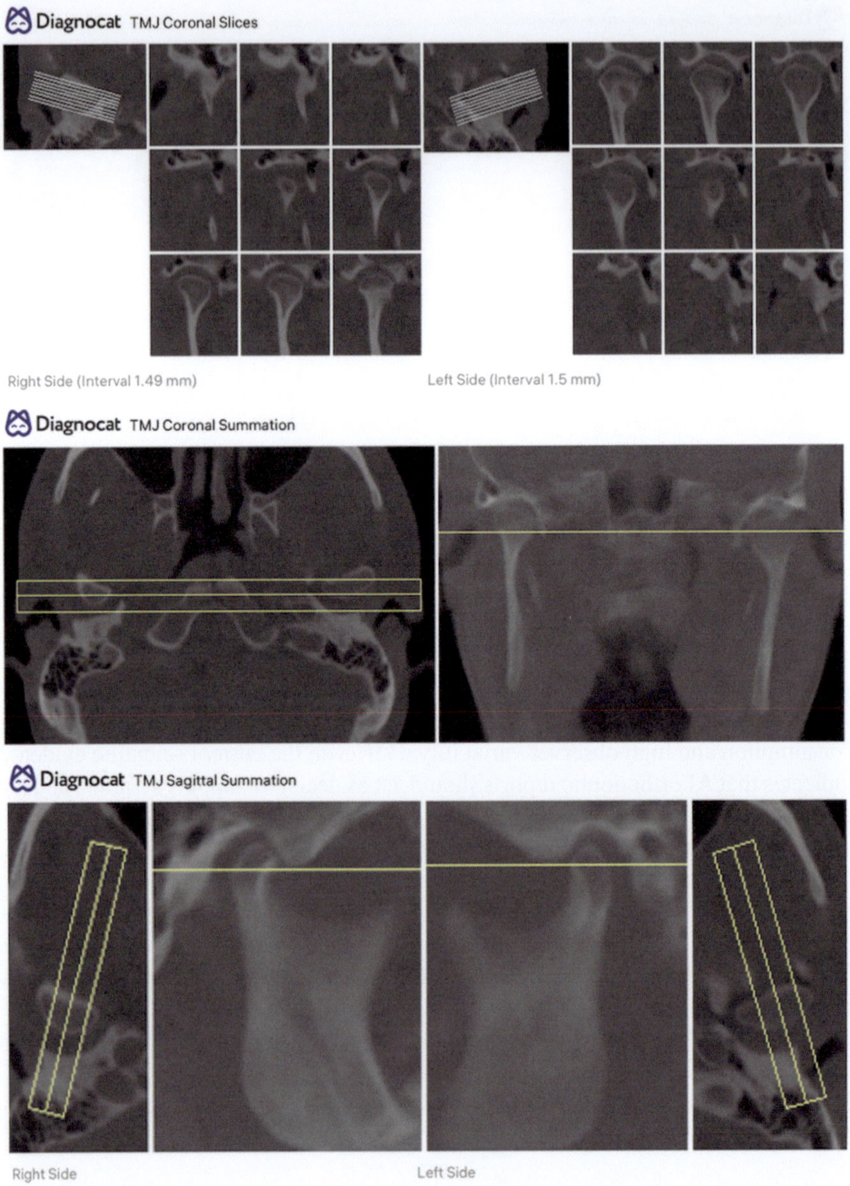

Fig. 8.5 Temporomandibular joint analysis with the Diagnocat software

A 14-year-old boy, with no known medical conditions, presented with a Class II division 1 malocclusion, severe crowding in both arches, a deep overbite, and unerupted upper canines. Extraction of all first premolars in the upper and lower arches was done to relieve significant crowding, provide space for alignment of the dentition, and facilitate the eruption and positioning of the maxillary canines.

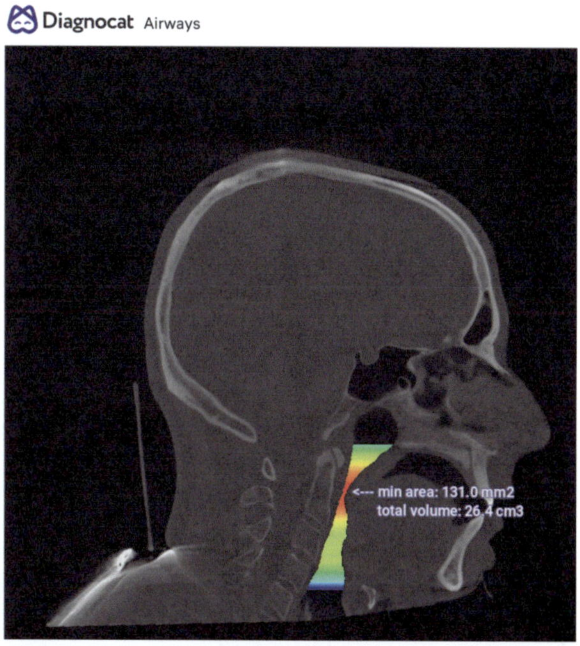

Fig. 8.6 AI-driven airway analysis of the Diagnocat software

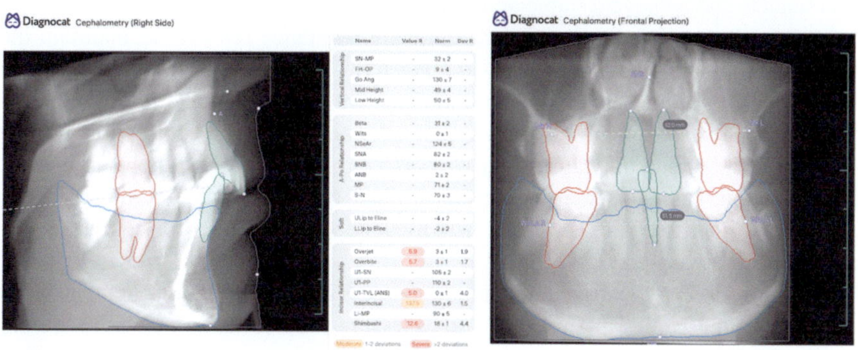

Fig. 8.7 AI-driven cephalometric analyses performed on a CBCT scan in occlusion, but with a smaller field-of-view (Diagnocat software). Note that most of the measurements could not be performed by the AI tool of the software since the cephalometric landmarks were not included in the volume of the field-of-view

Furthermore, both arches were bonded using pre-adjusted edgewise fixed appliances to achieve alignment and leveling of both arches, correction of the deep overbite, coordination of arch forms, and application of traction to the canines for guidance into the arch.

Surgical open exposure of the unerupted upper canines was done to allow their eruption into the dental arch using the fixed appliances. It also provided direct visualization and access for bonding. It also allowed the canines to erupt through keratinized tissue, which is associated with better gingival contour, increased width of attached gingiva, and lower risk of recession in the long term.

Initial alignment was carried out using round nickel titanium (NiTi) archwires to relieve crowding and begin leveling. This was followed by progression to rectangular NiTi archwires to enhance 3D control, improve incisor torque, and continue arch coordination prior to working wire mechanics. The archwires were advanced to rectangular stainless-steel wires to provide greater rigidity and improved 3D control.

This phase was followed by open surgical exposure of the unerupted maxillary canines, providing improved visualization of the crowns. The enhanced access allowed accurate bonding of attachments, facilitating controlled orthodontic traction and guided eruption into the arch.

Orthodontic traction using an elastomeric chain was applied to the exposed maxillary canines, guiding them into the line of the arch in a controlled manner while maintaining root parallelism and periodontal health. Once the maxillary canines were fully aligned in the arch, treatment progressed to finishing mechanics using light stainless-steel wires.

Final detailing of the case included adjustment of torque, tip, and rotational control of the canines and adjacent teeth; coordination of upper and lower arch forms; refinement of overjet and overbite; and correction of midlines and optimization of intercuspation. Light settling elastics were used in the final phase to improve occlusal contacts and achieve a stable and functional finish.

A retention regime was provided following appliance removal to maintain the corrected tooth positions and support long term stability. For the upper arch, a bonded palatal retainer was placed on the incisors, together with a removable vacuum formed retainer to maintain alignment, overjet, and overbite correction. For the lower arch, a bonded lingual retainer was placed canine to canine to preserve lower incisor alignment, particularly important given the pretreatment crowding. The patient was instructed on wear, care, and hygiene and scheduled for regular review to monitor retainer fit and stability.

Traditional 2D radiographic techniques possess critical limitations in the diagnosis of impacted canines, particularly in assessing their relationship with adjacent structures. These methods can produce image distortions and superimposition, masking important pathologies such as root resorption. As evidence of this limitation, approximately 37% of the lateral incisors undergoing root resorption appear normal on conventional 2D radiographs [13].

For this reason, CBCT is established as an adequate method for the diagnosis of impacted teeth. The diagnostic advantages of CBCT scans are significant for an effective treatment planning, including accurately identifying and locating the impacted tooth's precise three-dimensional position; assessing for possible damage, such as external root resorption, to adjacent teeth; and quantifying the amount of the surrounding bone to inform the surgical approach and the direction of orthodontic force application.

A correct clinical and imaging diagnosis is very important since untreated impacted canines can lead to numerous pathological alterations and clinical complications. A comprehensive risk assessment must consider the following potential sequelae: poor positioning of the impacted tooth; migration of adjacent teeth, leading to a loss of arch perimeter; internal resorption of the impacted tooth; external root resorption of both the impacted tooth and adjacent teeth; development of dentigerous cysts from the dental follicle; and infections and pain, mainly caused by partial eruptions.

Once a definitive diagnosis is established, the clinician must select from several distinct treatment pathways. This decision is driven by a careful evaluation of case-specific prognostic factors, where determinants such as patient age, impaction depth, tooth angulation, and available arch space dictate the most appropriate clinical course. The appropriate choice for cases with a better prognosis is usually the orthodontic traction of the impacted canines. This is particularly beneficial for growing patients without severe space deficiencies. The most common potential complications include bone loss, root resorption, and gingival recession.

The clinical execution of orthodontic traction demands a systematic, multistage approach. This protocol details the requisite steps for pre-traction preparation, surgical coordination, mechanical application, and final alignment to ensure predictable and periodontally sound outcomes.

Clear communication and close collaboration between the orthodontist and the surgeon are essential for a successful surgical phase. The chosen surgical technique is determined by the three-dimensional position of the impacted canine. Since the present case showed labially (or buccally) impacted canines (Figs. 8.8 and 8.9), the recommended surgical exposure methods include gingivectomy, an apically rotated flap, or the closed surgical approach, depending on the tooth's position relative to the mucogingival junction. During the surgical procedure, an orthodontic attachment, such as a hook with a metal chain, is bonded to the exposed crown. This allows for the application of orthodontic forces. In case of palatally impacted canines, the "closed approach" is strongly recommended for canines impacted in the middle or upper third of the alveolus. This technique is clinically superior as it aims to replicate the natural eruption path through keratinized tissue, thereby yielding optimal aesthetic and periodontal results.

As a final clinical recommendation, the status of third molars must be assessed at the conclusion of treatment. If their position poses a risk to the stability of the orthodontic result, their extraction should be prescribed.

8.5.2 AI Reports in Cases with Supernumerary Teeth

As briefly mentioned in Chap. 1, detecting supernumerary teeth may be a challenge especially on 2D radiographic images, which is clinically relevant in the field of orthodontics. Scientific evidence on the analysis of the AI's misclassifications revealed recurring patterns. Errors more frequent in cases involving mixed

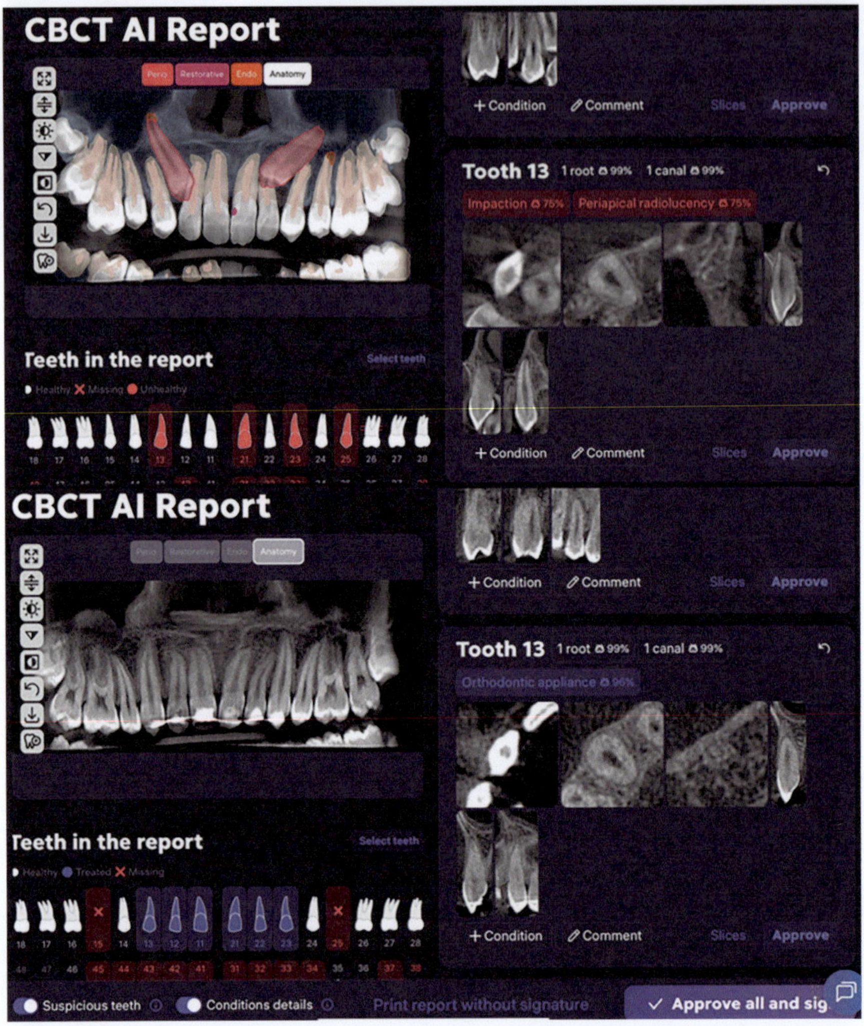

Fig. 8.8 Initial (top) and final (bottom, taken for additional reasons) CBCT AI reports of the case. Note that the AI tool identifies a periapical radiolucency on tooth 13, which was actually the space of the open apex

dentition, non-erupted teeth with suboptimal radiographic visibility, and teeth with ambiguous morphology. This challenge was particularly relevant to the study sample, as 59% of cases belonged to individuals in the mixed dentition category. Furthermore, the challenge of interpreting overlapping anatomical structures, which is a frequent occurrence with supernumerary teeth in two-dimensional radiographs, is known to reduce diagnostic accuracy in AI models and likely contributed to the

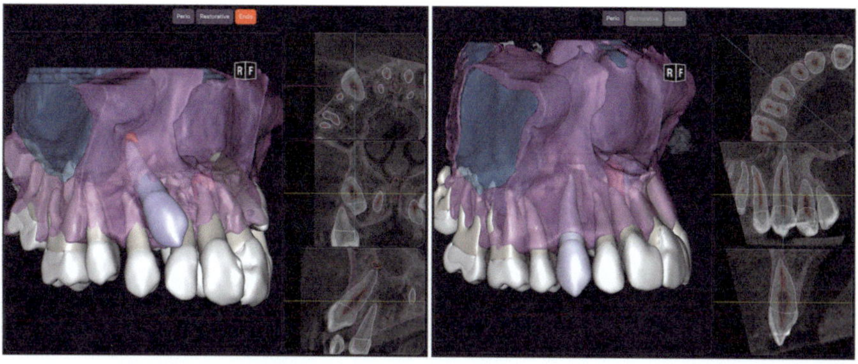

Fig. 8.9 Initial (left) and final (right, taken for additional reasons) CBCT 3D models. Note the remaining situation of the upper right third molar

low sensitivity for this anomaly [14]. These limitations highlight that clinical integration is contingent upon understanding the model's specific failure modes and establishing rigorous expert oversight protocols. Finally, it is important to remember that 3D multiplanar reconstruction from CBCT is required to precisely locate the position of impacted and supernumerary teeth, as shown in Fig. 8.10.

8.6 Conclusion

This scientific literature review of this chapter suggests that specialized AI models demonstrate significant potential and high accuracy for specific and well-defined tasks in orthodontic treatment planning. For complex decisions such as Class II treatment pathway selection and extraction prediction, advanced models such as random forest, SVM, and especially CNNs can achieve expert-level performance. The integration of explainability through XAI methods such as SHAP is a critical advancement, fostering the clinical trust necessary for adoption. This progress stands in contrast to the current capabilities of general-purpose generative AI, which has shown limited accuracy and consistency for visual diagnostic tasks such as dental crowding assessment. While the AI landscape is characterized by rapid evolution, the responsible and effective integration into clinical practice requires further continued research, greater standardization in model development and validation, and a clear understanding of its role as a supportive tool that could help to augment the indispensable expertise of the orthodontist.

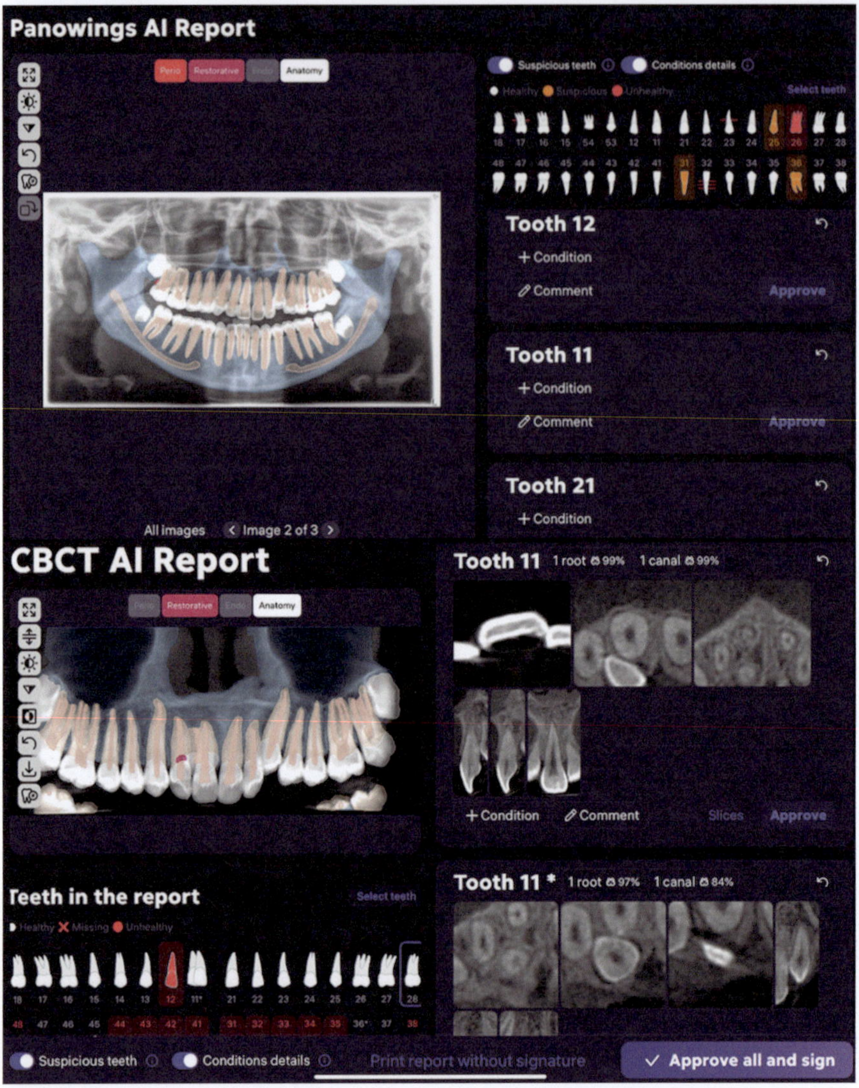

Fig. 8.10 Panoramic radiographic (top) and CBCT (bottom) AI reports of a case with a mesiodens. Note that the mesiodens was not identified or segmented in the OPG, but it was described as "tooth 11*" on the CBCT AI report and adequately segmented (case by Dr. Adriana Bartolo)

References

1. Kumar M, Kumar S, Agarwal M, Yadav E, Gandi S. Predicting treatment pathways in Class II malocclusion patients using machine learning: a comparative study of four algorithms for classifying camouflage, growth modulation, and surgical decisions. Int Orthod. 2025;24(1):101070. https://doi.org/10.1016/j.ortho.2025.101070.
2. Ziaei S, Samani D, Behjati M, Ravari AO, Salimi Y, Ahmadi S, Rajaei S, Alimohammadi F, Raji S, Deravi N, Fakhimi H. Accuracy of artificial intelligence in orthodontic extraction treatment planning: a systematic review and meta analysis. BMC Oral Health. 2025;25(1):1576. https://doi.org/10.1186/s12903-025-06880-9.
3. Trakulmututa S, Win KT. Machine learning in orthodontics: transforming Invisalign treatment planning through precision, interpretability, and ethical practices. Int J Med Inform. 2025;206:106139. https://doi.org/10.1016/j.ijmedinf.2025.106139.
4. Wafaie K, Basyouni ME, Bhattacharjee T, Prasad S, Daraqel B, Mohammed H. Diagnostic accuracy of generative large language artificial intelligence models for the assessment of dental crowding. BMC Oral Health. 2025;25(1):1558. https://doi.org/10.1186/s12903-025-06960-w.
5. Li S, Guo Z, Lin J, Ying S. Artificial intelligence for classifying and archiving orthodontic images. Biomed Res Int. 2022;2022:1473977. https://doi.org/10.1155/2022/1473977.
6. Seo H, Hwang J, Jeong T, Shin J. Comparison of deep learning models for cervical vertebral maturation stage classification on lateral cephalometric radiographs. J Clin Med. 2021;10(16):3591. https://doi.org/10.3390/jcm10163591.
7. Amasya H, Cesur E, Yıldırım D, Orhan K. Validation of cervical vertebral maturation stages: artificial intelligence vs human observer visual analysis. Am J Orthod Dentofacial Orthop. 2020;158(6):e173–9. https://doi.org/10.1016/j.ajodo.2020.08.014.
8. Yu HJ, Cho SR, Kim MJ, Kim WH, Kim JW, Choi J. Automated skeletal classification with lateral cephalometry based on artificial intelligence. J Dent Res. 2020;99(3):249–56. https://doi.org/10.1177/0022034520901715.
9. Jeong Y, Nang Y, Zhao Z. Automated evaluation of upper airway obstruction based on deep learning. Biomed Res Int. 2023;2023:8231425. https://doi.org/10.1155/2023/8231425.
10. Shujaat S, Jazil O, Willems H, Van Gerven A, Shaheen E, Politis C, Jacobs R. Automatic segmentation of the pharyngeal airway space with convolutional neural network. J Dent. 2021;111:103705. https://doi.org/10.1016/j.jdent.2021.103705.
11. Li C, Teixeira H, Tanna N, Zheng Z, Chen SHY, Zou M, Chung CH. The reliability of two- and three-dimensional cephalometric measurements: a CBCT study. Diagnostics (Basel). 2021;11(12):2292. https://doi.org/10.3390/diagnostics11122292.
12. Cruz RM. Orthodontic traction of impacted canines: concepts and clinical application. Dental Press J Orthod. 2019;24(1):74–87. https://doi.org/10.1590/2177-6709.24.1.074-087.bbo.
13. Ericson S, Kurol J. Resorption of maxillary lateral incisors caused by ectopic eruption of the canines. A clinical and radiographic analysis of predisposing factors. Am J Orthod Dentofacial Orthop. 1988;94(6):503–13. https://doi.org/10.1016/0889-5406(88)90008-x.
14. Makrygiannakis MA, Giannakopoulos K, Kavadella A, Paraskevis D, Kaklamanos EG. Diagnostic accuracy of an artificial intelligence-based software in detecting supernumerary and congenitally missing teeth in panoramic radiographs. Eur J Orthod. 2025;47(4):cjaf054. https://doi.org/10.1093/ejo/cjaf054.

Artificial Intelligence in Oral Surgical Planning

9

Otavio Henrique Pinhata-Baptista,
Mauricio Pesce Gomes da Costa,
Alan Jony de Moura e Costa, Shaban Burgoa,
Virgilio Gutierrez, Gino Kopp, Fernanda Kopp,
David Peñarrocha-Oltra, Jorge Alonso Perez-Barquero,
Miguel Peñarrocha-Diago, Adam Bartolo,
and Arthur Rodriguez Gonzalez Cortes

Oral implantology has become a primary domain for AI innovation in dentistry, with the influence of systems on several aspects, from initial presurgical planning and digital impression-taking to predicting long-term prognosis. Current evidence suggests that AI tools and models have the potential to enhance the precision, predictability, and time efficiency of implant therapy [1].

O. H. Pinhata-Baptista
Military Hospital of São Paulo Area (HMASP), São Paulo, Brazil

M. P. G. da Costa
Doc Digital Institute, São Paulo, Brazil

A. J. d. M. e. Costa · S. Burgoa · V. Gutierrez
GoBeyond Dental Courses, Houston, TX, USA

G. Kopp · F. Kopp
Kopp Dental Institute, Curitiba, Brazil

D. Peñarrocha-Oltra · J. A. Perez-Barquero · M. Peñarrocha-Diago
University of Valencia, Valencia, Spain

A. Bartolo · A. R. G. Cortes (✉)
Faculty of Dental Surgery, University of Malta, Msida, Malta
e-mail: adam.bartolo@um.edu.mt; arthur.nogueira@um.edu.mt

A. R. G. Cortes (ed.), *Dental Clinical Procedures using Artificial Intelligence*,
https://doi.org/10.1007/978-3-032-24895-4_9

9.1 AI in Implant Surgical Planning

AI algorithms have been used to provide fully automated virtual implant placement, generating comprehensive treatment plans in a fraction of the time required by human operators. Current scientific evidence suggests that AI-driven treatment plans are highly comparable to those created by experienced specialists [2, 3]. In a qualitative assessment by clinical experts, approximately 89% of AI-planned implants were judged as clinically acceptable, a rate comparable to the 93% acceptability for human-planned implants. This statistical finding suggests that AI-driven planning has reached a point of development where its outputs can be considered diagnostically equivalent to those of human specialists for standard cases [2].

As discussed in Chap. 7, the AI algorithms used in recent studies have demonstrated the ability to accurately segment the teeth, maxilla, mandible, mandibular canal, maxillary sinus, and even existing implant restorations, achieving accuracy rates between 92% and 99.7% [2, 3]. This automated segmentation is an important prerequisite for subsequent virtual patient creation and treatment planning, enabling tasks such as virtual implant placement and the digital design of custom surgical guides and components [3, 4].

Furthermore, advanced ML models, such as those combining an artificial neural network with particle swarm optimization (ANN-PSO), can perform complex biomechanical optimizations [5]. These models can rapidly recommend an ideal implant configuration designed to reduce periimplant bone stress, which is considered a critical factor for long-term success. The time efficiency gains are also substantial, as demonstrated by the study.

The substantial time reduction is coupled with perfect reproducibility (a median surface deviation of 0.00 mm), a level of consistency that is unattainable with manual methods, which exhibit significant intra- and inter-operator variability. AI systems can also augment clinical decision-making by automatically identifying cases with insufficient bone volume and recommending the need for adjunctive procedures, such as sinus lifting and bone grafting, to ensure a successful outcome.

Further than developed AI algorithms, automated implant planning can be performed by means of commercial dental AI software programs and AI tools in implant planning software programs. It is noteworthy that virtual implant planning should be prosthetically driven, which means that a digital crown is usually placed on the edentulous site before the virtual implant is positioned on the bone as shown by the CBCT reconstructed images. In the Diagnocat software, an initial dental crown and implant virtual positions are automatically suggested by the AI algorithm of the software (Fig. 9.1). This can be then corrected and optimized and should also be approved by the dental professional, who is responsible for the clinical treatment planning and subsequent execution. The following steps are performed in order and include the automated creation of an implant surgical guide based on the library of implant and components chosen. This surgical guide can be exported as an STL file and 3D-printed or milled to be used in a static computer-assisted implant surgery (s-CAIS).

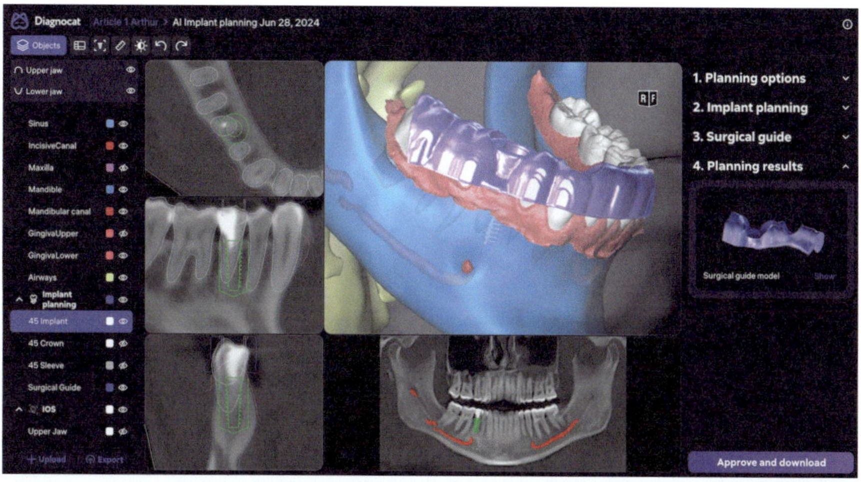

Fig. 9.1 AI implant planning with the Diagnocat software showing the automated implant position suggested by the AI algorithm of the software for an immediate implant placement to replace the tooth 45 (still without human amendments) and the subsequent automated generation of the resulting surgical guide

The following clinical case reports will illustrate and describe the role of AI-driven tools in clinical dental treatments with a focus on the surgical aspects. Clinical cases focused on the esthetic and prosthetic procedures of oral rehabilitations will be discussed in the next chapter.

9.1.1 Clinical Case Study with the Diagnocat Software (Case by Dr. Otavio Pinhata: Implant Planning Software Procedures by Prof. Arthur Cortes)

A 34-year-old female patient with no relevant medical conditions presented with a missing left mandibular first molar. The initial clinical and radiographic examinations revealed no major occlusal issues with all other teeth present in the mouth, as well as adequate alveolar bone and soft tissue volume and conditions. The patient agreed with the treatment plan involving a dental implant placement immediately loaded with a temporary crown. For this purpose, a commercial dental AI software program (Diagnocat, Diagnocat Ltd.) was used to perform automated prosthetically driven implant planning (Fig. 9.2). A crown shape and a BLX implant (Institut Straumann Ag) with 4.5 mm in diameter and 10 mm in length were selected from the software library and automatically placed on a suggested virtual position at the edentulous site. This position was further amended by the dental professional who was an oral implantologist.

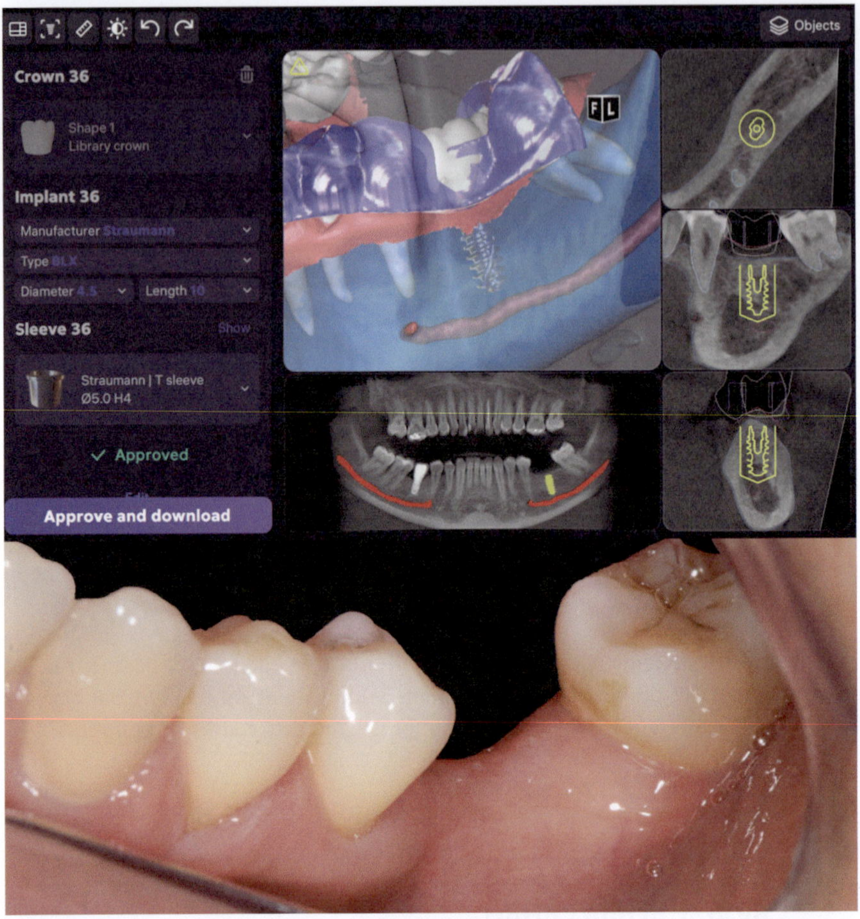

Fig. 9.2 AI implant planning with the Diagnocat software and respective automated generation of an implant surgical guide (top), to rehabilitate the implant site 36 (bottom)

The surgical guide was then manufactured using a polyjet 3D-printer (Objet30, Stratasys) before receiving the specific sleeves selected in the software library (Fig. 9.3). The surgical guide try-in confirmed its adequate adaptation on the dental arch of the patient.

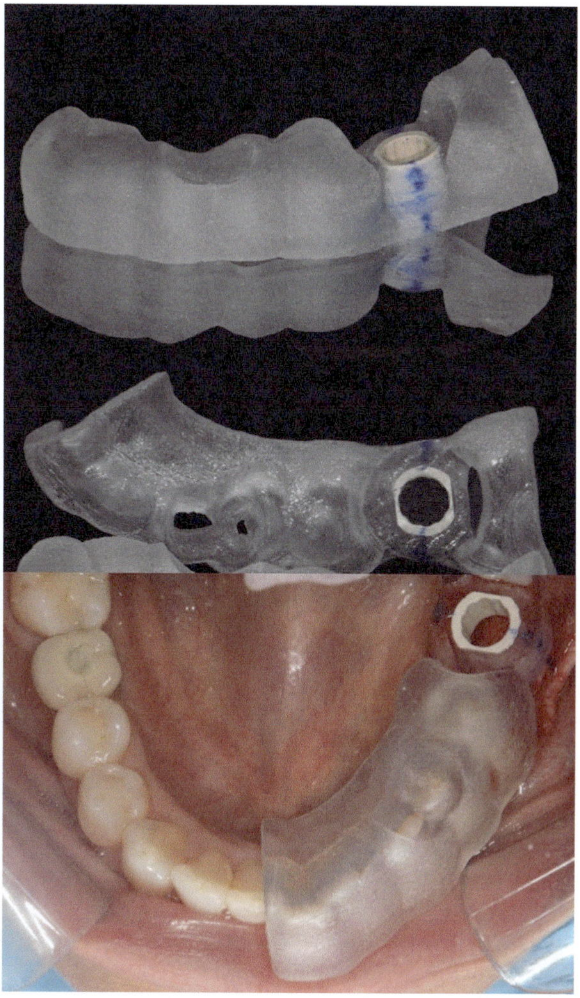

Fig. 9.3 Implant surgical guide (top) and try-in (bottom)

In order to improve the conditions and amount of keratinized tissue, a full-thickness flap was open to prepare the implant site and place the implant through the surgical guide, following usual static computer-assisted implant surgery guidelines (Fig. 9.4).

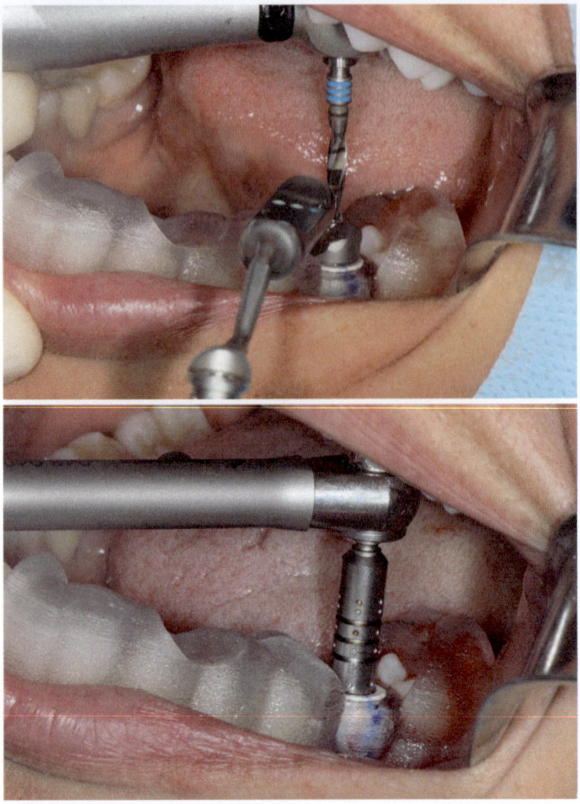

Fig. 9.4 Static computer-assisted implant site drilling (top) and placement (bottom) with the Straumann system

Within a few minutes, the planned dental implant was placed, followed by an abutment and the temporary crown to rehabilitate the site (Fig. 9.5). A postoperative periapical radiography revealed satisfactory implant conditions, which were also confirmed after the installation of a definitive implant-supported ceramic crown and a 3-month follow-up period.

9.1.2 Clinical Case Study with the coDiagnostiX and SmileCloud 3DNA Software Programs (Case by Dr. Otavio Pinhata: Treatment Planning Software Procedures by Dr. Mauricio Pesce Gomes da Costa)

A 58-year-old female patient with no relevant medical conditions presented with a chief complaint of unsatisfactory chewing ability after receiving a maxillary complete denture. A CBCT scan revealed adequate alveolar bone height but insufficient

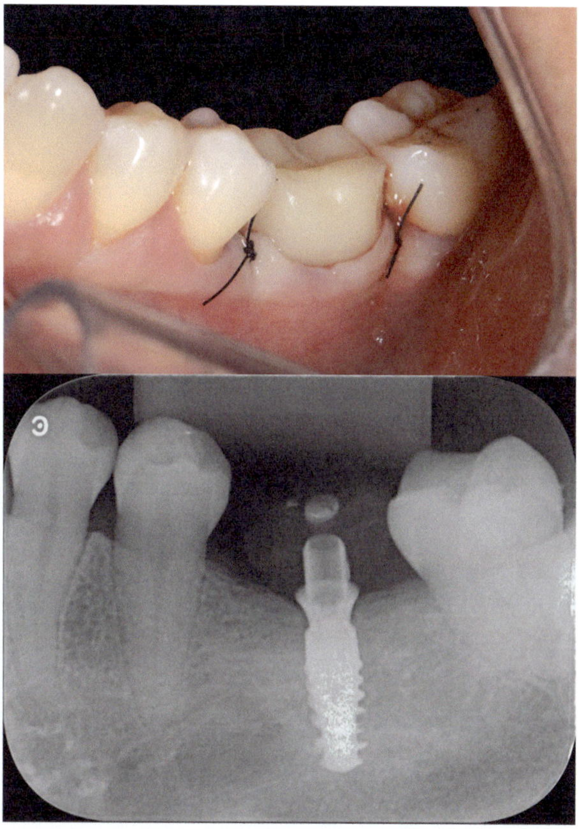

Fig. 9.5 Immediately loaded temporary crown (top) and postoperative periapical radiograph (bottom)

buccal-lingual bone width for conventional implant placement. The patient also underwent an initial intraoral scan (Trios 3, 3Shape A/S). Both CBCT and IOS images were imported into an AI-powered cloud-based treatment planning platform (SmileCloud 3DNA, SmileCloud SRL) in an integrated workflow with an implant planning software (coDiagnostiX, Dental Wings). The SmileCloud 3DNA performs a 2D smile design and a subsequent 3D prosthetic planning by means of an AI-driven cloud platform with the objective of ensuring a connection between initial aesthetic concepts and resulting functional restorations (Fig. 9.6). SmileCloud 3DNA uses a biometric library system, in which every 2D image of a tooth that is used in a design corresponds to a precise 3D model file (e.g., STL or OBJ). This helps the professional to decide if what is seen in the 2D smile design is actually clinically achievable in 3D.

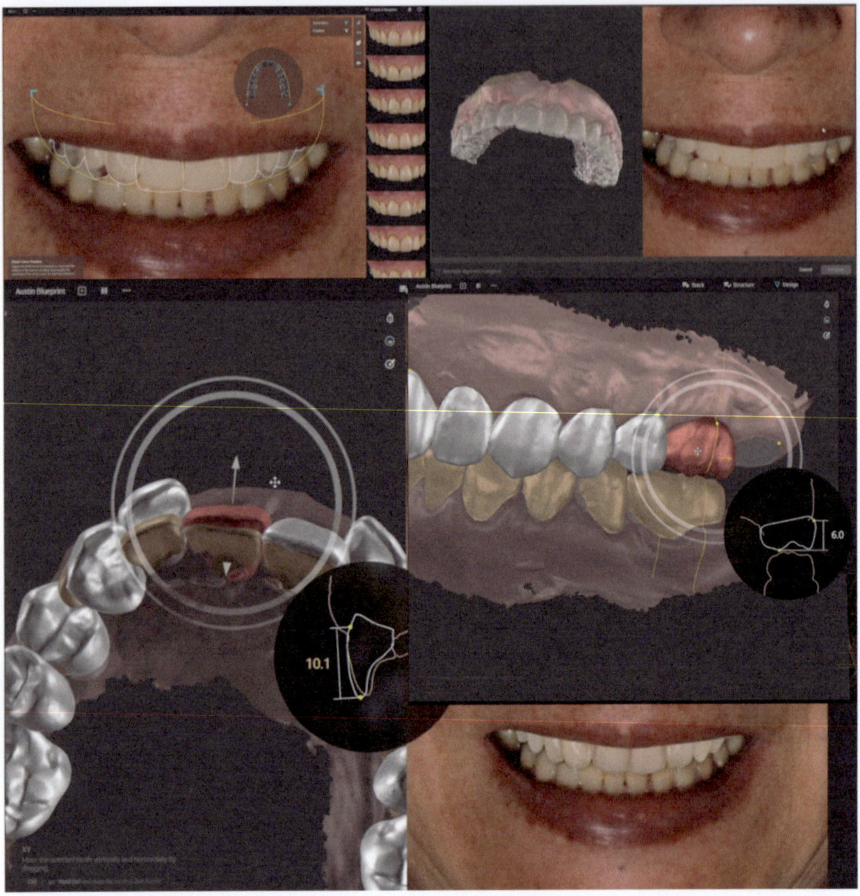

Fig. 9.6 Automated smile design and respective 3D digital prosthetic design (SmileCloud 3DNA)

Due to the lack of bone width, a surgical procedure of alveolar bone reduction followed by placement of four dental implants with 3.75 mm in diameter and 10 mm in length (BLX, Straumann) was planned (Figs. 9.7, 9.8, 9.9, 9.10 and 9.11). After a 3-month healing period, implant scanbodies (RevEX, Straumann) were screwed onto the implants and scanned with an intraoral scanner (Trios 3, 3Shape A/S). Four SRA implant abutments (Straumann; two anterior straight and two posterior angled abutments) were chosen. A temporary prosthesis was then milled in a polymeric material for trying-in and assessing occlusion and clinical esthetic parameters. The final implant-supported prosthesis was milled in PMMA with manual application of pink esthetics.

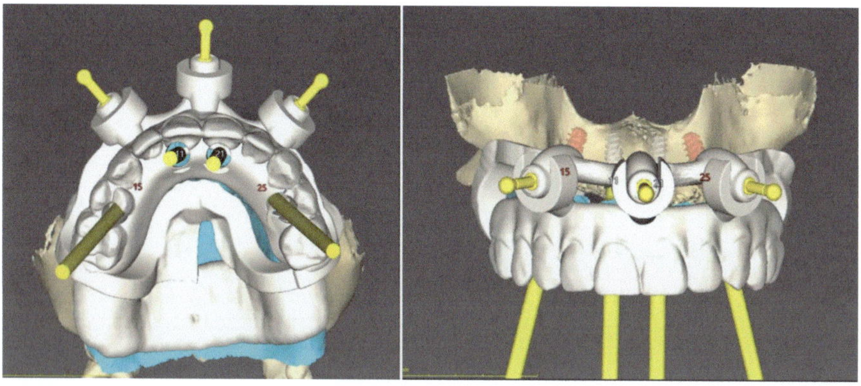

Fig. 9.7 Prosthetically driven surgical planning for alveolar bone reduction and subsequent implant placement, performed with the coDiagnostiX software

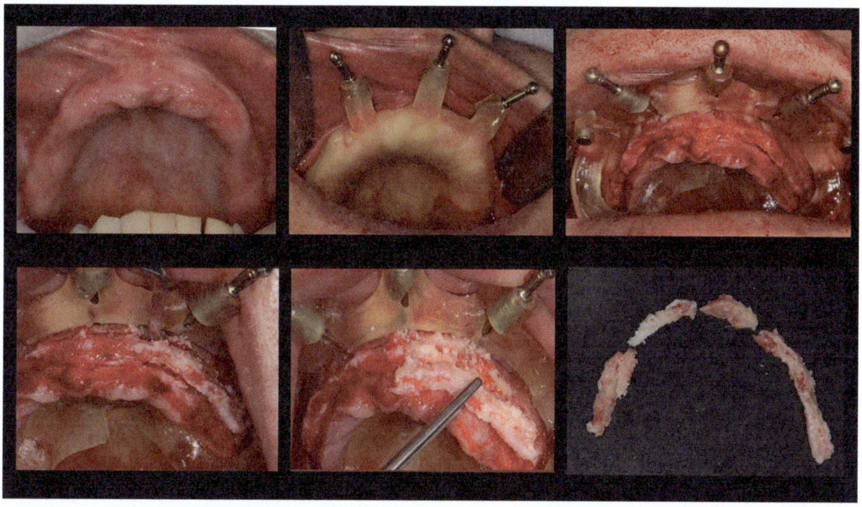

Fig. 9.8 Image-guided alveolar bone reduction

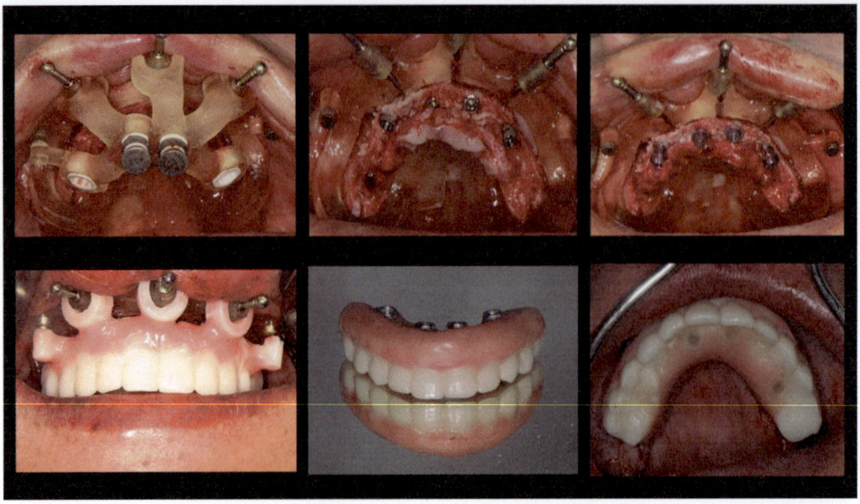

Fig. 9.9 Image-guided implant placement

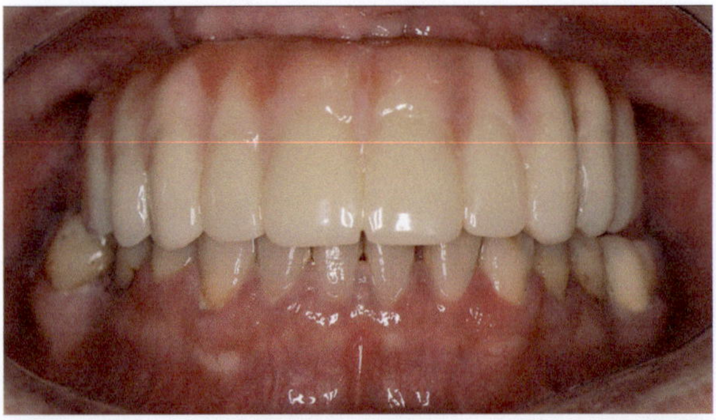

Fig. 9.10 Final full-arch implant-supported prosthesis

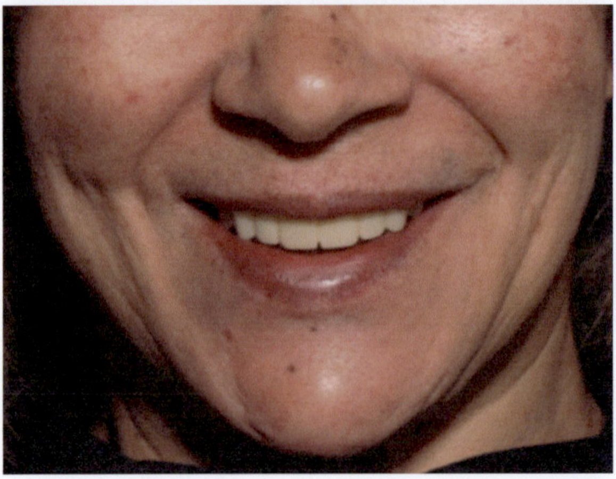

Fig. 9.11 Patient smile using the prosthesis

9.2 AI in Implant Digital Impressions and Prosthetic Design

The digital impression workflow, particularly for complete-arch implant cases, is another area benefiting from AI [6]. AI-assisted tools, such as the SmartX feature, have been introduced to improve the recognition of implant scanbodies (digital transfer abutments) and data alignment during intraoral scanning (digital impression). While research indicates these tools may not significantly improve the absolute accuracy of the final scan, they substantially enhance the consistency, reliability, and operator confidence of the process. This is especially valuable for novice users, as the AI guidance can help prevent scan failures and reduce inter-operator variability.

Furthermore, AI tools can also be used for digital design and fabrication of custom prosthetic components. AI algorithms assist in creating patient-specific crowns, surgical guides, and 3D-printed healing abutments that are precisely designed to replicate the natural emergence profile of the tooth being replaced [4], which is critical for achieving optimal aesthetic and biological outcomes.

9.2.1 Clinical Case Study Using AI-Powered Video of the Implant Prosthetic Design (Case by Dr. Alan Costa, Shaban Burgoa, and Vinicius Gutierrez)

A 62-year-old female patient presented with a failing remaining dentition. Before full-arch implant therapy, the AI video of Smilecloud software was used to analyze a patient's photo. The software uses an AI algorithm to generate a photorealistic and natural-looking smile design from a vast library of tooth shapes and then to subsequently animate these designs into dynamic "before and after" videos (namely "YES") that show the new smile in motion while the patient is artificially speaking. This allows for transforming a static image into a compelling visual story for patient acceptance and treatment planning. The process involves facial analysis, matching teeth to facial features, user customization (lip line, midline), and rendering 2D changes (Fig. 9.12) into a moving 3D simulation of the patient speaking (Fig. 9.13), creating a realistic preview without needing physical mockups.

In the present case, photographs, intraoral scans, and CBCT of the patient were sent to an international planning center (Beyond Digital Solutions, BDS3D), which performed a virtual surgical planning for alveolar bone reduction followed by immediate implant placement and loading (Fig. 9.14). AI-driven segmentations were also used in this case.

After alveolar bone reduction and implant placement surgery (Fig. 9.15), a temporary prosthesis was transferred from a 3D-printed cast to the mouth of the patient using a technique developed by the authors and published in a previous technique report [7]. The abutments chosen were then screwed to the implants and captured into the prosthesis by using bis-acrylic resin (Fig. 9.16). A definite prosthesis was installed after a 3-month healing period (Fig. 9.17).

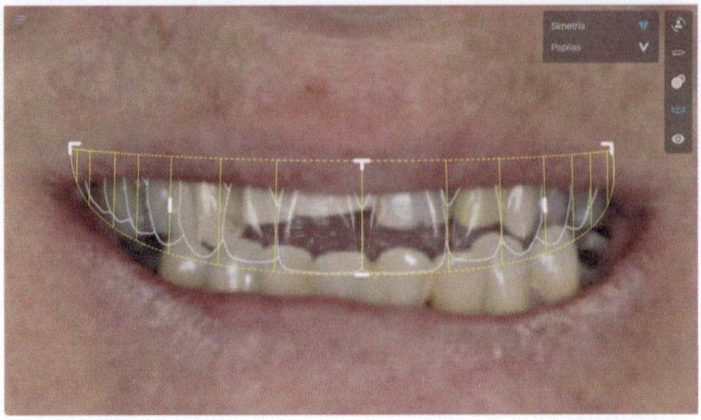

Fig. 9.12 AI-powered 2D smile design with the SmileCloud software

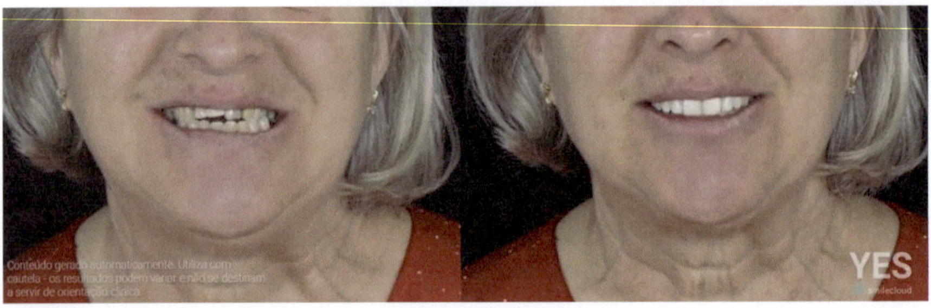

Fig. 9.13 AI-powered simulation of the patient speaking before the treatment (left) and with the planned implant prosthesis (right). The video contains instructions advising that the results may vary (depending on the clinical outcomes) and should not serve as an objective clinical orientation

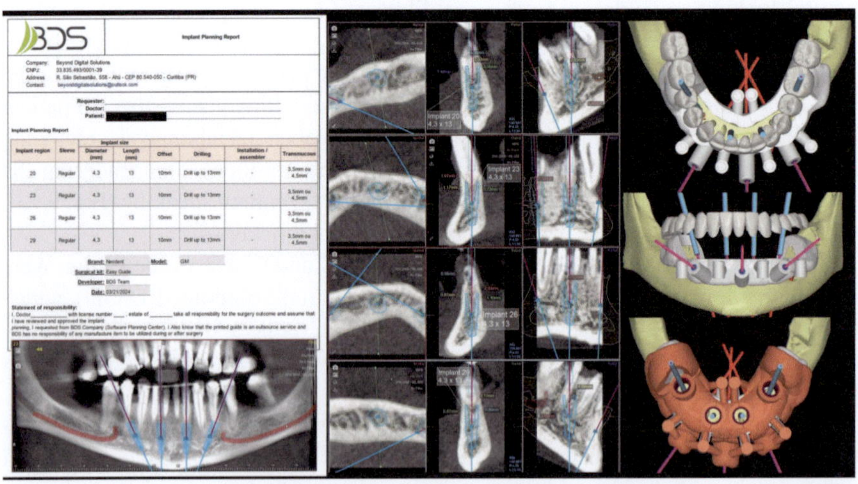

Fig. 9.14 Integrated treatment planning performed by the planning center BDS. Note that two magnetically connected surgical guides were created using the NemoStudio (Nemotec) software

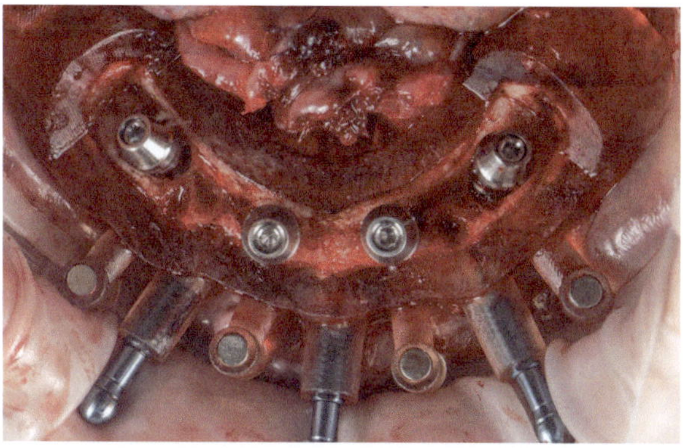

Fig. 9.15 Clinical aspect after alveolar bone reduction and subsequent implant placement

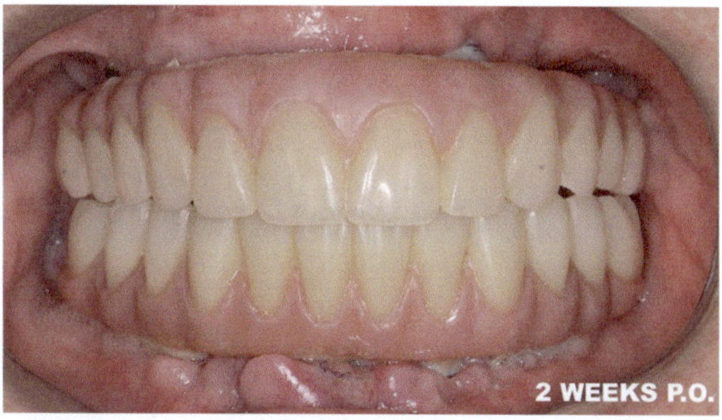

Fig. 9.16 Immediate loading result after a postoperative period of 2 weeks

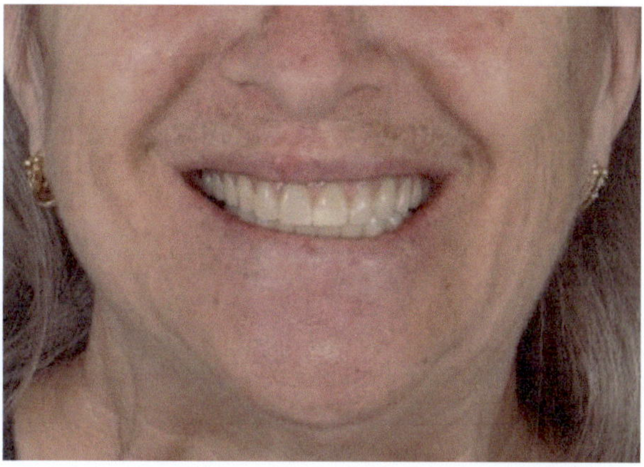

Fig. 9.17 Final smile of the patient

9.3 Postoperative Assessment and Prognosis Prediction

Specific AI models are proving effective in analyzing radiographic images to predict the long-term prognosis of dental implants [7, 8]. The aforementioned systematic reviews of the literature confirm that AI algorithms can be trained to identify subtle patterns that correlate with future clinical outcomes. Specific clinical outcomes that AI tools have shown potential to predict include periimplantitis, marginal bone loss, implant failure or success, degree of osseointegration, and implant stability.

The performance of these prognostic models is promising, with reported diagnostic accuracy rates ranging from 70% to as high as 99.76%. This capability allows for earlier interventions and the development of personalized patient maintenance protocols. From the highly structured domain of implantology, AI is also finding a role in the more unpredictable field of maxillofacial trauma.

9.4 The Use of AI-Powered Segmentation for Bone Graft Surgical Planning (Illustrated with a Clinical Case Study by David Peñarrocha-Oltra Y Miguel Peñarrocha-Diago Dr. Jorge A. Perez-Barquero)

Following tooth extraction or trauma, the alveolar bone naturally undergoes a remodeling process that frequently leads to significant vertical and horizontal bone loss. This reduction in bone volume presents a major clinical challenge, especially in the anterior maxilla. Inadequate bone architecture can compromise the ideal placement of dental implants, jeopardize their long-term stability, and negatively impact the surrounding soft tissue contours. The ultimate result can be an unfavorable aesthetic outcome that fails to meet patient expectations, leading to dissatisfaction and complicating functional rehabilitation.

Among the main solutions are bone grafts, which can be basically particulate or blocks. The latter is an appropriate option for severe bone atrophies, with a large area of buccal-lingual width loss. Autogenous onlay block grafts have satisfactory osteoinductive and osteoconductive properties and can be retrieved from areas of the mandible such as the ramus. In this context, a precise segmentation and automated alignment of CBCT and intraoral scans enable guided surgical planning and volume calculation of the block graft (Fig. 9.18) [9]. Automating these procedures with AI has three main objectives: precise dimensional control of the graft, optimized donor site selection, and facilitation of an exact and stable graft fixation.

The virtual shape of the required autogenous bone graft is used to identify a suitable donor site, typically in the mandible. The CAD software helps match the required width, length, and curvature of the onlay bone graft to the donor anatomy. Once the optimal site is selected, a custom surgical harvesting guide can be designed,

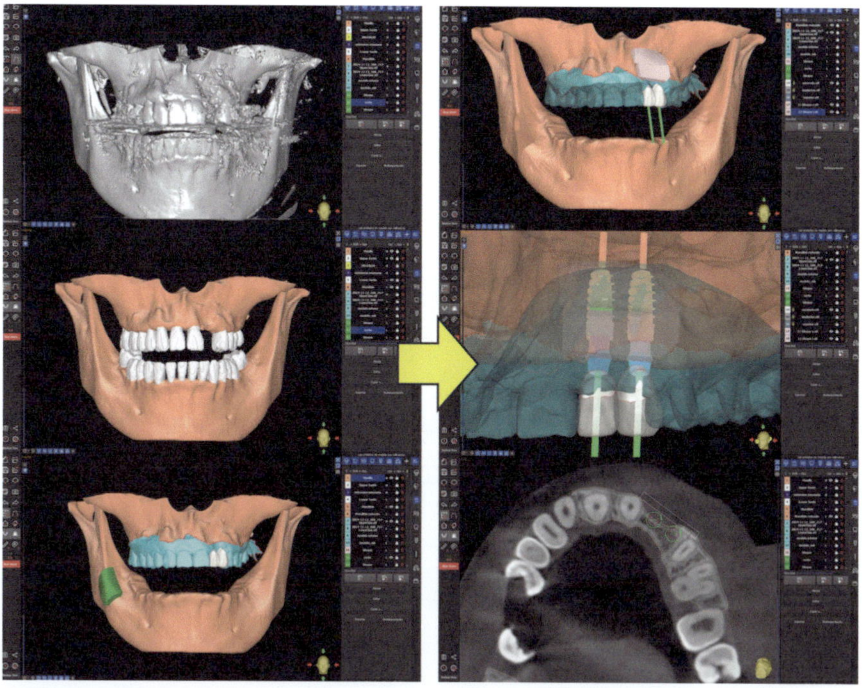

Fig. 9.18 Automated segmentation and alignment of CBCT and intraoral scan with a digital ramus bone graft and prosthetic plan (left column), as well as the subsequent prosthetically driven implant planning of the case performed with the software 3D Exacto (Galimplant)

exported as an STL file, and 3D-printed ideally with a resin specifically used for surgical guides. Then, the surgical guide should undergo a process of finishing, polishing, and disinfection to prepare it for the sterile surgical environment. An initial surgical procedure with a full-thickness flap is then performed to retrieve and install the autogenous block graft on the atrophic edentulous sites to achieve adequate lateral alveolar ridge augmentation (Fig. 9.19).

After a 6-month healing period (depending on the follow-up conditions), a new CBCT is taken to confirm adequate graft healing conditions and to perform image-guided implant surgical planning and the corresponding surgical procedure (Fig. 9.20), following the theories of digital implantology discussed previously in this chapter. If needed, guided-bone regeneration for immediate buccal wall grafting can also be performed. After confirming clinical satisfactory conditions, an implant-supported temporary crown can be then placed, before proceeding with imaging and clinical follow-up (Fig. 9.21).

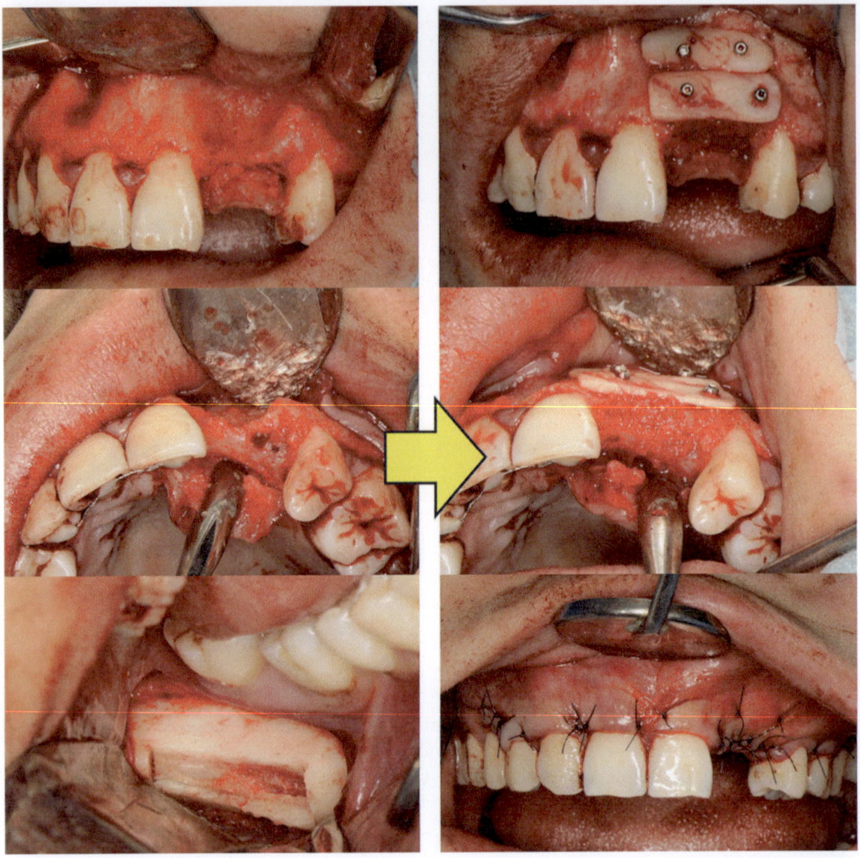

Fig. 9.19 Surgical procedure to retrieve the ramus bone graft with a piezoelectric surgical device (left column) and the subsequent installation of the autogenous block graft on the edentulous sites, before filling the remaining gaps with particulate autogenous bone (right column). Note that the horizontal incision was long enough to avoid the need of releasing incisions in the esthetic region

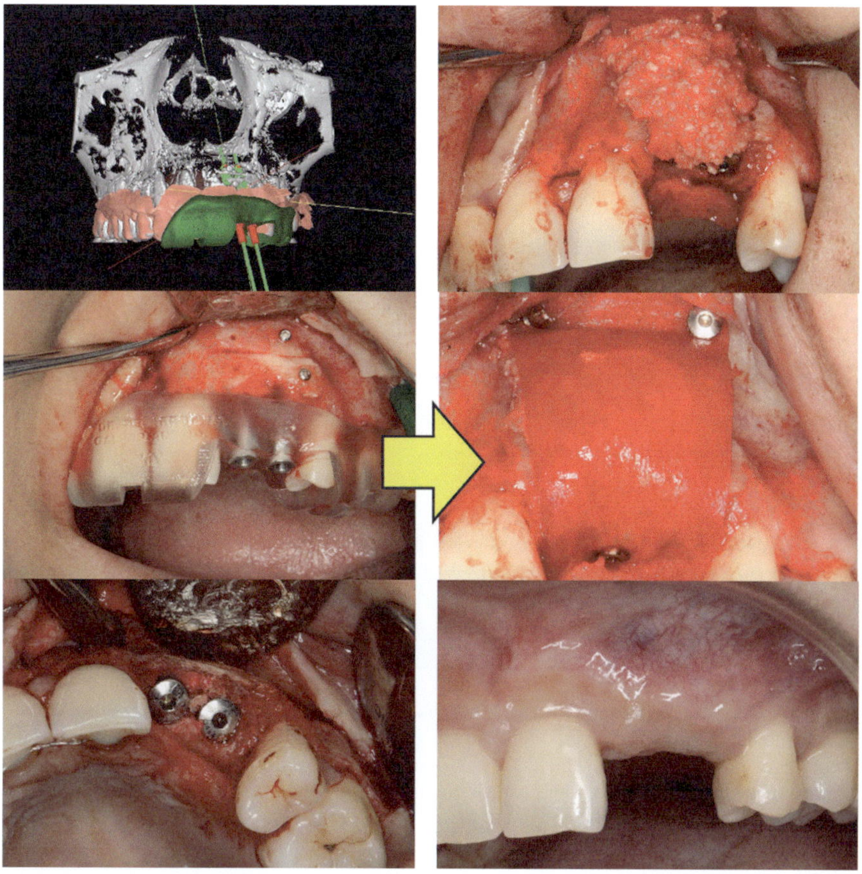

Fig. 9.20 Image-guided implant placement procedure (left column) with a particulate allograft material followed by a collagen membrane (Lyoplant, Aesculap AG) and subsequent immediate guided-bone regeneration to graft the periimplant buccal wall (right column). Two dental implants 3.5 mm in diameter (IPX, Galimplant) were satisfactorily placed

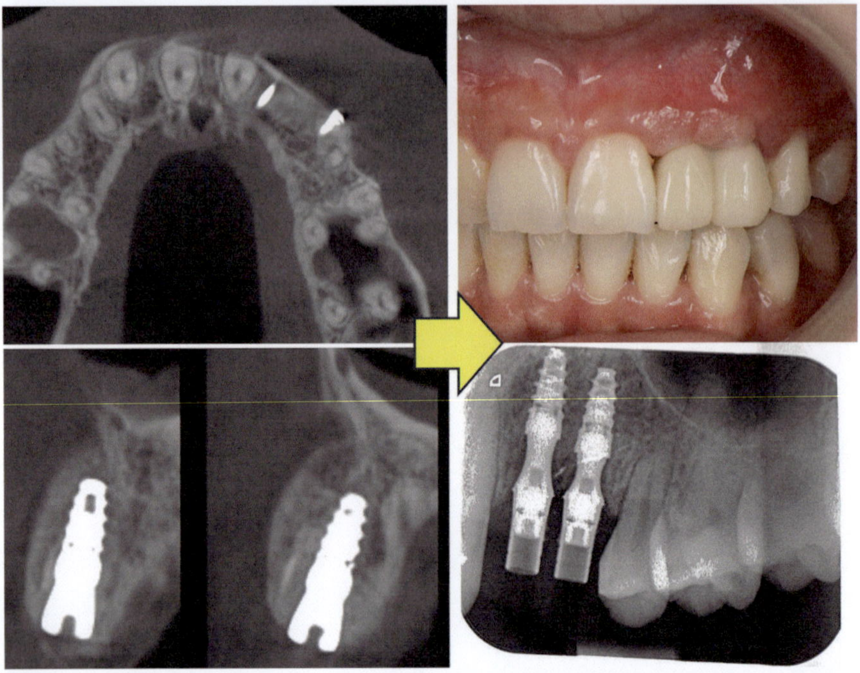

Fig. 9.21 Comparison between the CBCT taken after a 6-month graft healing period (top left) to plan the implants and a CBCT taken during the implant follow-up period (bottom left), confirming adequate lateral augmentation, which allowed for obtaining satisfactory clinical outcomes with the implant-supported temporary crowns (right column)

9.5 Full-Arch Static Computer-Assisted Implant Surgery (Illustrated with a Clinical Case Study: Smart Guided Surgery as an Innovative Concept for the Precise Placement of Dental Implants in Different Clinical Scenarios—A 2.5-Year Follow-Up Case Report)

The rehabilitation of fully edentulous maxillae remains a clinical challenge requiring accurate diagnosis, precise planning (Fig. 9.22), seamless integration between surgical and prosthetic phases, and predictable long-term outcomes. As previously discussed in this chapter, S-CAIS allows prosthetically driven implant positioning to reduce surgical deviations and enhance procedural safety.

When associated with immediate loading protocols, s-CAIS aims to provide functional and psychological benefits to the patient. Furthermore, the adoption of a full digital workflow optimizes clinical efficiency, reduces the number of appointments, and improves control over laboratory procedures [9].

The Smart Guided concept, developed in Brazil, was designed to overcome limitations commonly associated with conventional guided surgery systems by offering increased clinical versatility with variable offsets and integration with prefabricated

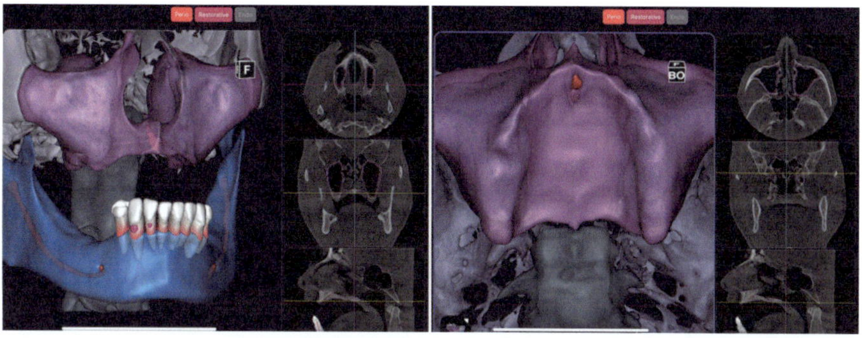

Fig. 9.22 AI-driven assessment of mandibular alveolar bone loss (left) and maxillary atrophy (right) of the case with the Diagnocat software

prosthetic components. The concept is particularly useful for cases with restricted mouth opening and limited working space for implant drilling. For this purpose, the Smart Guided surgical system (Kopp) achieves offset control by means of a calibrated interaction among digitally defined sleeve height, variable-offset guide components, and depth-limiting drilling instruments. This configuration enables precise control of the apico-coronal position of the implant during static computer-guided surgery, particularly in mucosa-supported protocols.

In this case report, a 67-year-old male patient presented to a dental institute (Curitiba, Brazil) reporting masticatory impairment and esthetic dissatisfaction with his maxillary complete denture. Clinical and radiographic examinations revealed a fully edentulous maxilla with moderate alveolar ridge atrophy, sufficient vertical and horizontal bone volume, and a thick, healthy band of keratinized mucosa. A treatment plan for the upper arch was proposed, consisting of full-arch maxillary rehabilitation with six immediately loaded implants using the Smart Guided surgical protocol. The patient signed an informed consent form.

An initial conventional impression was obtained to fabricate a temporary prosthesis, which served as the reference for prosthetically driven planning. Digital photographs were used for Digital Smile Design analysis, considering smile line, occlusal plane, and facial symmetry. The temporary prosthesis was duplicated to fabricate the radiographic guide. A dual-scan CBCT protocol was performed, consisting of one scan of the patient using the prosthesis and one separate scan of the prosthesis. The resulting DICOM datasets were aligned on an implant planning software (Dental Slice, Bioparts). Digital waxing and virtual prosthetic setup were performed (DentalCAD, Exocad, Align Technology), enabling prosthetically driven implant positioning (Fig. 9.23).

A magnetic mucosa-supported surgical guide [10], a capture guide, and the prefabricated PMMA provisional fixed prosthesis were manufactured prior to surgery according to the Smart Guided protocol. Surgical and prosthetic procedures were then conducted in a single clinical appointment. After antisepsis and local anesthesia, surgery began with adaptation of the magnetic mucosa-supported surgical guide. Implant site osteotomies were performed using the Smart Guided Pilot 4.0 drill with an 11 mm offset, following the planned drilling sequence.

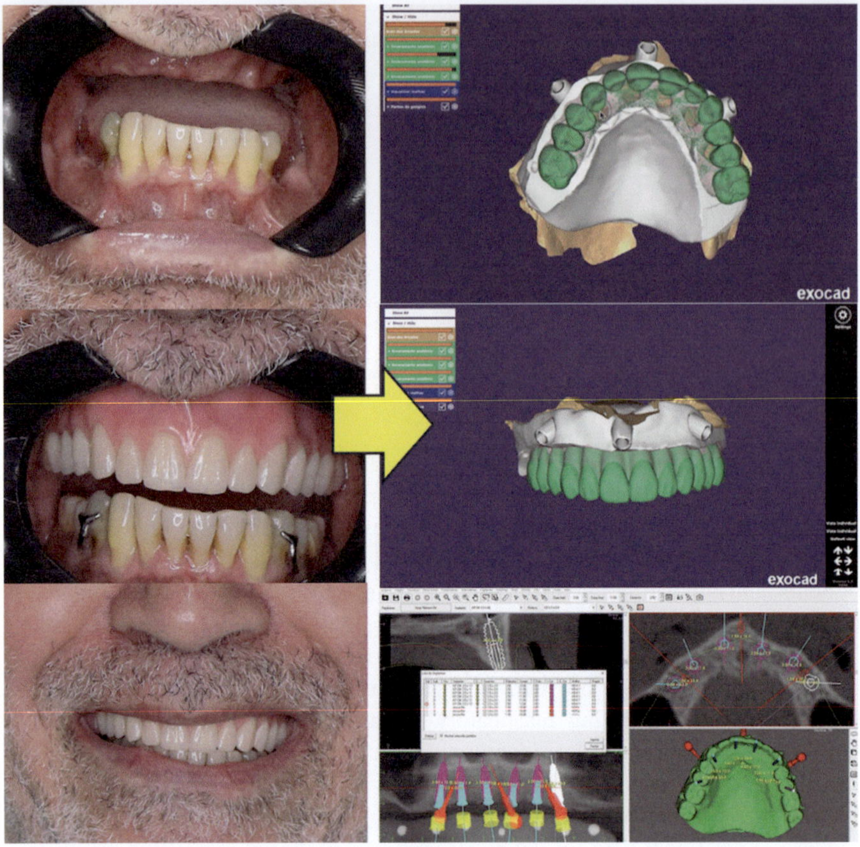

Fig. 9.23 Prosthetically driven implant planning of the case

Six Cone Morse Platinum implants (Kopp Implantes) were placed, all achieving insertion torque values higher than 45 Ncm. Prosthetic mini-abutments were installed, and the prefabricated PMMA provisional fixed prosthesis was captured and screw-retained, enabling immediate loading (Fig. 9.24).

The patient was monitored clinically and radiographically for 2.5 years postoperatively. Throughout the follow-up period, periimplant bone stability, absence of soft tissue inflammation, maintenance of masticatory function, and adequate adaptation of the fixed prosthesis were observed. Radiographic evaluations demonstrated preservation of alveolar crestal bone levels around all implants, confirming the success of the surgical and prosthetic approach (Fig. 9.25).

The results of this case suggest that s-CAIS combined with immediate loading can achieve successful outcomes when properly indicated. The Smart Guided concept differs from most conventional systems by allowing offset adjustments and improved control of the relationship between the guide, bone, and soft tissues, thereby enhancing surgical accuracy.

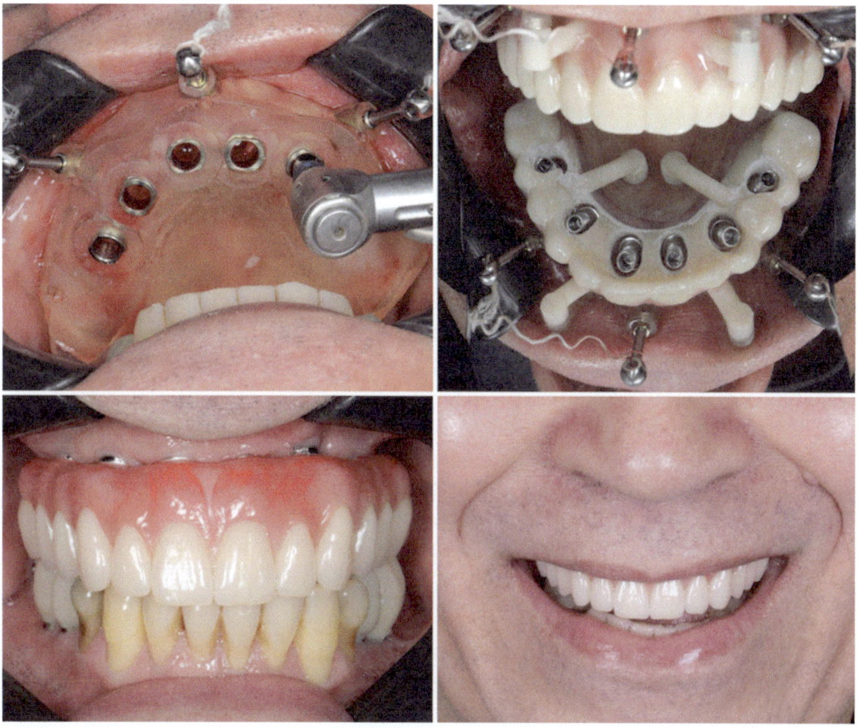

Fig. 9.24 Implant rehabilitation. Top: Implant placement and abutments capture using magnetic guides (BDS planning center) with the Smart Guided System (Kopp). Bottom: Final outcome of the final full-arch implant-supported fixed prothesis

Fig. 9.25 Final follow-up panoramic radiographic image

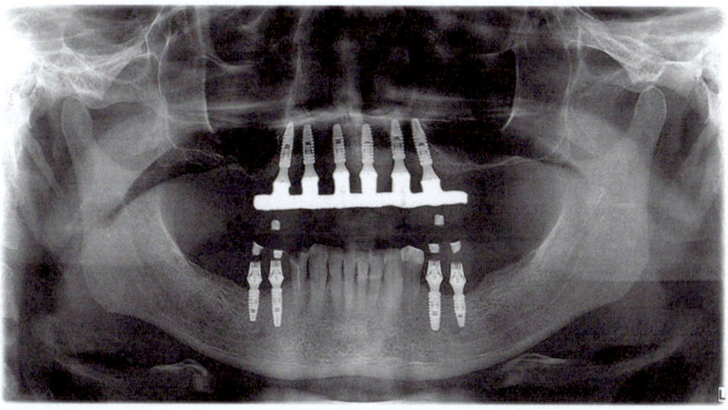

9.6 AI in Maxillofacial Trauma and Fracture Management

In the context of maxillofacial trauma, the application of AI is taking a different form. Rather than AI surgical planning tools, large language models (LLMs, also known as AI chatbots) are emerging as supplementary tools for knowledge dissemination, patient education, and clinical support [11, 12].

The related studies have evaluated the performance of various LLMs by testing their knowledge of traumatic dental injuries (TDIs), which include complex conditions such as tooth fractures and luxations. The findings indicate that while LLMs can achieve moderate to high accuracy, their performance is often inconsistent, particularly for complex clinical scenarios such as luxation injuries, in which the accuracy across all models was notably lower.

Similarly, LLMs have shown mixed results to address patient-generated frequently asked questions (FAQs) regarding treatments such as maxillomandibular fixation (MMF). The information provided is often factually accurate, but its clinical utility is frequently undermined by poor readability. The linguistic complexity as measured by Flesch-Kincaid Grade Level scores often far exceeds the comprehension level of an average patient, with some models generating text requiring a postgraduate-level understanding.

This reinforces a consistent finding described throughout the literature: current AI systems and LLMs should be viewed as adjunctive educational and clinical tools. Algorithms are not a replacement for the nuanced expertise, critical thinking, and communication skills of a qualified surgeon, who remains essential for interpreting information and guiding patient care.

9.7 Comparative Performance Analysis: Efficiency, Consistency, and Accuracy

To critically evaluate the true clinical value of AI, it is essential to benchmark its performance against human intelligence and conventional methods [1–3]. This comparison reveals AI's core strengths in efficiency and consistency while also highlighting its current limitations in terms of autonomous accuracy and reliability.

The most significant and consistently demonstrated benefit of AI in oral surgery is a significant improvement in speed and workflow efficiency. Across a range of applications, AI automates repetitive and time-consuming tasks, allowing clinicians to focus on higher-level decision-making. In virtual implant planning, for instance, AI-assisted systems have been shown to reduce planning time by more than half, from 406 s to 187 s. In regard to biomechanical analyses, advanced ML models can complete complex optimizations in seconds, a process that would require days using traditional finite element analysis (FEA). AI also exhibits superior consistency. In repetitive tasks such as virtual implant placement, AI demonstrates perfect reproducibility with 100% consistency. This stands in contrast to the inherent variability of human performance, which was quantified in one study measuring median surface deviation (MSD) in implant placement [2]. In this study, the AI achieved an MSD of 0.00 mm, whereas human operators showed an MSD of 0.33 mm (0.14) for intra-operator performance and 0.56 mm (0.34) for inter-operator performance.

Nevertheless, the limitations discussed in Chap. 5 and the current lack of robust clinical research on several AI applications should also be considered to interpret the findings discussed above. Based on all results shown, the accuracy of AI systems should still be considered variable and context dependent. Very high accuracy rates up to 99.76% have been reported for well-defined tasks such as radiographic prognosis prediction for dental implants [2]. However, the reliability of LLMs for knowledge-based tasks in trauma management is less consistent, with performance varying between models and scenarios.

An important finding is that AI-generated surgical plans are often clinically acceptable and statistically comparable to those produced by experienced human specialists. This ability to mimic expert-level decision-making was highlighted in a form of "Turing test," in which clinical experts evaluated a series of implant plans. The experts were unable to distinguish an AI-generated plan from a human-generated one in 58% of cases. This inability for experts to reliably distinguish between AI and human outputs in a majority of cases is a powerful indicator of the potential of some AI algorithms to replicate the nuanced decision-making patterns inherent in expert-level surgical planning.

9.8 Conclusion

Despite the significant potential demonstrated in the literature, the widespread and autonomous clinical adoption of AI faces the considerable technical, ethical, and practical challenges discussed in the previous chapters. A critical understanding of these limitations is necessary to guide responsible innovation and implementation.

The clinical cases analyzed and the findings of the scientific literature raised herein indicate that AI is a transformative technology in oral and maxillofacial surgery. Its primary, proven value lies in enhancing operational efficiency and consistency by automating time-consuming and repetitive tasks in diagnostics, digital data preparation, and virtual surgical planning. While AI models often achieve accuracy levels comparable to, and in some metrics exceeding, those of human experts, their current role is best defined as that of a powerful adjunctive tool. AI can assist but does not replace the indispensable critical judgment, nuanced clinical understanding, and ethical responsibility of the human clinician, who remains at the center of patient care.

References

1. Schiavon L, Benkeser SM, Settecase E, Jung RE, Zitzmann NU, Joda T. Can AI assistants improve time efficiency in digital dataset preparation in virtual implant planning? A comparative study. J Dent. 2025; https://doi.org/10.1016/j.jdent.2025.106152.
2. Elgarba BM, Fontenele RC, Du X, Mureşanu S, Tarce M, Meeus J, Jacobs R. Artificial intelligence versus human intelligence in presurgical implant planning: a preclinical validation. Clin Oral Implants Res. 2025; https://doi.org/10.1111/clr.14429.
3. Ma H, Wu Y, Bai H, Xu Z, Ding P, Deng X, Tang Z. Preclinical Investigation of artificial intelligence-assisted implant surgery planning for single tooth defects: a case series study. J Oral Rehabil. 2025; https://doi.org/10.1111/joor.14009.
4. de Moura e Costa AJ, de Campos WG, Burgoa S, Gutierrez V, Gonzalez Cortes AR. A digital workflow combining root submergence, a definitive intermediate abutment, and a custom 3D printed healing abutment for a natural peri-implant emergence profile. J Prosthet Dent. 2025; https://doi.org/10.1016/j.prosdent.2025.08.026.

5. Chen YC, Lin JW, Wang KH, Lin CL. Real-time optimization of prosthetic design for complete arch implant-supported treatments using finite element-based machine learning. J Prosthet Dent. 2024; https://doi.org/10.1016/j.prosdent.2024.06.012.
6. Tallarico M, Qaddomi M, De Rosa E, Cacciò C, Meloni SM, Gendviliene I, Att W, Bourgi R, Lumbau AM, Cervino G. Effectiveness of an AI-assisted digital workflow for complete-arch implant impressions: an in vitro comparative study. Dent J (Basel). 2025;13(10):462. https://doi.org/10.3390/dj13100462.
7. Alqutaibi AY, Algabri RS, Alamri AS, Alhazmi LS, Almadani SM, Alturkistani AM, Almutairi AG. Advancements of artificial intelligence algorithms in predicting dental implant prognosis from radiographic images: a systematic review. J Prosthet Dent. 2024; https://doi.org/10.1016/j.prosdent.2024.10.036.
8. Mugri MH. Accuracy of artificial intelligence models in detecting peri-implant bone loss: a systematic review. Diagnostics (Basel). 2025;15(6):655. https://doi.org/10.3390/diagnostics15060655.
9. Cortes ARG. Digital dentistry: a step-by-step guide and case atlas. Hoboken, NJ: Wiley; 2022. https://doi.org/10.1002/9781119852025.
10. Costa AJM, Teixeira Neto AD, Burgoa S, Gutierrez V, Cortes ARG. Fully digital workflow with magnetically connected guides for full-arch implant rehabilitation following guided alveolar ridge reduction. J Prosthodont. 2020;29(3):272–6. https://doi.org/10.1111/jopr.13150.
11. Termteerapornpimol K, Kulvitit S, Prommanee S, Khurshid Z, Porntaveetus T. Comparative benchmark of seven large language models for traumatic dental injury knowledge. Eur J Dent. 2025; https://doi.org/10.1055/s-0045-1812064.
12. Alagarsamy R, Lal B, Chawla J, Arangaraju R, Mohanty S, Fatima K, Barathi A. Evaluating the effectiveness of large language models in addressing patient queries regarding maxillomandibular fixation for maxillofacial fractures. J Oral Maxillofac Surg. 2025; https://doi.org/10.1016/j.joms.2025.09.016.

Artificial Intelligence in Prosthodontics

10

José Lincoln de Queirós Jr., Ji Yong Han, Newton Sesma, Lisya Vizotto de Barros, Sergio Candido Dias, Bruno B. R. Matias, Marcelo Lucchesi Teixeira, Laura Althea Cuschieri, Arthur Rodriguez Gonzalez Cortes, Guilherme Saavedra, Tatiana Cursino Pereira, Fernando Antonio Reis Laurino, Roberto Adrian Markarian, and Jorge Alonso Perez-Barquero

10.1 Introduction

Over the past two decades, prosthodontics has undergone consistent developments driven by digital technologies such as computer-aided design and computer-aided manufacturing (CAD-CAM). The advent of this technology has shown several benefits to the clinical workflow in restorative dentistry, such as improved efficiency,

J. L. de Queirós Jr.
ClickDent, Brasilia, Brazil

J. Y. Han
Seoul National University, Seoul, South Korea
e-mail: jiyong@snu.ac.kr

N. Sesma · L. V. de Barros · B. B. R. Matias · M. L. Teixeira
University of São Paulo, São Paulo, Brazil
e-mail: sesma@usp.br

S. C. Dias
Private Practice, Msida, Malta

L. A. Cuschieri · A. R. G. Cortes (✉)
Faculty of Dental Surgery, University of Malta, Msida, Malta
e-mail: lcusc01@um.edu.mt; arthur.nogueira@um.edu.mt

G. Saavedra · T. C. Pereira · F. A. R. Laurino
São Paulo State University—UNESP, São Paulo, Brazil
e-mail: guilherme.saavedra@unesp.br

R. A. Markarian
Clínica Implart, São Paulo, Brazil

J. A. Perez-Barquero
University of Valencia, Valencia, Spain

A. R. G. Cortes (ed.), *Dental Clinical Procedures using Artificial Intelligence*,
https://doi.org/10.1007/978-3-032-24895-4_10

predictability of outcomes, and communication among professionals, with satisfactory accuracy and esthetic outcomes [1, 2]. Despite these benefits, many aspects of the digital workflow remain labor-intensive and time-consuming, often requiring extensive manual adjustments by skilled dental technicians. Artificial intelligence (AI) has recently emerged as the next evolutionary step, potentially addressing these remaining challenges [3, 4].

10.2 Main Applications of AI in Prosthetic Design and Treatment Planning

The integration of AI into prosthodontics represents a rapidly expanding range of possibilities. Current algorithms have potential to undergo an evolution from automating routine tasks such as single-unit restorations to an emerging role as an indispensable tool in complex and interdisciplinary rehabilitations. For this purpose, the current performance of AI algorithms should be compared with established clinical standards, in order to identify advantages and specific challenges inherent to each stage of prosthetic design and treatment planning.

10.2.1 Automated Design of Single-Unit Restorations

The design of single-unit restorations is one of the most developed areas for AI application, offering significant potential to streamline daily clinical workflows. Recent comparative studies have shown that AI can design full crowns with an overall morphology comparable to that of experienced dental technicians [5]. The aforementioned study found that while designs from both groups (AI and dental technicians) produced larger buccal cusp angles than natural teeth, AI-designed crowns demonstrated superior dimensional accuracy. Buccal-lingual and mesial-distal measurements of AI crowns closely matched those of natural teeth, whereas technician-designed crowns were often dimensionally smaller or different.

The primary limitation identified in current AI systems is their inability to accurately reproduce functional cusp wear facets and occlusal contact areas. In contrast, technician designs showed greater accuracy in this task, despite sometimes overcompensating for wear [5]. Regarding time efficiency, however, the AI system tested can generate a crown design in an average time of 10–20 s, compared to approximately 6 min for an experienced dental technician. To address morphological limitations, advanced AI models like 3D deep convolutional generative adversarial networks (3D-DCGAN) and point-to-mesh transformers (DCrownFormer) are being developed to improve the generation of fine anatomical details and create complete 3D meshes directly from scan data [6–8].

One of the AI models of the aforementioned citations adopts an end-to-end framework designed to directly generate high-fidelity dental crown meshes from

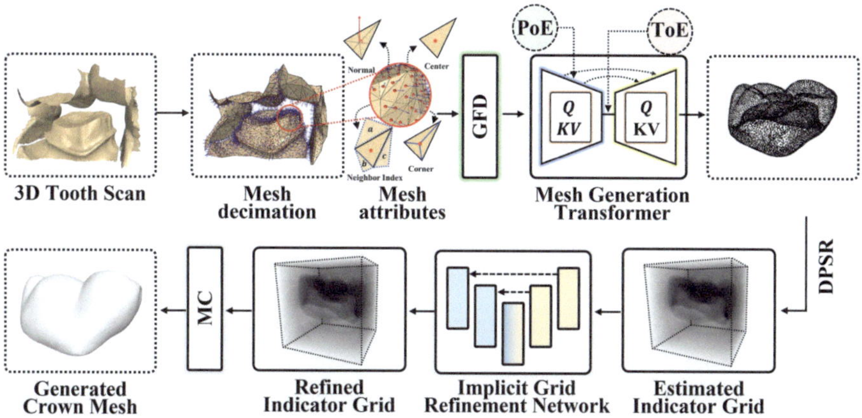

Fig. 10.1 Overview of our DCrownFormer+. GFD, DPSR, and MC are the geometric feature attention descriptor, differentiable Poisson surface reconstruction, and marching cube, respectively. PoE and ToE indicate positional conditioning and tooth-type encoding. The fire symbol within circles means trainable parameters

three-dimensional scan data of preparation and antagonist teeth [8]. Rather than decoupling point generation and mesh reconstruction into separate pipelines, the framework integrates these steps into a unified architecture. The overall process consists of three key stages: extraction of rich geometric features from mesh inputs, transformer-based generation of crown points and normal, and implicit surface reconstruction and refinement for mesh generation [9]. This integrated design reduces error propagation between stages and enables joint optimization of general shape and local surface details (Fig. 10.1).

10.2.1.1 Clinical Case Study: Automated Single Crown Design (Case by Dr. Roberto A. Markarian)

This case report describes the prosthetic rehabilitation of a 55-year-old female patient presenting with a compromised monolithic zirconia crown on a molar. The indication for replacement was diagnosed as secondary caries associated with marginal infiltration. The primary clinical objective was to restore function and aesthetics using a lithium disilicate restoration (Ivoclar IPS e.max CAD). This case represents the first clinical evaluation of an AI module integrated into the CAD software, to test the feasibility, accuracy, and efficiency of a fully automated design workflow, compared with the traditional manual digital design used in the clinic. The accompanying documentation includes patient's history, initial intraoral photographs, panoramic and periapical radiographs, screen recordings of the design and editing phases, and photographs of the final cementation. The patient signed an informed consent.

Following the acquisition of intraoral scans using a TRIOS 3 intraoral scanner (3Shape A/S), the digital workflow was initiated within the 3Shape Dental Designer (2025 version). Instead of the conventional manual design protocol, a newly integrated AI tool was utilized (3Shape Automate). Upon case creation, the scan data was uploaded directly to the manufacturer's cloud-based server via a dedicated interface. The processing time for the automated design generation ranged between 5 and 15 min. Upon notification of completion, the system presented a 3D proposal of the restoration, including the automatically detected finish line (margin) and anatomical contours. The workflow allows for two distinct pathways: direct approval or manual editing.

To rigorously test capabilities of this AI tool, the initial AI-driven crown design was approved for manufacturing without any manual intervention. However, intraoral evaluation of this first crown revealed a discrepancy in the marginal integrity. Specifically, the restoration was under-extended at the vestibular (buccal) margin, exposing the preparation (Fig. 10.2).

The system provides a "verification" stage where the operator can inspect the automated proposal in a 3D environment before manufacturing. If the proposal is suboptimal, the software seamlessly transitions to standard CAD tools for manual refinement. Consequently, the project was reopened in the software's standard CAD editor. The marginal line was redefined to correct the vestibular deficiency, and minor adjustments were made to the anatomy and contours. The corrected design was then exported and milled using a Sirona MC XL milling unit utilizing Ivoclar IPS e.max CAD block, followed by crystallization according to the manufacturer's instructions (Fig. 10.3).

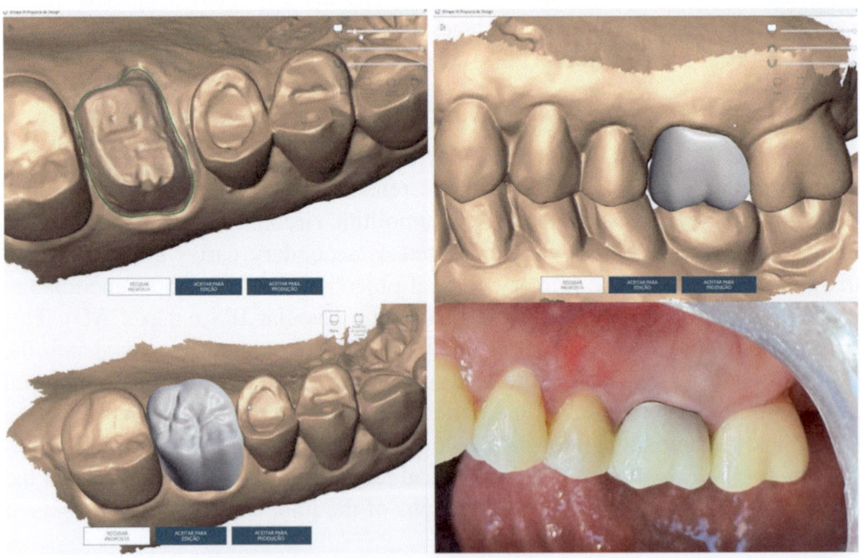

Fig. 10.2 CAD-CAM single crown designed by the AI tool of 3Shape Automate (left and top right images) without any human manual intervention and the respective clinical try-in result (bottom right image), showing unsatisfactory marginal adaptation at the buccal aspect of the crown

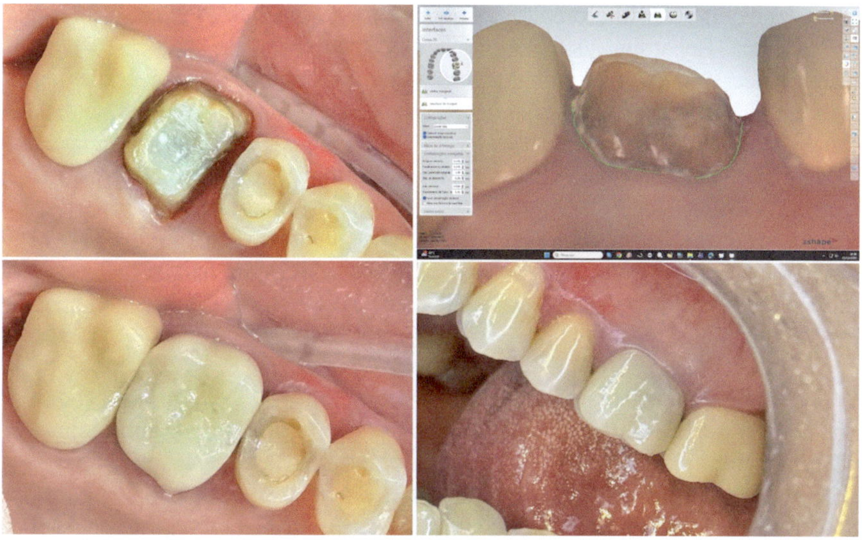

Fig. 10.3 Final clinical result of the CAD-CAM single crown designed by the AI tool after correction by human manual intervention on the design, which included optimization of the crown margin design (top right image)

The present AI tool functions by segmenting the scan data and proposing a complete design via remote cloud processing. The AI algorithm is programmed to strictly adhere to predefined design parameters set within the software's control panel. Variables such as cement spacer thickness, drill radius compensation, minimum thickness, and marginal ramp width are established by the operator prior to the workflow. The AI tool respects these constraints while autonomously generating the variable anatomy and marginal fit. It is noteworthy that at the time of this procedure, the AI feature was in a progressive implementation phase. Its scope is currently limited to single units or short-span fixed partial dentures (up to three crowns or veneers simultaneously). Complex rehabilitations are not yet supported by this specific AI module.

Clinically, the final restoration was functional and well-adapted. A minor aesthetic discrepancy was noted, as the ceramic shade presented slightly higher value (lighter) than the adjacent natural dentition. However, due to the limited availability of the patient for corrections, the restoration was cemented with the full approval of the patient, who confirmed satisfaction. Despite the remaining need of human oversight, the laboratory protocol was updated to adopt the use of this AI-driven design tool as the standard operating procedure for eligible cases of the present clinic because of the faster and more effective workflow for short-span prosthetic rehabilitations.

Finally, it is important to address the commercial accessibility of this technology. This AI tool is not an open-platform solution but is deeply integrated into the proprietary 3Shape Dental System ecosystem. Access necessitates a comprehensive annual subscription, representing a significant financial investment that effectively limits its availability to professional laboratories or specialized clinics rather than casual users. Regarding technical scalability, the current iteration restricts automated processing to a maximum of three simultaneous units. However, the manufacturer has indicated a developmental roadmap to progressively expand these capabilities, aiming to include a wider array of restorative indications and accommodate more extensive rehabilitation scenarios in future software updates.

In conclusion, while the system can autonomously remove visual interference (soft tissue artifacts) and propose digital designs, human oversight remains mandatory. The present AI tool can be defined as an assistive tool to handle routinely performed tasks, allowing the professional to focus on complex aesthetic and functional aspects of the oral rehabilitation.

10.2.1.2 AI-Driven Design of Inlay Restorations

For inlay restorations, deep learning workflows have also significantly improved time efficiency, particularly for beginner-level users, which effectively narrows the skill gap. A previous related study demonstrated that an AI-driven DL-based workflow without manual optimization could produce designs quickly but often resulted in a high frequency of heavy premature occlusal contacts and suboptimal contour quality [10]. This finding highlights that human expertise remains crucial in prosthetic and restorative dental treatments. Technician intervention was necessary to modify the initial AI-generated designs to achieve clinically acceptable occlusal contacts, proximal contacts, and contours. Therefore, in the context of inlay design, it is suggested that AI can currently be used as a powerful tool along with dental technician skills to improve outcomes and boost efficiency, rather than as a fully autonomous replacement for human oversight and clinical judgment.

10.2.1.3 Clinical Case Study: AI-Driven Design of Onlay Restorations (Clinical Case by Dr. Roberto A. Markarian)

This case describes the restorative treatment of a 25-year-old female patient presenting with a compromised mandibular right first molar. The tooth exhibited a history of recurrent marginal leakage and secondary caries associated with extensive preexisting class II composite resin restorations. Due to the significant volumetric loss of tooth structure and the need for biomechanical reinforcement, the treatment plan indicated a transition from direct restoration to an indirect partial ceramic coverage (onlay). The primary objective was to arrest the carious progression and restore function while preserving the tooth's vitality.

The clinical procedure began with the removal of the defective restorations. Careful tactile exploration (probing) of the cavity floor confirmed the complete removal of carious tissue. The pulp vitality was preserved, and no endodontic therapy was required. The preparation followed conventional guidelines for ceramic onlays, ensuring adequate reduction and smooth internal line angles.

A digital workflow was performed, starting with an intraoral digital impression, which was captured using the TRIOS 3 scanner (3Shape A/S). Utilizing the "one-click" feature within the 3Shape Dental System, the scan data was uploaded

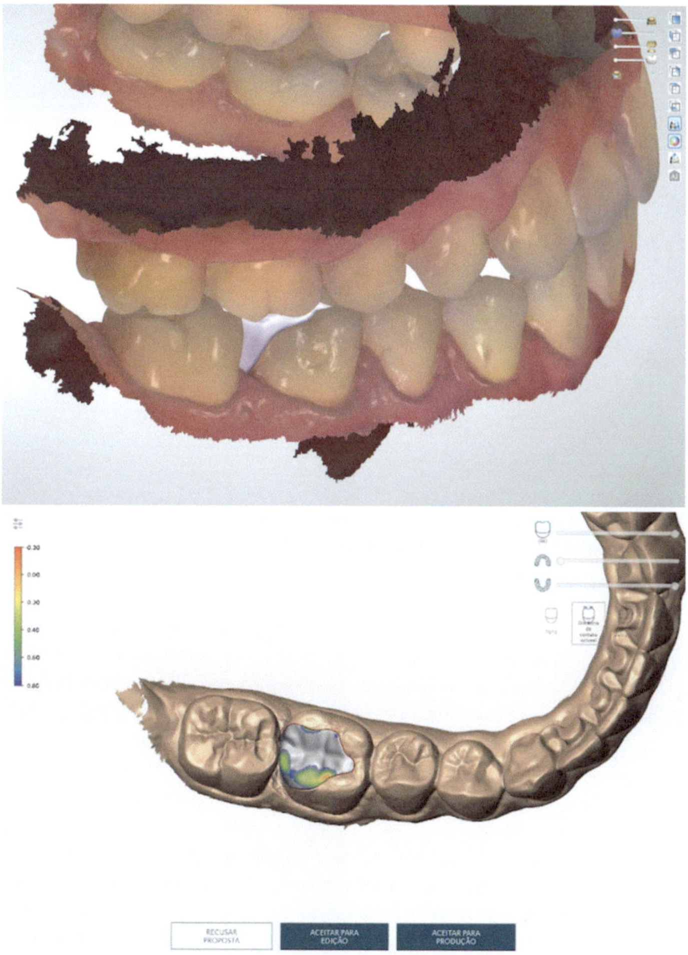

Fig. 10.4 CAD-CAM onlay restoration designed by the AI tool of 3Shape Automate (left and top right images). Initial aspect before any human manual intervention

directly to the cloud-based AI service (3Shape Automate). Approximately 10 min post-submission, the system returned a fully modeled restoration proposal (Fig. 10.4). The proposed AI-driven onlay design was reviewed collaboratively by the dental technician and the clinician. Minor manual adjustments were applied via the CAD editor to optimize margin limits, the contact points, and occlusal anatomy (Fig. 10.5). Upon approval, the file was exported for CAM processing. The restoration was milled from a lithium disilicate block (Ivoclar IPS e.max CAD) using a Sirona MC XL milling unit (Fig. 10.6) and luted on the preparation with a resin cement (Ivoclar Variolink).

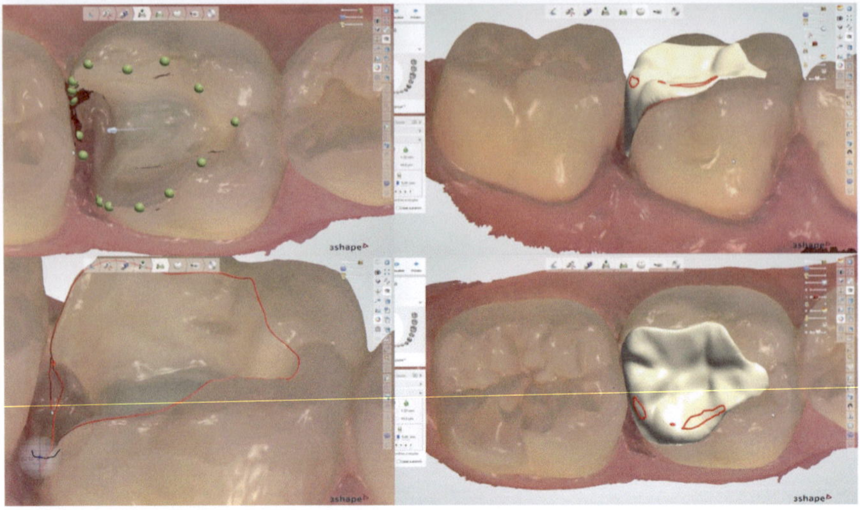

Fig. 10.5 Optimization of the onlay design on the CAD software, performed by a certified dental technician

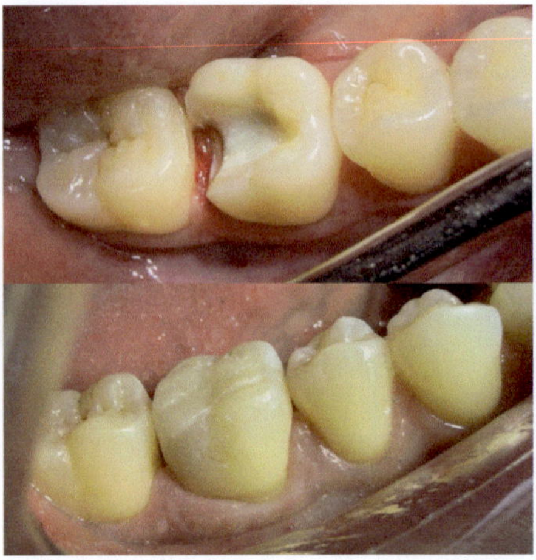

Fig. 10.6 Preparation (top) and final clinical result of the CAD-CAM onlay restoration designed by the AI tool after correction by human manual intervention (bottom)

While the AI provided a viable baseline design within a short timeframe (10 min), the software architecture allowed for seamless manual intervention. As discussed in the previous case study of a single crown, this hybrid approach ensured that the algorithmic proposal could be further improved to meet specific clinical preferences before manufacturing.

10.2.2 AI in Occlusal Analysis and Devices

Beyond single restorations, AI is being applied to more complex occlusal challenges, including determining maxillomandibular relationships and fabricating occlusal devices. AI-based programs such as Bite-Finder (Bite-Finder company) can automatically articulate non-articulated intraoral scans to establish the maximum intercuspal position (MIP) with satisfactory performance [11] and simulate excursive movements (Fig. 10.7). In this context, findings from the aforementioned study have suggested that these AI programs can achieve an MIP accuracy that is comparable to or even better than the native software of some intraoral scanners.

Nevertheless, the performance of this AI software is significantly impacted by the specific IOS system used to acquire the initial scans. For instance, using an AI tool to correct occlusal collisions improved MIP trueness for scans acquired with some systems (e.g., iTero, PrimeScan) but actually decreased trueness for others (e.g., TRIOS 4, i700). Satisfactory results can also be obtained using AI tools of CAD software programs to correct the occlusion on intraoral scans mounted on virtual articulators, as shown in Chap. 7 with the Zirkonzahn Modifier software. All these findings highlight a complex interaction between scanning technology and AI algorithms, indicating that results are not universally consistent across different hardware and software combinations [11].

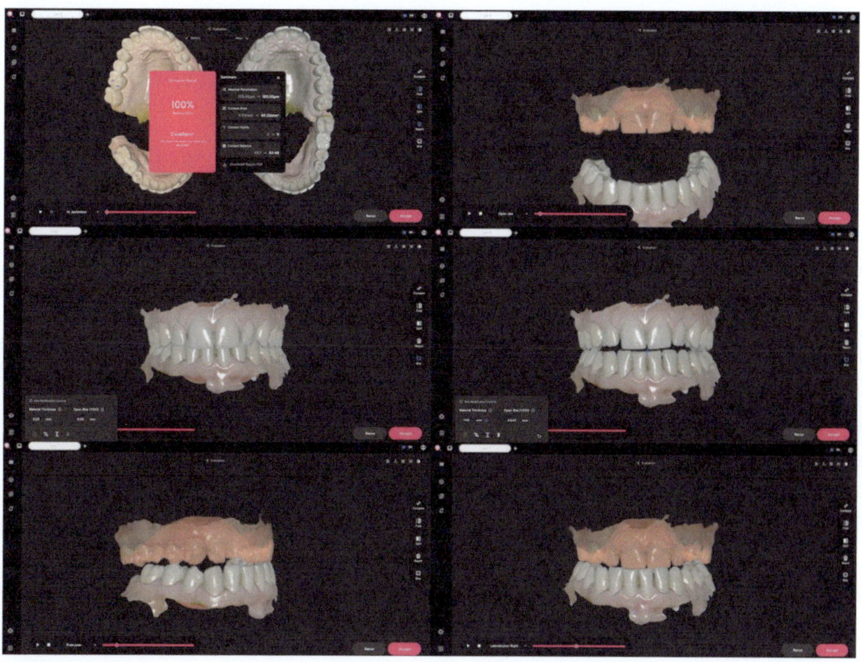

Fig. 10.7 Screenshots of the Bite-Finder AI tool performing automated articulation of intraoral scans and simulation of occlusal movements

Regarding the automated design of occlusal devices, AI has demonstrated high repeatability but notable differences when compared to human experts. A previous study compared occlusal devices designed by an experienced dental technician with those generated by two AI software programs (Medit Splints and 3Shape Automate). The results showed significant discrepancies in the overall, intaglio (internal), and occlusal surfaces between the AI-generated devices and the technician-designed reference [9]. This suggests that the some of the underlying design principles, such as the path of insertion and occlusal patterns, determined by the AI algorithms may be fundamentally different from those applied by a human expert. While the AI designs were highly consistent, the clinical impact of these discrepancies is not yet understood and requires further investigation to determine their suitability for patient care.

10.3 AI in Esthetic and Interdisciplinary Rehabilitation

AI-based digital smile design (DSD) tools, such as SmileCloud (presented for prosthetically driven implant planning in the previous chapter), REBEL, and Invisalign SmileView, have been shown to significantly improve facial esthetic outcomes. A recent systematic review reported a high pooled patient and clinician satisfaction prevalence of 58% when using these tools [12]. AI algorithms analyze facial images and dental features to provide personalized treatment strategies that enhance smile symmetry, harmonize lip arcs, and optimize incisal edge visibility [12, 13]. Furthermore, as mentioned in the previous chapter, AI-powered software programs such as SmileCloud 3DNA (SmileCloud SRL) can generate realistic 2D and 3D simulations of treatment outcomes (Fig. 10.8). This capability dramatically

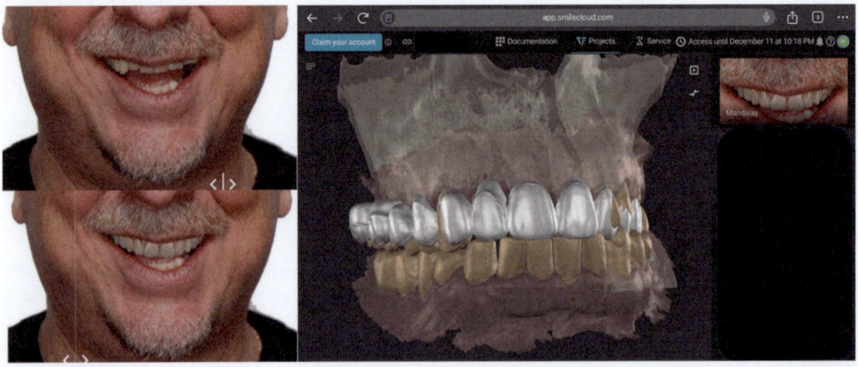

Fig. 10.8 AI-driven smile design (left) and screen capture of the corresponding 3D virtual mock-up (right) using the SmileCloud 3DNA platform (treatment planning performed by Dr. Mauricio Pesce Gomes da Costa, from Doc Labs Digital, São Paulo, Brazil). The screen capture shows the interface by which dentists can receive the case in the cloud-based platform from the dental laboratories. A chat window for discussion about the case among the professionals is also available in the platform

enhances patient-dentist communication, allows for informed decision-making before any irreversible procedures begin, and ultimately increases treatment acceptance rates [14, 15]. Furthermore, the impact of AI in prosthetic rehabilitations has been assessed by several studies [16–18].

10.3.1 Clinical Case Study: The Use of AI in a Prosthetically Driven Implant Therapy (Case by Prof. Newton Sesma, Dr. Lisya Vizotto de Barros, Dr. Sergio Candido Dias, Dr. Bruno B. R. Matias, and Dr. Marcelo Lucchesi Teixeira)

A 54-year-old female patient presented with esthetic and functional impairment, reporting masticatory difficulty and instability of a provisional maxillary removable partial denture. Clinical examination indicated loss of occlusal stability, compromised smile harmony, and the need for fixed implant-supported rehabilitation to restore function and vertical dimension.

A complete digital diagnostic workflow was performed, including extraoral and intraoral photographs, intraoral scanning (STL files), cone beam computed tomography (CBCT, DICOM files), and panoramic radiography. Both maxillary and mandibular scans were automatically aligned in occlusion and analyzed using the AI tool of Bite-Finder (Bite-Finder AG). Digital smile design and three-dimensional diagnostic waxing were conducted using Smilecloud software (Smilecloud Biometrics, Spain), which employs artificial intelligence algorithms to correlate occlusion, smile line, and gingival contours (Fig. 10.9). The digital wax-up was transferred to coDiagnostiX software (Dental Wings, Straumann Group, Switzerland) for STL-DICOM data fusion and prosthetically guided implant planning. The treatment plan included preservation of posterior molars for later indirect restorations, extraction of teeth 14 and 24, and implant placement in the anterior and premolar regions. Straumann BLX implants (Straumann AG, Basel, Switzerland) and screw-retained abutments (SRA, Straumann) were selected.

Surgical and prosthetic procedures were performed using a stackable guide system composed of three guides, despite the presence of remaining teeth. This approach was selected to ensure that the provisional prosthesis would be positioned exactly as defined during digital smile planning and that implant access openings would precisely coincide with the planned implant positions [19, 20]. A fully mucosa-supported base guide was designed to serve as a stable reference for the prosthetic phase. A tooth-supported positioning guide was then used to accurately seat and fix the base guide with transosseous pins, ensuring reproducible positioning. All subsequent guides were supported by this base guide, preserving the spatial relationship between surgical and prosthetic phases.

Following stabilization of the base guide, tooth extraction was performed, and a surgical guide was attached using the stackable system. Fully guided implant placement was carried out with Straumann BLX implants at positions 15 and 25

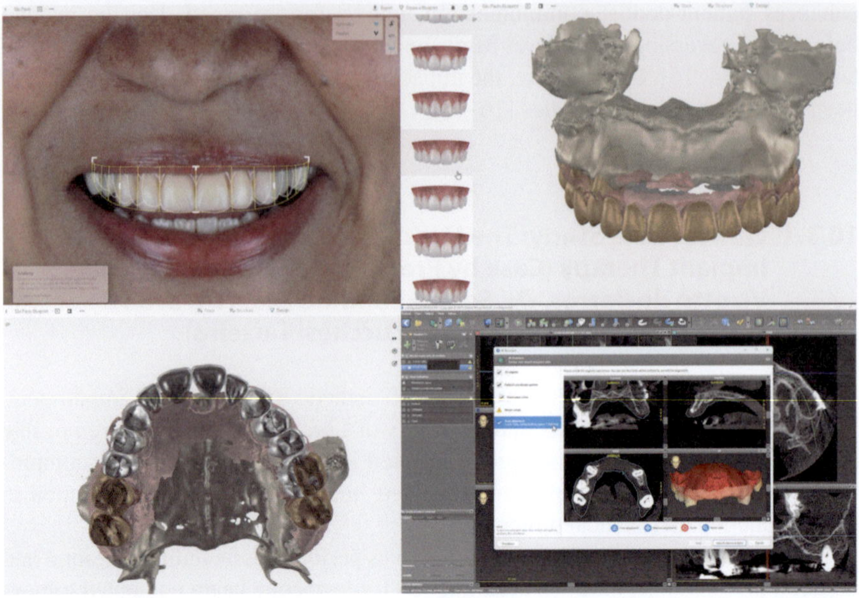

Fig. 10.9 AI-driven digital 2D (top left) and 3D prosthetic design (bottom left and top right) with SmileCloud and AI-powered automated alignment of CBCT and intraoral scans on the coDiagnostiX software (bottom right)

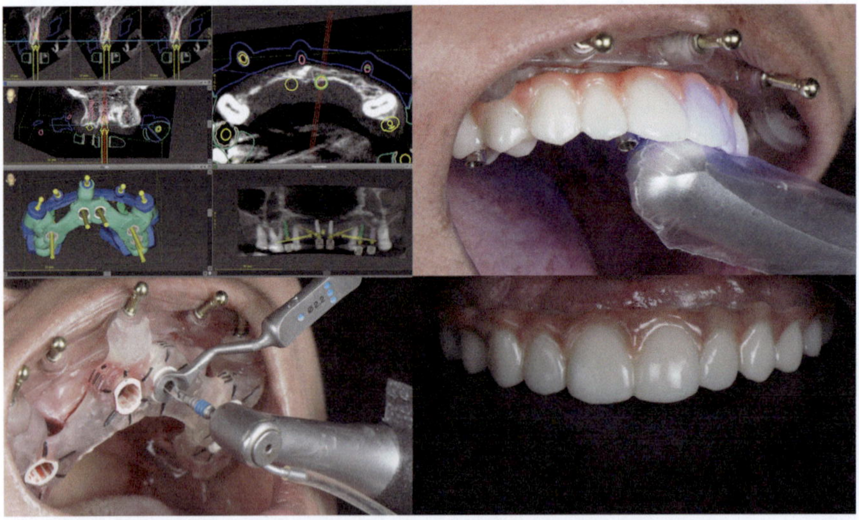

Fig. 10.10 Prosthetically driven implant therapy

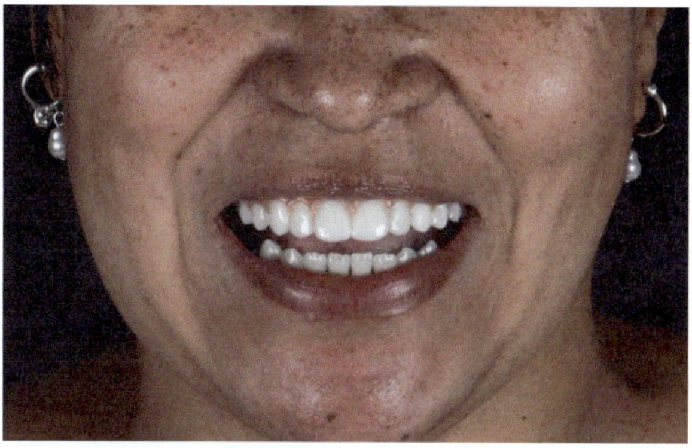

Fig. 10.11 Final clinical result of the patient's smile

(4.5 × 12 mm, SLActive), 12 and 22 (3.5 × 12 mm, SLActive), and 26 (5.0 × 8 mm, SLActive), followed by immediate connection of SRA abutments (Fig. 10.10).

The provisional prosthesis, digitally designed in Smilecloud, was fabricated by 3D printing (Espectra Printer, Straumann Group) using Yller Cosmos Plus Full-Arch resin (Yller Biomaterials, Brazil; 65% ceramic filler). A capture guide was used to position the prosthesis onto the base guide, ensuring passive fit and accurate occlusal positioning. The prosthetic cylinders were finally captured using flowable bulk-fill composite resin (Opus Bulk Fill Flow, FGM, Brazil), followed by finishing and polishing (Fig. 10.11).

The choice of a tooth-supported positioning guide combined with a mucosa-supported base guide in this partially edentulous case was based on well-established evidence regarding the influence of guide support on implant placement accuracy. Previous studies and systematic reviews have consistently demonstrated that tooth-supported surgical guides exhibit lower linear and angular deviations when compared with mucosa-supported guides, particularly due to their superior mechanical stability and resistance to displacement during drilling. In contrast, mucosa-supported guides may be affected by soft tissue resilience and compression, resulting in reduced precision, especially in situations requiring high prosthetic accuracy [21, 22]. By using a tooth-supported guide to position and stabilize the base guide, this workflow capitalized on the accuracy advantages of dental support while maintaining a stable reference for the subsequent surgical and prosthetic phases. This strategy is supported by the current literature and is particularly relevant in cases requiring immediate or highly precise prosthetic capture. Thereby, this digitally integrated workflow enabled precise surgical execution and prosthetic accuracy, illustrating the clinical value of AI-assisted planning combined with stackable guided systems, even in partially edentulous situations.

This integrated AI-assisted approach ensures high predictability and fidelity between the virtual plan and the final clinical result. It also streamlines communication and coordination among different dental specialists, ensuring all phases of treatment are aligned with the initial esthetic goal. This level of integration represents a significant step forward in managing complex restorative cases.

10.3.2 Clinical Case Study: The Use of AI in the Rehabilitation of the Esthetic Area (Case by Dr. Lincoln Queirós)

The patient sought treatment for the final stages of orthodontic treatment. Initial clinical examination revealed a conical maxillary right lateral incisor (tooth 12), partial loss of canine guidance, and small incisal fractures on teeth 11 and 21 (Fig. 10.12). The first use of artificial intelligence (AI) in this case was to evaluate the occlusion. Using the Medit Occlusion Analyzer app (Medit), it was possible to analyze the patient's occlusion aesthetically and dynamically (Fig. 10.13).

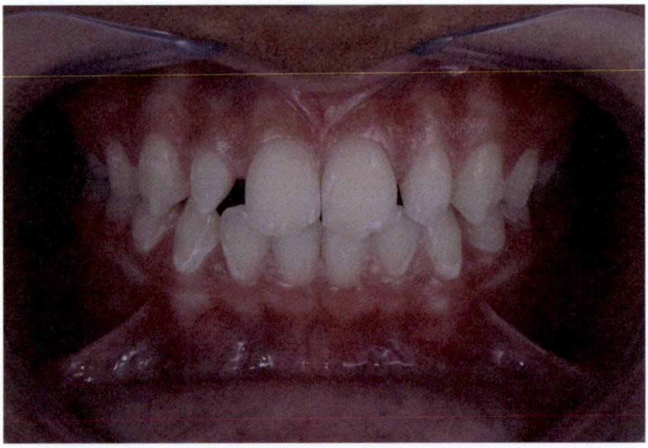

Fig. 10.12 Initial clinical intraoral aspect

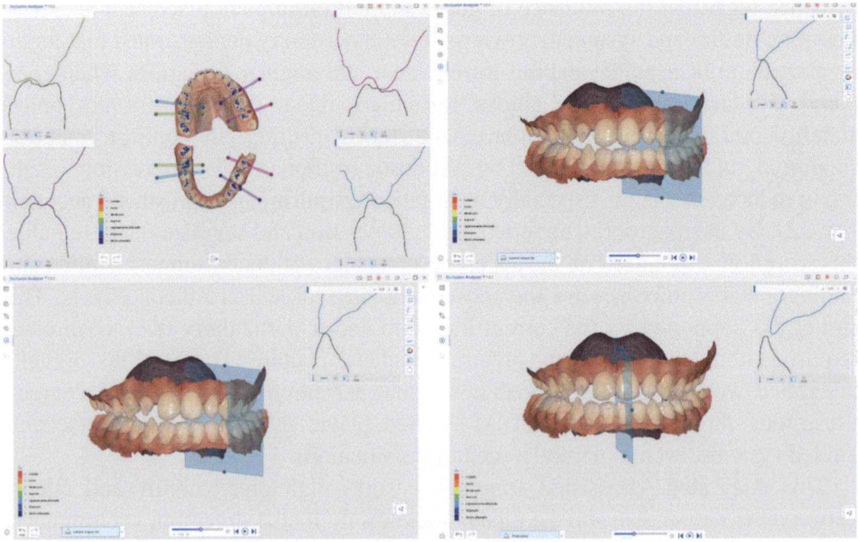

Fig. 10.13 Automated occlusion analysis (Medit Occlusion Analyzer app) in centric (top left) and lateral excursion (bottom left and top right) and protrusion (bottom right)

The patient's natural occlusal movements, recorded with the i900 intraoral scanner (Medit), allowed for the evaluation of the absence of partial contact on the left lateral movement, total contact on the right, and protrusive contact. The patient's 3D data was recorded according to the virtual patient technique described in the previous book, and the digital diagnostic wax-up was performed in DentalCAD (Exocad, Align Technology), taking into account the specific mandibular movement as a starting point and correcting it with the re-anatomization of teeth 13–23 (Fig. 10.14).

After the aesthetic restorative mock-up (performed with bis-acrylic resin) was approved (Fig. 10.15), preparations and a working intraoral scan were performed. The technique used was then the double scanning with the use of AI auxiliary intelligent scanning filters (Fig. 10.16). These allow for a more fluid digital procedure, with fewer interruptions and less variations of scanner head movements, which, according to the literature, favors greater precision in the final digital model [22, 23]. An important detail was that the original diagnostic wax-up file was imported as a supplementary file, which was aligned with the reference model (mock-up scan) and used for the final design in DentalCAD (Exocad) as the reference model

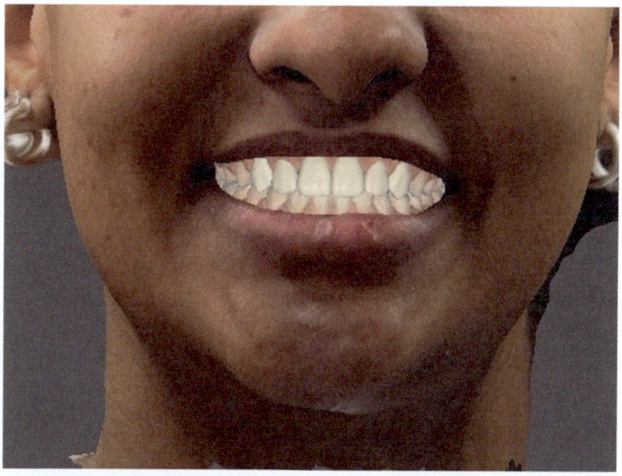

Fig. 10.14 Digital mock-up (Exocad)

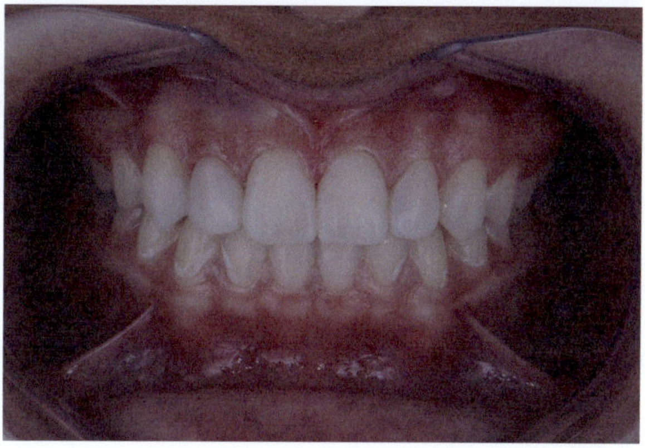

Fig. 10.15 Mock-up try-in

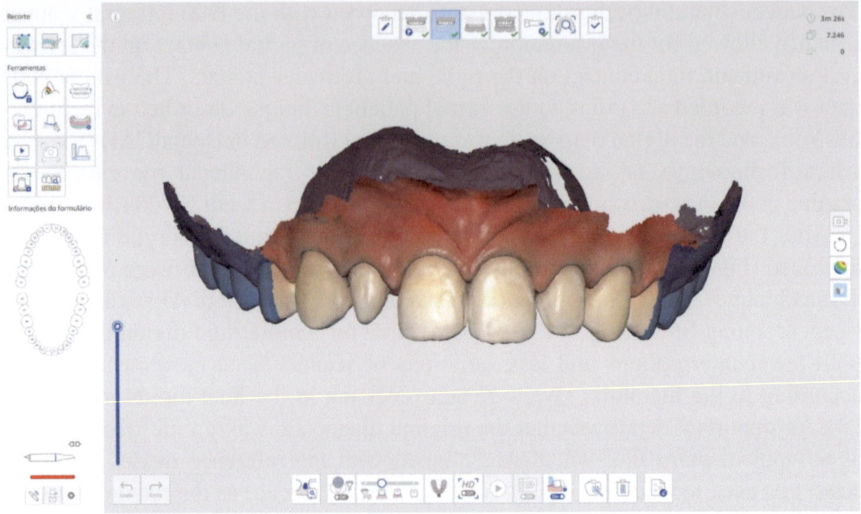

Fig. 10.16 Preparations and the use of AI filter (Medit i900)

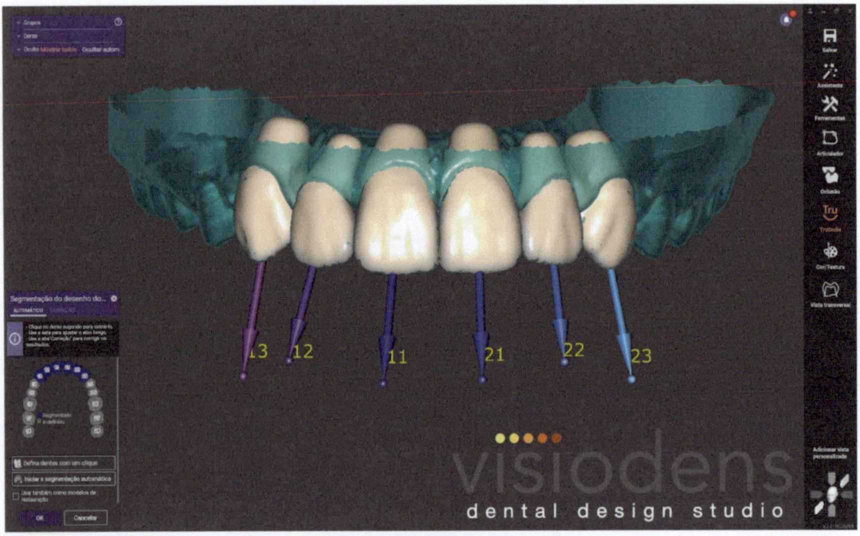

Fig. 10.17 Automated segmentation used during digital wax-up (Exocad)

itself. This makes possible the precision of yet another AI-assisted step: digital dental segmentation for copying the anatomy of the wax-up (Fig. 10.17). Within Exocad, this feature allows AI-assisted segmentation of the anatomy of the diagnostic wax-up, and the software allows the use of this segmentation as the anatomy of the final restoration (Fig. 10.18). This provides a faithful copy of the design, including in proximal regions, which significantly reduces design time and increases the precision and fidelity of the final restoration.

Once the restorations were designed, the milling, finishing, and pigmentation of the lithium disilicate veneers followed (Fig. 10.19). At the end of the trials and cementation, it was possible to observe improved outcomes using AI resources (Fig. 10.20), as well as a reduction in chairside occlusal adjustments and faster patient adaptation to the work performed. In conclusion, AI can be an important ally in improving the experience of patients and the clinical team, optimizing processes and improving clinical steps.

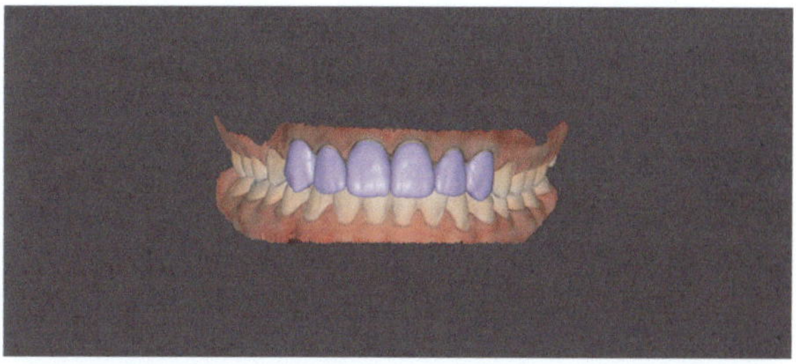

Fig. 10.18 Final digital designs

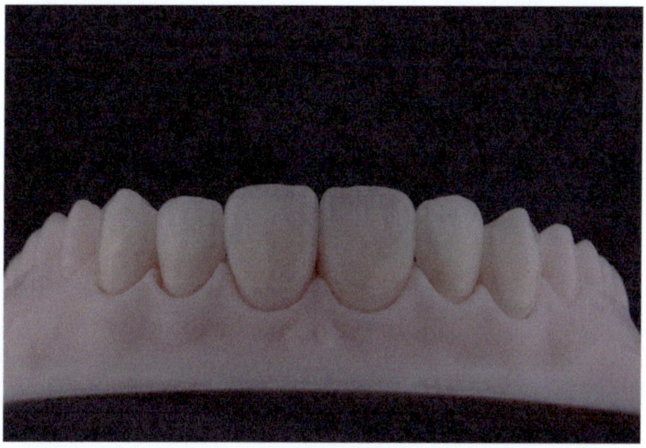

Fig. 10.19 Final CAD-CAM restorations on the 3D-printed dental cast

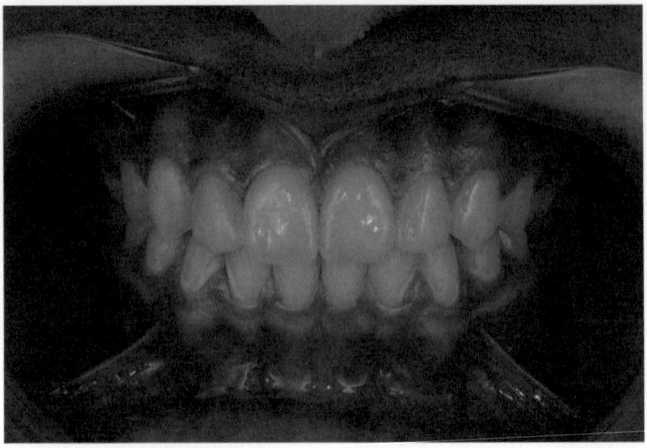

Fig. 10.20 Final clinical result of the case

10.4 AI-Driven Occlusal Splint Design

In the near future, AI workflows are expected to assist all stages of the occlusal splint design. Currently, the assistance of most AI systems enables peripheral delimitation based on patient-specific dental anatomy, reducing operator-dependent variability and improving appliance adaptation and comfort. In addition, AI supports standardized adjustment of centric occlusal contacts, promoting balanced force distribution and enhancing static mandibular stability. During eccentric movements, AI-assisted analysis minimizes occlusal interferences along protrusive and lateral trajectories, thereby contributing to dynamic mandibular stability and protection of the temporomandibular joints. By digitally optimizing both static and dynamic occlusal contacts, artificial intelligence reduces the need for extensive chairside adjustments, shortens clinical time, and improves reproducibility across cases. Furthermore, this technology enables the reproduction of average mandibular movements and inclinations while allowing subsequent personalization according to individual functional requirements. Importantly, AI functions as a decision-support tool integrated within the digital workflow, enhancing the implementation of established occlusal principles without replacing clinical judgment.

10.4.1 Clinical Case Study: Occlusal Splint with AI-Assisted Design and Functional Occlusal Adjustment

In this case, an occlusal splint workflow was conducted entirely within the iTero Design Suite (Align Technology, Israel) software environment, starting with the creation of a digital work order (Fig. 10.21). Patient's intraoral scans served as the primary dataset for occlusal splint planning, providing accurate three-dimensional representations of the dental arches. Following data import, the anteroposterior insertion axis of the occlusal splint was defined to ensure appropriate path of insertion and seating of the appliance. Subsequently, artificial intelligence was employed to automatically define the peripheral delimitation of the occlusal splint. This

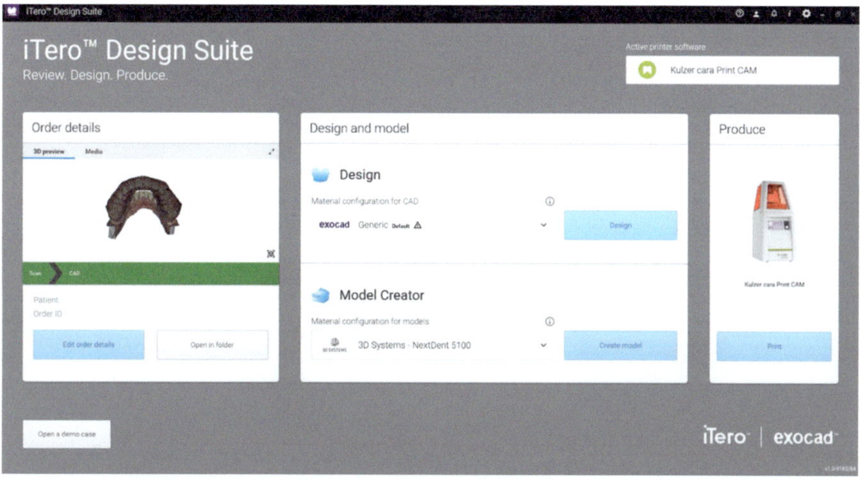

Fig. 10.21 Initial screen of the iTero Design Suite software displaying the work order for occlusal splint planning based on the patient's intraoral scans

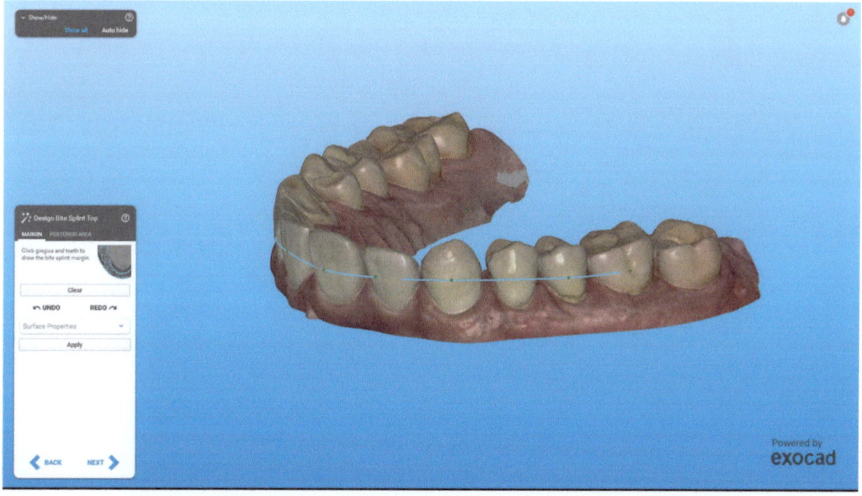

Fig. 10.22 Artificial intelligence-based initial peripheral delimitation of the occlusal splint, enabling the professional to complement the design

AI-based margin definition was initially generated according to the patient's individual dental anatomy (Fig. 10.22). Based on this peripheral delimitation, the occlusal splint design was generated and visualized in both frontal (vestibular) and occlusal views, allowing verification of overall morphology and extension.

After initial design, artificial intelligence was used to adjust occlusal contacts in centric relation (Fig. 10.23). Contact points were analyzed and optimized to promote balanced force distribution, ensuring static mandibular stability. The occlusal

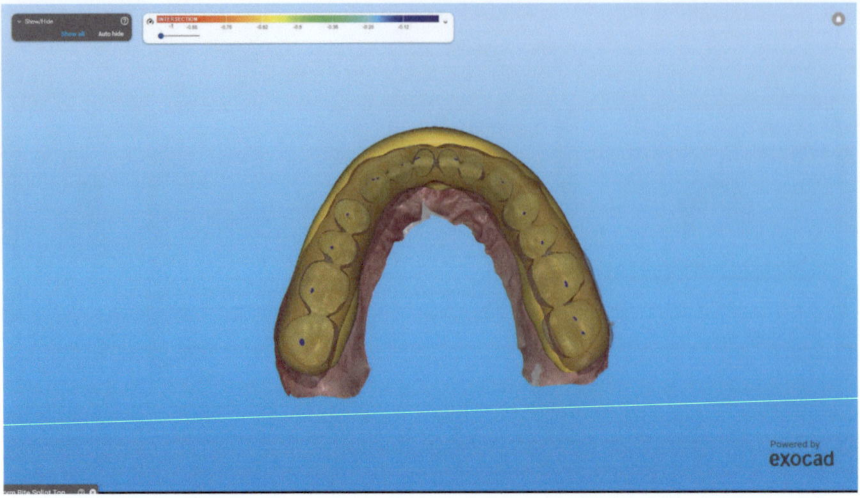

Fig. 10.23 Centric relation contact points adjusted by artificial intelligence; occlusal view

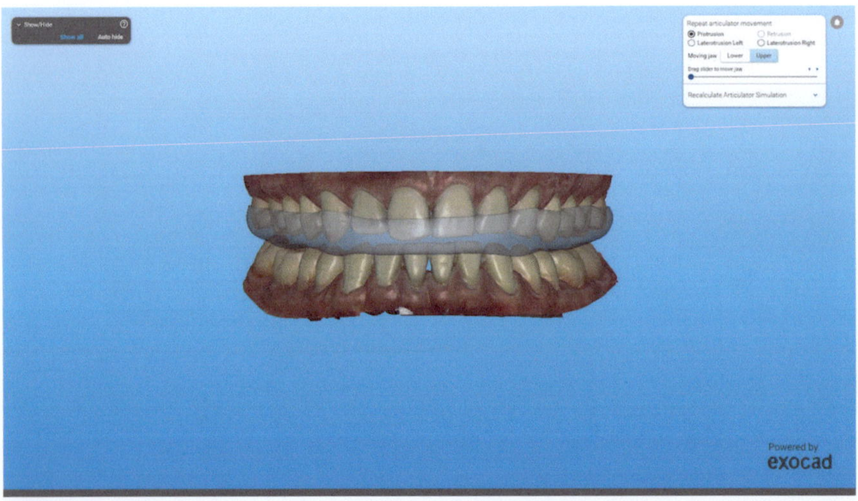

Fig. 10.24 Occlusal splint design in centric relation after occlusal adjustments performed by artificial intelligence; frontal/vestibular view

contacts were then further refined by means of AI-assisted adjustments during functional mandibular movements. Protrusive movement contacts were evaluated and optimized to minimize interferences, followed by similar adjustments during left and right lateral excursions. These steps aimed to enhance dynamic mandibular stability by controlling contact patterns throughout eccentric movements. Once occlusal adjustments were completed, the final occlusal splint design was evaluated in centric relation (Fig. 10.24) as well as during protrusive and lateral movements,

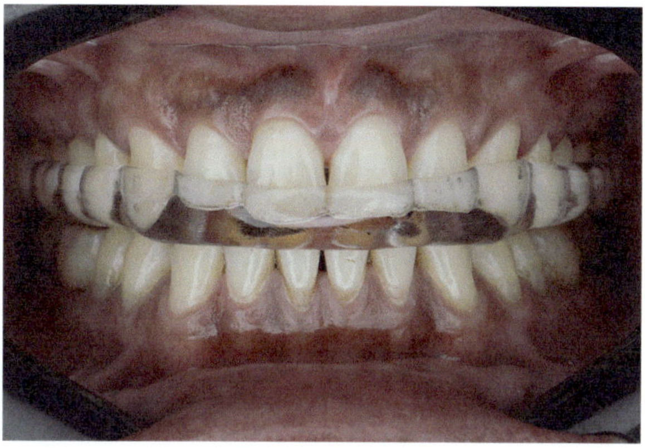

Fig. 10.25 Final intraoral photograph of the occlusal splint try-in

with frontal and occlusal visualizations confirming the consistency of the occlusal scheme across static and dynamic conditions. The finalized design was then manufactured by milling from a transparent PMMA ProArt CAD Splint disc (Ivoclar, Lichtenstein). Finally, the occlusal splint was clinically delivered, and its fit and adaptation were documented with an intraoral photograph (Fig. 10.25).

10.4.2 Clinical Case Study: AI-Automated Design of an Occlusal Splint for TMD Management (Case by Dr. Roberto A. Markarian)

This is a clinical report of the management of a 24-year-old female patient presenting with clinical signs and symptoms of temporomandibular disorder (TMD) associated with nocturnal parafunctional habits (sleep bruxism). The patient's chief complaint included morning tension headaches and masticatory muscle fatigue. The therapeutic objective was to fabricate a rigid occlusal stabilization splint (night guard) to alleviate muscle hyperactivity, reprogram the mandibular position, and increase the vertical dimension of occlusion.

The digital workflow commenced with intraoral data acquisition using a TRIOS 3 scanner (3Shape A/S). An important feature of this phase was the recording of functional mandibular movements, allowing the digital design to account for the patient's specific dynamic envelope of motion. The scan data was converted to STL format and uploaded to the HeyGears Cloud platform for automated planning.

During the setup, specific design parameters were defined, including minimum thickness, offset settings, and the desired degree of intercuspation (Fig. 10.26). A "flat plane" occlusion with minimal, well-distributed contacts was selected. Approximately 10 min post-submission, the system performed AI generation and returned a complete design proposal without prior manual interaction. Upon inspection, the AI proposal was deemed structurally sound but geometrically simplified, as it utilized a plane device without any protrusive and laterality considerations.

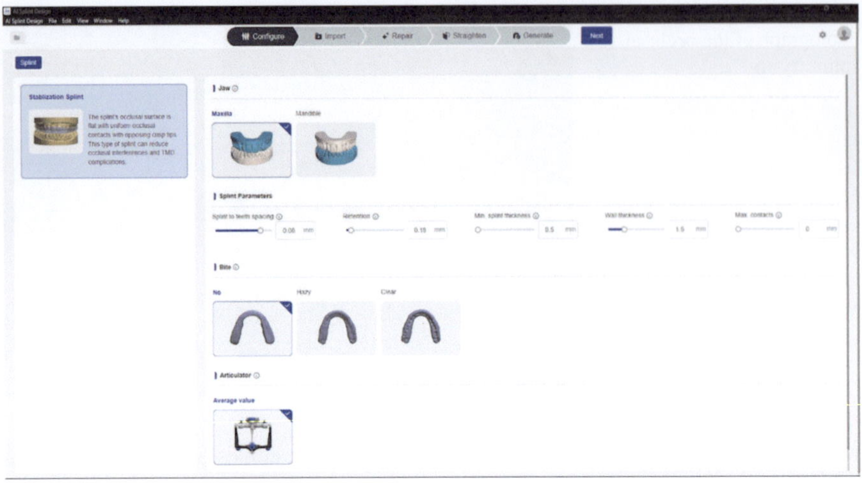

Fig. 10.26 AI splint design setup (HeyGears)

Consequently, a manual editing step was performed within the same software interface to create ramps to refine and ensure the presence of these guidance functional features (Figs. 10.27 and 10.28).

Following approval, the file was sent for additive manufacturing on a HeyGears UltraCraft Chairside Pro 3D printer. The material selected was Keystone KeySplint Soft. Intraoral evaluation revealed optimal internal adaptation requiring no internal adjustments. Occlusal adjustments were minimal and comparable to conventional workflows. The splint was then polished and delivered (Fig. 10.29).

This AI system demonstrated high efficiency (intuitive interface, rapid 10-min generation). However, the automated output exhibited a tendency toward oversimplified occlusal schemes (ramps). The platform's integrated editor proved essential, allowing the clinician to easily modify the design to incorporate specific functional guidance, demonstrating a flexible workflow that combines automation with clinical customization.

An important aspect of this case was the material performance. Although KeySplint Soft is classified as a rigid resin at room temperature, it possesses thermoplastic properties. This allows for a unique "thermo-adaptation" using warm water for fine-tuning while providing a tactile feel that is less brittle and harsh than conventional polymethyl methacrylate (PMMA) acrylics.

At the 30-day follow-up, the clinical outcome was highly favorable. The patient reported total remission of morning symptoms and explicitly noted that the device was significantly more comfortable than previous appliances she had utilized. This case, supported by previous pilot tests conducted by our team under a temporary license, confirms the reliability of the system. The combination of AI-driven design efficiency and advanced resin materials is suggested to provide a predictable, comfortable, and clinically effective solution for TMD management.

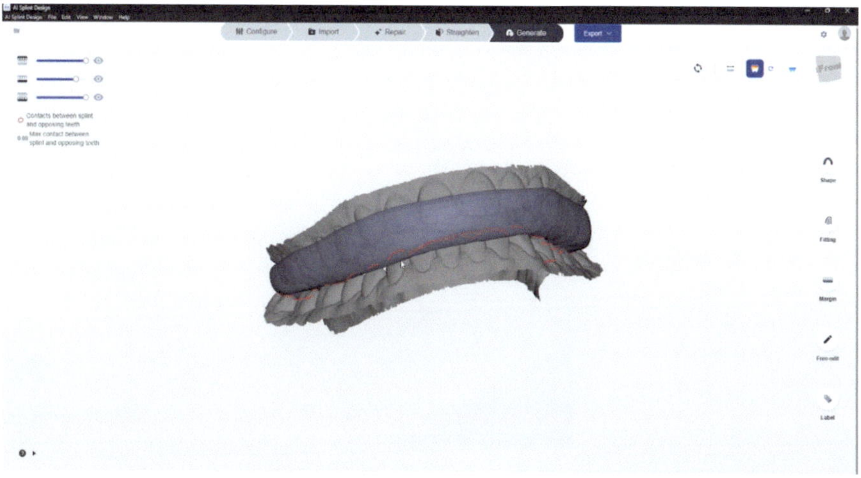

Fig. 10.27 AI splint design (HeyGears)

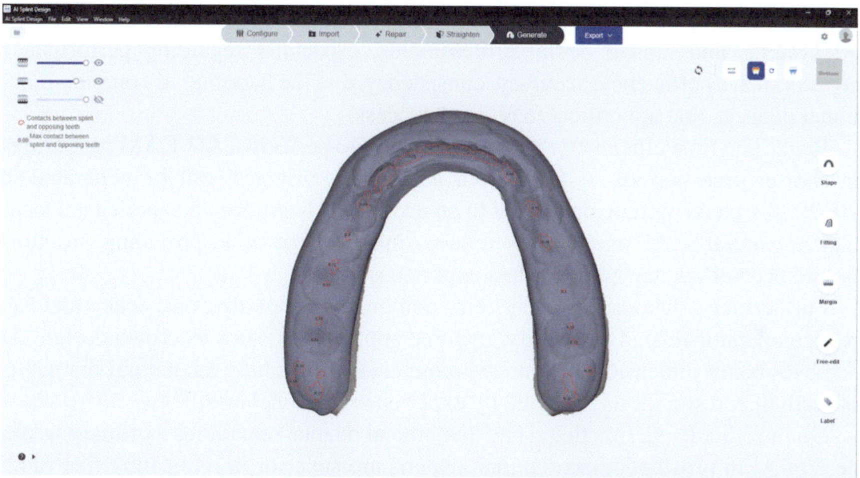

Fig. 10.28 Occlusal contacts assessment of the AI splint design (HeyGears)

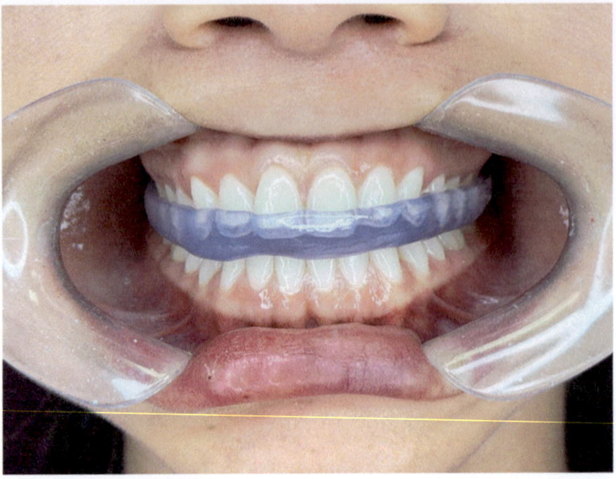

Fig. 10.29 Final clinical view of the occlusal splint

10.5 Comparative Analysis: AI Versus Human Expertise

It is important to understand and follow up research on direct comparisons between AI systems and human dental professionals, especially regarding performance aspects such as efficiency, accuracy, consistency, and the handling of complex functional nuances that are critical to clinical success.

Regarding time efficiency, AI tools contribute to perform CAD-CAM procedures in shorter time periods. A full crown design, for instance, can be generated in 10–20 s by an AI system, compared to an average of 6 min for an experienced technician. Similarly, AI significantly reduces inlay design time, providing the most pronounced efficiency gains for less experienced users.

Furthermore, data-driven AI systems demonstrate superior consistency and can reduce operator-related variability. In some applications, such as crown design, AI achieves better dimensional accuracy, more closely matching the natural diameters of teeth than restorations designed by experienced technicians.

On the other hand, functional and anatomical nuance remains as a primary weakness of AI in prosthodontics. Human experts are superior in replicating fine functional details such as cusp wear facets. Human intervention is also essential for optimizing occlusal and proximal contacts, which AI systems may generate suboptimally, leading to remaining premature contacts. Furthermore, human dental technicians can make intentional important clinical modifications based on patient-specific context, such as reducing the buccolingual dimension of a crown to decrease occlusal load in a patient with periodontitis. Current AI systems lack this level of contextual clinical judgment and require human correction to meet qualitative standards. These limitations suggest that the role of AI lies in its ability to augment but not replace the skills of the dental professional, particularly when addressing complex clinical variables.

10.6 Future Research Directions

To overcome the limitations discussed in the previous chapters in the field of prosthodontics, future research could focus on several important aspects. Future models must be trained on datasets that include patient-specific records of mandibular movement or dynamic bite patterns to improve the clinical fidelity and functional accuracy of the designs. In addition, research must move beyond in vitro design comparisons to evaluate the long-term durability, clinical success, and patient-reported outcomes of AI-fabricated restorations. The economic impact of integrating AI tools into dental practice also needs to be rigorously evaluated to understand the return on investment for clinicians and healthcare systems. Finally, there is significant heterogeneity in the metrics used across studies. The development of consensus-based performance standards for AI-generated designs is needed to allow for more reliable and valid comparisons between different systems and studies. Addressing these areas will be crucial for the continued evolution of AI from a promising technology into an indispensable, collaborative tool in daily dental practice.

10.7 Conclusion

Artificial intelligence and artificial neural networks have demonstrated significant potential to transform the field of prosthodontics. By dramatically increasing efficiency, improving design consistency, and aiding in complex interdisciplinary treatment planning, these technologies are already beginning to reshape digital workflows. However, the evidence synthesized in this review leads to a clear and consistent conclusion: current AI technology functions most effectively as a "copilot" or a sophisticated assistant rather than a full replacement for the dental professional.

The clinical judgment, artistic sensibility, and nuanced functional understanding of an experienced clinician or technician remain indispensable for achieving optimal, patient-specific outcomes. The ability to adapt a design to unique biological contexts, correct for algorithmic shortcomings, and ensure functional harmony is a uniquely human skill set that AI cannot yet replicate. The future of prosthodontics will not be a contest of AI versus human but rather a collaboration. The synergy between data-driven artificial intelligence and human expertise will define the next generation of restorative and esthetic dentistry, leading to more predictable, efficient, and personalized patient care.

References

1. Cortes ARG. Digital dentistry: a step-by-step guide and case atlas. Hoboken, NJ: Wiley; 2022. https://doi.org/10.1002/9781119852025.
2. Padrós RP, Giner L, Herrero-Climent M, Falcao-Costa C. Influence of the CAD-CAM systems on the marginal accuracy and mechanical properties of dental restorations. Int J Environ Res Public Health. 2020;17:4276.

3. Yeslam HE, von Maltzahn NF, Nassar HM. Revolutionizing CAD/CAM-based restorative dental processes and materials with artificial intelligence: a concise narrative review. PeerJ. 2024;12:e17793.
4. Ille CE, Jivănescu A, Pop D, et al. Exploring the properties and indications of chairside CAD/CAM materials in restorative dentistry. J Funct Biomater. 2025;16:46.
5. Wang Y, Li Y, Xu M, Liu F. Comparative analysis of full crown morphology designed by artificial intelligence and dental technicians. J Dent. 2025. https://doi.org/10.1016/j.jdent.2025.106131.
6. Ding H, Cui Z, Maghami E, et al. Morphology and mechanical performance of dental crown designed by 3D-DCGAN. Dent Mater. 2023;39:320–32.
7. Yang S, Han J, Lim SH, et al. DCrownFormer: morphology-aware point-to-mesh generation transformer for dental crown prosthesis from 3D scan data of antagonist and preparation teeth. In: Linguraru MG, et al., editors. MICCAI 2024. LNCS 15006. Springer; 2024. p. 109–19.
8. Yang S, Han JY, Lim SH, Kim S, Lee J, Kim KS, Kim JM, Yi WJ. DCrownFormer+: morphology-aware mesh generation and refinement transformer for dental crown prosthesis from 3D scan data of preparation and antagonist teeth. Med Image Anal. 2025;105:103717. https://doi.org/10.1016/j.media.2025.103717.
9. Kois JC, Zeitler JM, Barmak AB, et al. Discrepancies in the occlusal devices designed by an experienced dental laboratory technician and by 2 artificial intelligence-based automatic programs. J Prosthet Dent. 2025;134:214–21.
10. Cho JH, Yoon HI, Yilmaz B, Schimmel M. Benchmarking deep learning-designed inlay restorations across operator experience: an in vitro comparison of time efficiency, contact intensity, and contour quality. J Dent. 2025;162:106083.
11. Revilla-León M, Fernández-Estevan L, Barmak AB, Kois JC, Pérez-Barquero JA. Accuracy of maximum intercuspal position located by using four intraoral scanners and an artificial intelligence-based program. J Prosthet Dent. 2025;134:1242–50.
12. Saini RS, Kaur K, Gurumurthy V, et al. Impact of artificial intelligence-based digital smile design on patient and clinician satisfaction and facial esthetic outcomes: a systematic review and meta-analysis. Digit Health. 2025;11:20552076251388392.
13. Ceylan G, et al. Evaluating the facial esthetic outcomes of digital smile designs generated by artificial intelligence and dental professionals. Appl Sci. 2023;13:9001.
14. Fonseca FJPO, Matias BBR, Pacheco P, et al. Artificial intelligence-assisted treatment planning in an interdisciplinary rehabilitation in the esthetic zone. J Esthet Restor Dent. 2025. https://doi.org/10.1111/jerd.70034.
15. Matias BBR, Fonseca FJPO, Cordeiro JVC, Bohner L, Sesma N. Realistic esthetic virtual simulation and reverse scan body technique for complete mouth implant supported rehabilitation: a dental technique. J Prosthet Dent. 2025. https://doi.org/10.1016/j.prosdent.2025.08.050.
16. Chen Y, Lee JKY, Kwong G, Pow EHN, Tsoi JKH. Morphology and fracture behavior of lithium disilicate dental crowns designed by human and knowledge-based AI. J Mech Behav Biomed Mater. 2022;131:105256.
17. Tian S, Wang M, Dai N, et al. DCPR-GAN: dental crown prosthesis restoration using two-stage generative adversarial networks. IEEE J Biomed Health Inform. 2022;26:151–60.
18. Bobeică O, Iorga D. Artificial neural networks development in prosthodontics—a systematic mapping review. J Dent. 2024;151:105385.
19. Yang JW, Liu Q, Yue ZG, Hou JX, Afrashtehfar KI. Digital workflow for full-arch immediate implant placement using a stackable surgical guide fabricated using SLM technology. J Prosthodont. 2021;30(8):645–50. https://doi.org/10.1111/jopr.13375.
20. García-Sala Bonmati F, Pérez-Barquero JA, Ilzarbe Ripoll LM, Labaig Rueda C, Fernandez-Estevan L, Revilla-León M. An additively manufactured, magnetically retained, and stackable implant surgical guide: a dental technique. J Prosthet Dent. 2023;130(4):444–52. https://doi.org/10.1016/j.prosdent.2021.09.037.

21. Shi Y, Wang J, Ma C, Shen J, Dong X, Lin D. A systematic review of the accuracy of digital surgical guides for dental implantation. Int J Implant Dent. 2023;9(1):38. Published 2023 Oct 25. https://doi.org/10.1186/s40729-023-00507-w.
22. Markiewicz M, Nowicki AA. Accuracy of computer-guided dental implant placement: a clinical comparison of three surgical guide types. J Clin Med. 2025;14(24):8652. https://doi.org/10.3390/jcm14248652.
23. Nulty AB. An in vivo comparison of trueness and precision of two novel methods for improving edentulous full arch implant scanning accuracy: a pilot study. Dent J (Basel). 2024;12(11):367. https://doi.org/10.3390/dj12110367.

Part III

Dental Treatment Execution

Artificial Intelligence in Robotic Dental Treatments

11

Clifford Camilleri, Baoluo Xing Gao, Rui Xie, Shizhu Bai, Jiani Liu, Jesus Torres Garcia-Denche, Guillermo Pradies, and Arthur Rodriguez Gonzalez Cortes

The high global prevalence of oral diseases underscores the critical need for more accessible, predictable, and effective treatments [1]. For this purpose, dentistry has strategically embraced technological innovation to meet this demand. Dental fields of study have been progressing from digital workflows and CAD-CAM technologies to the integration of artificial intelligence (AI) as a foundation for modern robotic applications [2]. Such systems aim to further refine surgical precision, streamline complex procedures, and improve clinical outcomes. In this context, it is important to understand the current research on this topic to analyze the performance of AI-driven robotic systems across various dental surgical treatments and critically evaluate both their established benefits and developmental challenges.

C. Camilleri
Master of Oral Implantology, Goethe University Frankfurt a.M., Frankfurt am Main, Germany
e-mail: clifford@stpaulsdental.com

B. Xing Gao
Afonso X el Sabio University, Madrid, Spain

Complutense University of Madrid, Madrid, Spain

R. Xie · S. Bai · J. Liu
State Key Laboratory of Oral & Maxillofacial Reconstruction and Regeneration, Xi'an, China

National Clinical Research Center for Oral Diseases, Xi'an, China

Digital Center, School of Stomatology, The Fourth Military Medical University, Xi'an, China

J. T. Garcia-Denche · G. Pradies
Complutense University of Madrid, Madrid, Spain
e-mail: Gjpradie@ucm.es

A. R. G. Cortes (✉)
Faculty of Dental Surgery, University of Malta, Msida, Malta
e-mail: arthur.nogueira@um.edu.mt

A. R. G. Cortes (ed.), *Dental Clinical Procedures using Artificial Intelligence*,
https://doi.org/10.1007/978-3-032-24895-4_11

11.1 Robot-Assisted Dental Implantology

Computer-assisted implant surgery (CAIS) represents a foundational advancement in implant dentistry, developed to achieve the precise implant positioning that is a prerequisite for successful long-term functional and aesthetic outcomes [3]. This technology has evolved in different modalities designed to address the limitations of their predecessors in the pursuit of enhanced surgical accuracy and flexibility.

Static computer-aided surgery (s-CAIS) was the first method developed to translate a preoperative digital plan into a physical and patient-specific surgical guide to orient the respective implant site drilling procedure, generally fabricated using 3D printing or milling. Although initially used for guiding implant osteotomies, the applications of these guides have expanded significantly to include alveolar bone reduction, stabilization of temporary prostheses, and guidance for specialized procedures such as sinus lift and apicoectomies. In this context, AI is increasingly being used to streamline both the planning of implant placement and the automated design and manufacturing of these guides, as explained in Chap. 9. Despite its widespread use, s-CAIS has two primary limitations: its inflexibility, as any intraoperative plan alteration renders the guide unusable, and the time delay between planning and execution, which usually requires a couple of hours even with in-office systems.

To overcome the critical limitations of intraoperative inflexibility and time delays associated with static guides, dynamic computer-aided surgery (d-CAIS) was developed. This approach utilizes real-time tracking of the anatomy of the patient and the surgical handpiece to provide visual navigation without physical constraints [4]. The surgeon views a monitor that displays an overlay of the real-time position of the implant drill, relative to the preoperative CBCT scan of the patient. As a result, d-CAIS has an important advantage over its static counterpart, which is the ability to perform continuous intraoperative adjustments. However, the high costs of acquisition and training, along with a lack of physical rigidity during drilling, have remained significant barriers to its widespread adoption.

Robotic computer-aided surgery (r-CAIS) represents the next evolutionary step, synthesizing the main advantages of its predecessors to address their respective shortcomings. Adapted from other medical fields, r-CAIS combines the intraoperative versatility of d-CAIS with the physical rigidity of s-CAIS [5–8]. In this approach, a robotic arm follows a preplanned surgical trajectory, providing versatile guidance while ensuring the same physical stability during osteotomy preparation that is achieved with a static guide. These systems are being engineered to address specific challenges, such as patient movements and maneuvering in restricted surgical fields [7, 8]. Therefore, this fusion of technologies provides the foundation for the advanced robotic systems currently being implemented in clinical practice.

11.1.1 Technical Foundations of Robotic Systems in Dentistry

To properly evaluate the clinical applicability and potential of dental robotic systems, it is crucial to understand their hardware, software, and operational principles.

These technical foundations dictate their capabilities, from the precision of their movements to their level of clinical autonomy.

A typical dental robotic system is composed of four main components: a manipulator (the mechanical robotic arm), control software, sensors, and tracking devices that monitor the positions of the patient and surgical instruments in real time [9]. Based on how these components interact and the degree of surgeon intervention required, r-CAIS systems can be classified by their level of autonomy [10]:

1. Passive robots: These systems provide physical or haptic constraints to guide the surgeon, who still manually controls the instrument. The Yomi® system (Neocis) is a primary example.
2. Semiautonomous robots: These systems assist the surgeon with partial autonomy for specific tasks, such as drilling, but require constant surgeon supervision. Many of these systems offer dual-mode functionality, providing both passive and semiautonomous guidance.
3. Task-autonomous robots: These robots can execute a specific and preprogrammed surgical plan with the surgeon providing oversight for safety. The YakeBot (Beijing Yakebot Technology Co., Ltd.) is classified at this level.
4. Fully autonomous robots: Capable of performing the entire workflow from planning to execution without human intervention, these systems are not yet commercially available.

The manipulator, or robotic arm, is responsible for executing the planned movements. The two primary types described in the dental literature are serial and hybrid manipulators. The former are conventional industrial robotic arms that have been modified for surgical use. They are the most common type used in current dental systems [8, 11, 12]. The latter combine serial and parallel mechanisms to enhance versatility and rigidity. While theoretically expected to provide greater accuracy, current research does not yet support their superiority over serial robots [7, 13, 14].

Another important factor related to robotic implant surgeries is the tracking technology. Tracking is a critical function in both d-CAIS and r-CAIS, allowing the system to correlate the real-time position of the patient with the virtual surgical plan. The three main tracking methods currently utilized are optical, electromagnetic, and coordinate measuring machine (CMM) tracking.

Optical tracking is a well-established method evolved from d-CAIS systems—this technique uses cameras to track reflective markers placed on the patient and instruments [8, 13, 15, 16].

In contrast, electromagnetic tracking uses an electromagnetic field to determine the position of sensors. As it does not require a direct line of sight, it is particularly suitable for procedures in areas with restricted vision, such as zygomatic implant placement or mandibular angle osteotomies [16, 17]. Finally, CMM is the tracking method used by the Yomi system, which employs a second robotic arm connected to the patient. This arm continuously registers the spatial position of the patient, allowing the primary robotic arm to immediately compensate for any movement [11].

Implant site preparation can be executed by the system using robot-guided mechanical or laser osteotomy. The mechanical method is the most commonly used and involves a robotic arm guiding a conventional drill for implant site preparation. Multiple systems, including Yomi and YakeBot, have been validated for this purpose, consistently demonstrating the ability to translate a virtual plan to the clinical site with submillimeter precision [6, 18, 19]. Laser osteotomy is novel alternative to mechanical drilling offered by the Cold Ablation Robot-Guided Laser Osteotome (CARLO®) system. This technology utilizes an Erbium-doped Yttrium Aluminium Garnet (Er:YAG) laser to cut bone tissue through photoablation, without direct mechanical contact. This approach offers significant biological advantages, including minimal thermal damage, reduced surgical debris, and better preservation of the native bone architecture, which may promote faster and more robust osseointegration [20].

11.1.2 Clinical Case Studies: AI-Driven Robotic Implant Surgeries (Cases by Dr. Rui Xie, Dr. Shizhu Bai, Dr. Jiani Liu, and Dr. Baoluo Xing Gao)

Three clinical cases performed using the YakeBot autonomous robotic system are presented. The first case involves a single implant placement to rehabilitate the site of a maxillary right first molar, representing one of the earliest dental implants performed using robotic surgery in Europe, conducted at the Complutense University of Madrid within the Master's Program in Restorative Dentistry Based on New Technologies. The second case consists of a transcrestal sinus floor elevation and immediate implant placement, while the third case represents the first fully autonomous robotic surgery performed for a full-arch rehabilitation worldwide. These latter two procedures were carried out in Xi'an, China, at the Fourth Military Medical University.

11.1.2.1 Case Study: AI-Driven Robotic Single Implant Placement

A 62-year-old male patient classified as ASA 1 with no relevant systemic comorbidities presented for treatment. No drug allergies were reported. The patient lost the maxillary right first molar 7 years ago due to a root fracture (Fig. 11.1).

Preoperative planning was performed using DentalNavi software (YakeBot). This software is also used for the surgical workflow of the YakeBot system. By integrating and aligning the patient's cone-beam computed tomography (CBCT) data with the intraoral scans, a prosthetically driven surgical plan is generated. Once the implant position is defined, the drilling protocol is planned, including detailed drilling depth, rotational speed (rpm), and the robotic arm's entry angulation for the procedure (Fig. 11.2).

Based on the resulting surgical plan, two surgical guides were designed using the DentalNavi software. The anterior guide is worn throughout the entire procedure, as it stabilizes the reference marker, enabling the ADIR system's infrared camera to track the patient's spatial position in real time. The other guide is specific for the

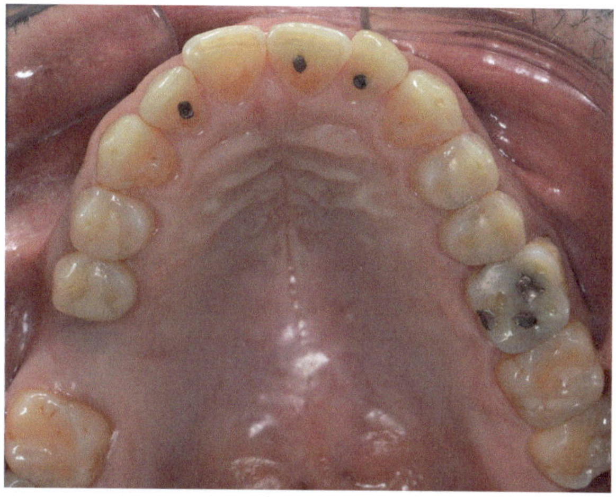

Fig. 11.1 Baseline intraoral photograph

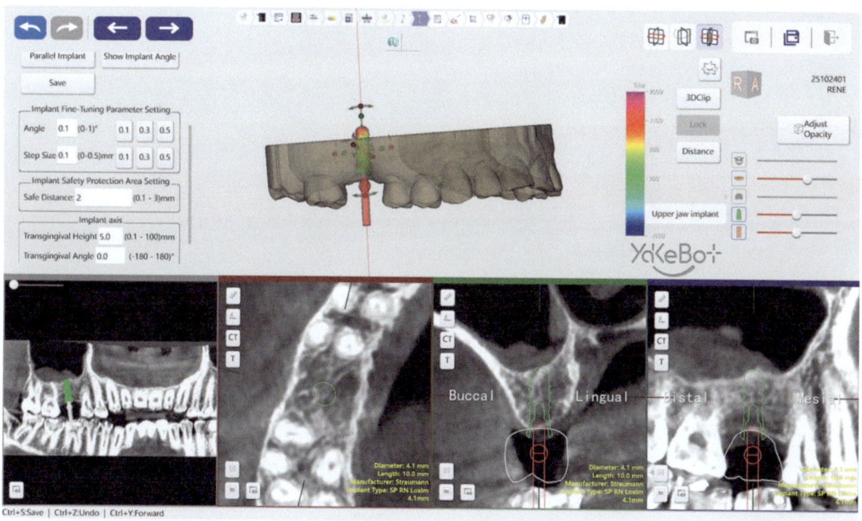

Fig. 11.2 Robotic dental implant planning

dental arch quadrant of the implant site and is used exclusively for the initial accuracy verification. This guide includes a targeting hole that allows clinical assessment of the positional accuracy of the pilot (needle) drill (Fig. 11.3).

Local anesthesia was administered by the dental clinician for implant placement in the right posterior maxilla. The robotic arm was manually guided to the operative field, after which the system autonomously positioned itself for implant drilling. An extraoral resting position was defined, allowing the robotic arm to consistently return to this position throughout the procedure to facilitate drill changes. A soft-tissue punch was used by the robot to remove the keratinized gingiva at the planned osteotomy site. Subsequently, the standard drilling sequence for the maxillary

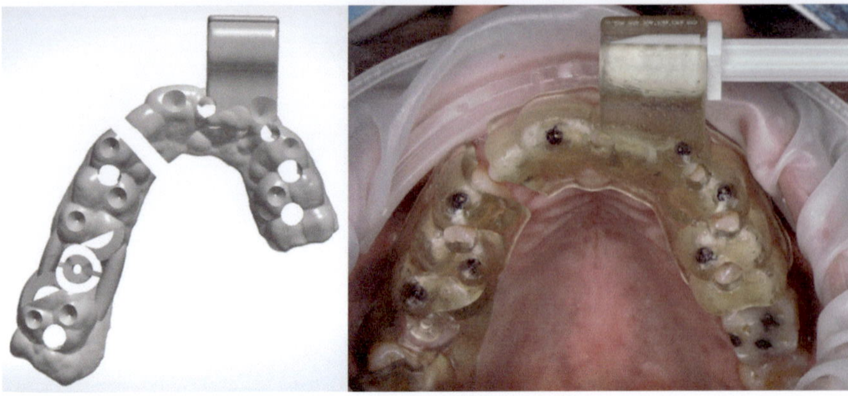

Fig. 11.3 Surgical guides with accuracy checkers painted in black

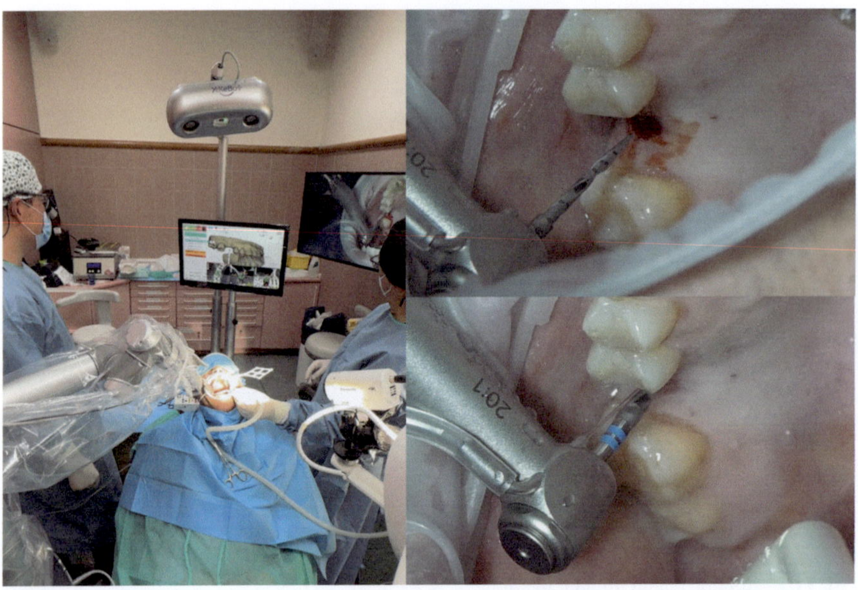

Fig. 11.4 Surgical room and drilling sequence

alveolar bone was performed for placement of a dental implant (Straumann SP, 4.1 mm in diameter and 10 mm in length, Institut Straumann) (Fig. 11.4).

The implant was autonomously inserted by the robotic arm and achieved an insertion torque of 35 Ncm. A compatible healing abutment was then selected and placed (Fig. 11.5).

One of the most relevant aspects of the ADIR robotic assistance systems is the extensive integration of AI-based tools within the software interface and ecosystem, in which the self-assessment module plays an important role. Posteriorly, another

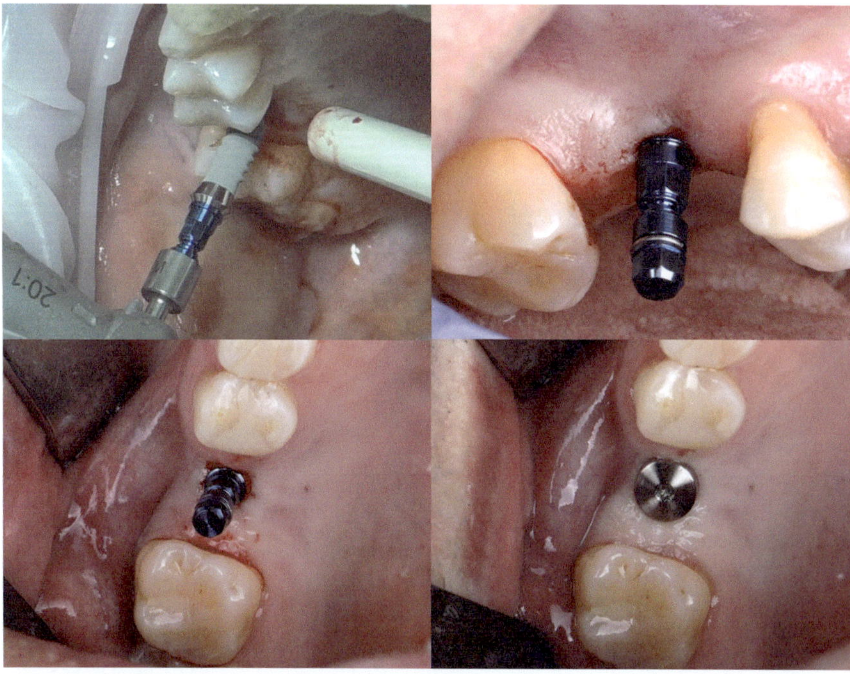

Fig. 11.5 Implant placement and postoperative result

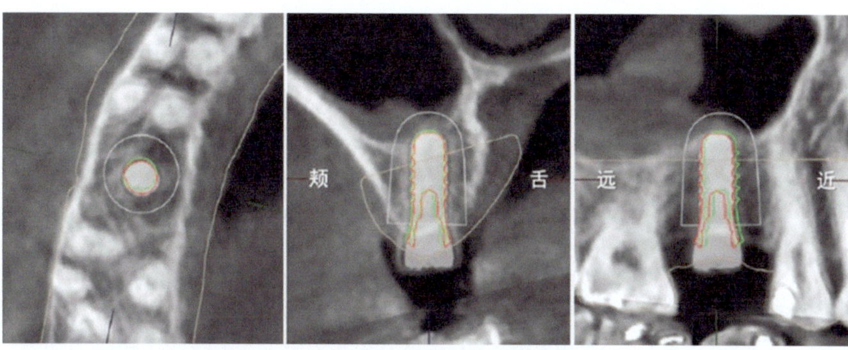

Fig. 11.6 Overlay between planned position and actual position

CBCT scan taken after the surgery enabled the DentalNavi software to automatically register and overlay the preoperative CBCT and planned workflow with the postoperative CBCT containing the final actual implant position, generating a detailed report on surgical accuracy (Fig. 11.6).

The postoperative report provides a three-dimensional assessment of the positional discrepancy. In this case, the coronal deviation was 0.293 mm in the buccolingual direction, 0.110 mm mesiodistally, and 0.135 mm in depth. At the apical

#46	颊舌侧	近远中	深度
颈部距离(mm)	舌 0.293	近 0.110	浅 0.135
根部距离(mm)	舌 0.240	远 0.042	浅 0.136

#46	误差信息
① 颈部误差	0.341
② 根部误差	0.279
③ 植体角度误差	0.921
④ 颈部水平误差	舌 0.293; 近 0.110
⑤ 根部水平误差	舌 0.240; 远 0.042
⑥ 颈部深度误差	浅 0.135
⑦ 根部深度误差	浅 0.136

#46	颊舌侧	近远中	总角度
角度(deg)	0.300	0.871	0.921

#46	颈部(mm)	根部(mm)	角度(deg)
总误差	0.341	0.279	0.921

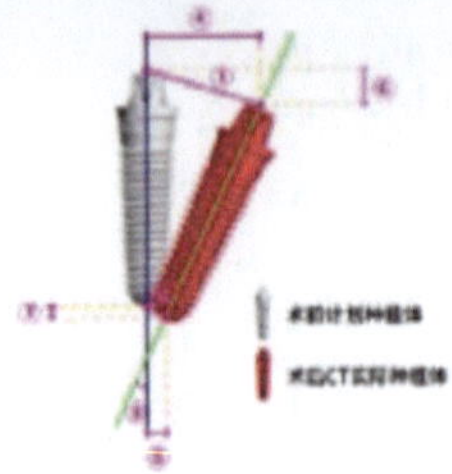

Fig. 11.7 DentalNavi accuracy assessment

level, the deviation was 0.240 mm buccolingually, 0.042 mm mesiodistally, and 0.136 mm in depth. The resulting combined deviation was 0.341 mm coronally and 0.279 mm apically, with an angular deviation of 0.921° (Fig. 11.7).

This case was performed in 2025, when robot-assisted implant surgery began to be performed in Europe, with the Complutense University of Madrid (UCM) pioneering this field. The learning curve is substantial and relies on solid expertise in digital planning, static guided surgery, and dynamic navigation systems. Following a series of clinical cases performed with the YakeBot system, improved operative ergonomics could be observed, together with a level of accuracy surpassing that of conventional guided and navigated approaches.

An important aspect of this method is that clinicians must relearn how to interpret intraoperative feedback, as tactile perception is markedly reduced. Surgical monitoring is therefore shifted toward visual and auditory cues. Visually, the surgeon must continuously assess real-time force diagrams displayed on the screen, which indicate the implant drilling forces acting on the robotic arm as well as the implant insertion torque. From an auditory perspective, attention must be paid to YakeBot's acoustic alerts, which provide critical information at important specific operative stages, such as confirmation of accurate drill-point positioning, in addition to the intraoperative sounds generated during implant osteotomy preparation.

11.1.2.2 Case Study: AI-Driven Robotic Sinus-Lift Surgery

Edentulous posterior maxillae pose unique anatomical challenges for dental implant placement, with inadequate residual bone height (RBH) being a prominent issue primarily due to maxillary sinus pneumatization. To address this issue, sinus floor elevation (SFE) has become an indispensable intervention, and transcrestal sinus floor elevation (TSFE) has gained widespread acceptance as a minimally invasive alternative to the lateral approach, offering comparable long-term success rates while reducing surgical trauma. Despite its procedural simplicity, TSFE outcomes are heavily contingent on the clinician's manual dexterity and clinical judgment, as the posterior maxillary region is often characterized by limited surgical access, variable bone quality, and complex sinus anatomy. These factors collectively increase the risk of intraoperative complications, with maxillary sinus membrane perforation being the most frequently encountered adverse event that may compromise surgical success. In addition, imprecise implant positioning such as deviations in angulation and spatial location may adversely affect implant osseointegration or even complicate the subsequent implant-supported restoration. Although digital computer-aided implant surgery (d-CAIS) has also improved placement accuracy in TSFE procedures, its performance remains susceptible to human variables such as operator fatigue and hand tremors. Recent evidence highlighted outcomes of robot-assisted implant surgery in comparison with static and dynamic navigation, as further discussed in this chapter. It has been suggested that there is a need for more robust and less operator-dependent guidance systems to optimize TSFE outcomes.

An autonomous dental implant robot (ADIR) has been developed, characterized by the merits of precision, minimal invasiveness, safety, and efficiency. The present case report of maxillary transcrestal sinus floor elevation was conducted with the employment of an autonomous dental implant robotic ADIR system (YakeRobot Technology Ltd., Beijing, China), in September 2024, as part of a study that was carried out in accordance with the principles of the Helsinki Declaration and approval by the Medical Ethics Committee of the Fourth Military Medical University (Approval No. IRB-REV-2022012), and written informed consent was obtained from patient.

A 71-year-old patient presented with a chief complaint of missing right maxillary posterior teeth for several months. The patient's dental history revealed that the previous diagnosis of this tooth included an endo-perio lesion, for which root canal therapy was also performed but yielding unsatisfactory outcomes and ultimately leading to the extraction of the tooth. The patient also had a history of periodontitis and had undergone sequential periodontal therapy. Systemically, the patient reported a medical history of hypertension and coronary heart disease while denying a history of diabetes mellitus as well as infectious diseases (including hepatitis and acquired immunodeficiency syndrome). There were no drug allergies to penicillins, cephalosporins, or other antibiotics. A history of sulfonamide allergy was self-reported by the patient.

Intraoral examination revealed missing maxillary right first molar (tooth 16) and left second molar (tooth 27), with mesial inclination of the former. Teeth 26, 36, and 46 exhibited percussion tenderness positive, no response to cold vitality testing, grade I mobility, and root exposure. General oral hygiene was deemed fair (Fig. 11.8).

Imaging examinations demonstrated horizontal bone loss, which was also related to the absence of tooth 16. Severe endo-perio lesions were observed on teeth 36 and 46, whereas chronic periodontitis was observed on tooth 26. Thickening of the left maxillary sinus mucosa was noted. CBCT revealed that the alveolar ridge height at the missing tooth 16 site was 6.3 mm and the residual alveolar ridge width at the edentulous area was 12.6 mm (Fig. 11.9).

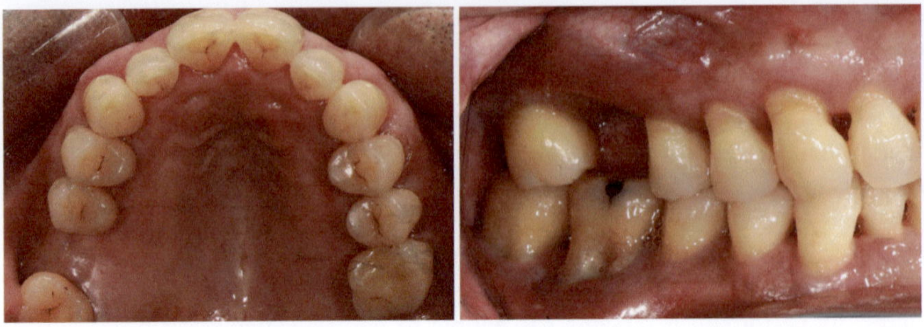

Fig. 11.8 Preoperative intraoral photographs. Occlusal (left) and buccal (right) views before surgery

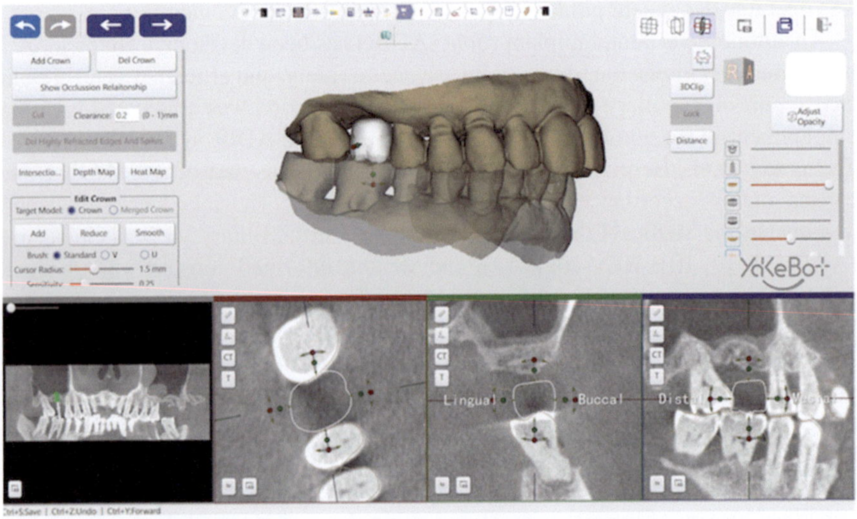

Fig. 11.9 Preoperative auxiliary examinations: CBCT axial (red), coronal (green), and sagittal images (blue)

CBCT data and the intraoral scanning data of the patient were imported into the software of the dental implant robot (DentalNavi) for 3D model reconstruction and trimming. The intraoral scanning model was superimposed to the CBCT space based on dental feature points, and the data alignment accuracy was verified (Fig. 11.10).

Implant position planning and robotic implantation were the next steps. An appropriate implant brand and model were selected, and precise implant positioning was planned. A prosthetically driven position of implant was digitally planned. The sequence of implant drills for osteotomies was determined following the surgical guidelines and according to the bone quality of the edentulous area. In the surgical planning, the use of an osteotome was programmed to first create an elevation pathway, preserving 1 mm of cortical bone at the sinus floor. Subsequently, the robotic

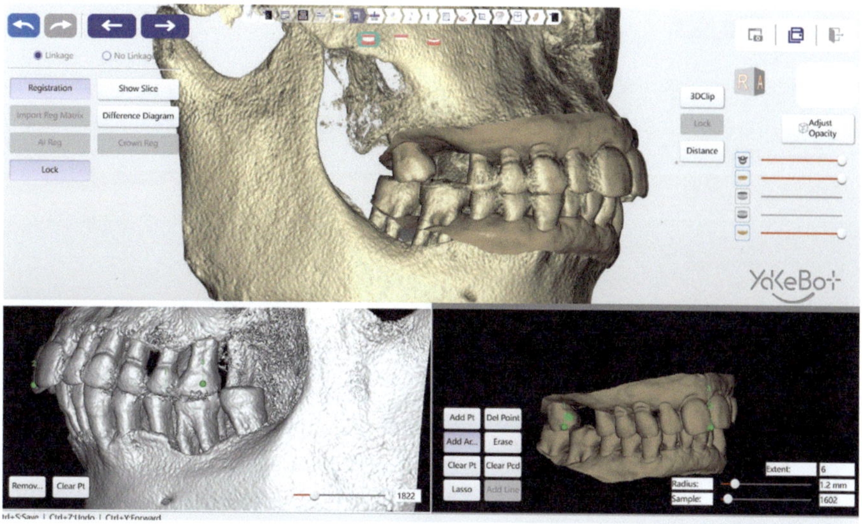

Fig. 11.10 Alignment of CBCT and intraoral scans in the planning software

elevation mode was activated to perform the actual sinus floor elevation. Upon completion of elevation, the final shaping of the implant socket was also conducted. The entire robotic implantation protocol was scheduled in strict accordance with the procedural sequence by robot (Fig. 11.11).

A customized positioning plate (surgical guide) suitable for the posterior maxillary region was designed. Surgical accessories were also designed before surgery, including a holder to connect the surgical marker, a prop to assist mouth opening, and a suction tray to evacuate blood and saline during drilling. Registration holes were designed in the marker holder and suction tray for intraoperative registration. The guide plate material was also selected. Then, the customized positioning plate was fabricated using three-dimensional (3D) printing technology (Pro S95; SprintRay) (Fig. 11.12).

Under robotic assistance, the implant socket was prepared in a stepwise manner. Subsequently, the maxillary sinus floor bone was elevated by the robot under the maxillary transcrestal sinus elevation module, and finally, the implant was placed with robot autonomously. Ultimately, the autonomous dental implant robot (ADIR) successfully placed the implant (Straumann BL 4.1 mm in diameter and 8 mm in length; Institut Straumann, Switzerland) at the preplanned position. In this case, the Z-axis direction, aligned with the drill axis, was selected to analyze the force-feedback data from the drill bit when it contacted the cortical bone until it passed through the sinus floor. The final implantation torque was 50 Ncm, and the surgical events executed by the robot are illustrated below (Fig. 11.13). During the surgical procedure, the surgeon could control the robotic arm via a foot pedal, and the force-feedback data were calculated by the software and displayed on the screen.

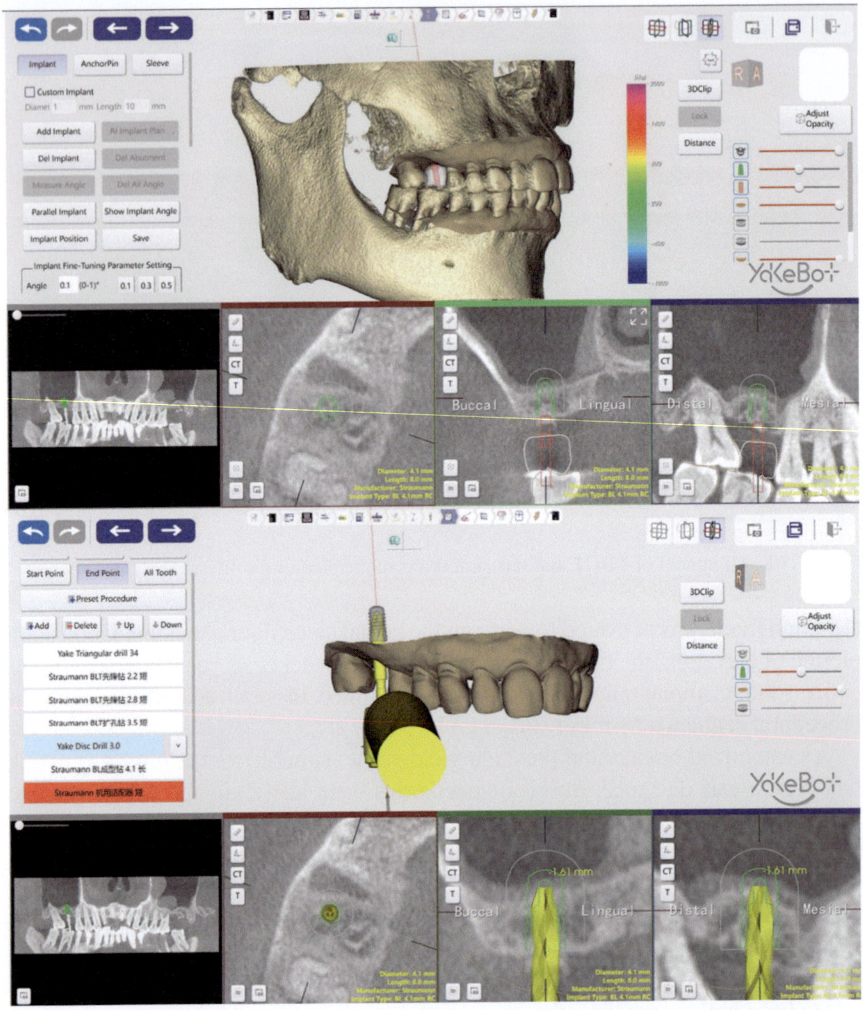

Fig. 11.11 Implant position planning. Top: a planning position with restoration oriented. Bottom: implant location and drill sequence of osteotomies designed in robotic software

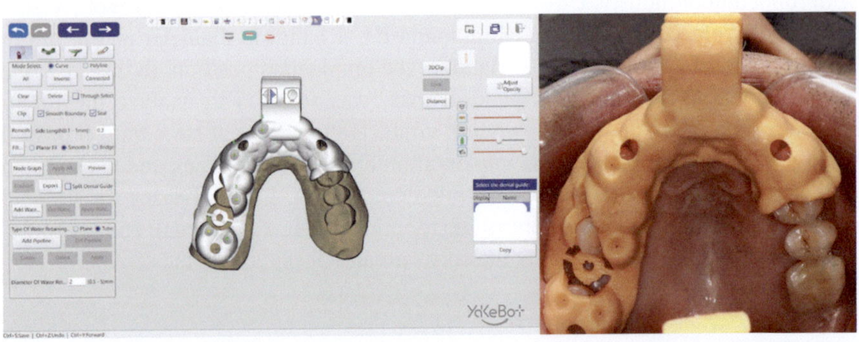

Fig. 11.12 Fabrication of a customized positioning plate, generating positioning plates and adding accessories (left) and 3D-printed accessories tried intraorally (right)

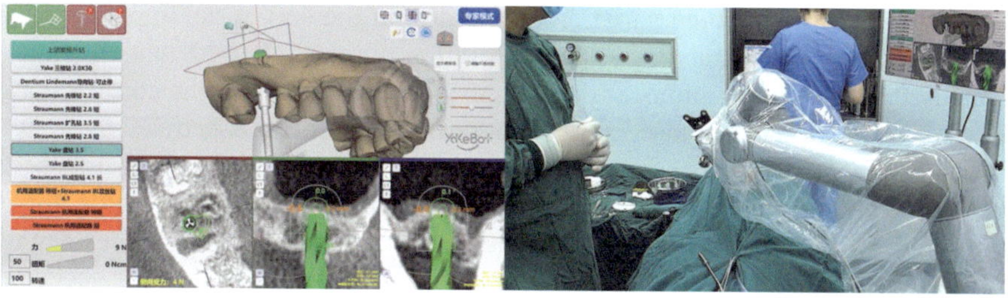

Fig. 11.13 Digital clinical workflow. Autonomous maxillary sinus floor elevation (left) performed by autonomous implant robot in conjunction with disk-up sinus reamer. Surgical scenario of dental implant placement surgery with autonomous dental implant robot (right)

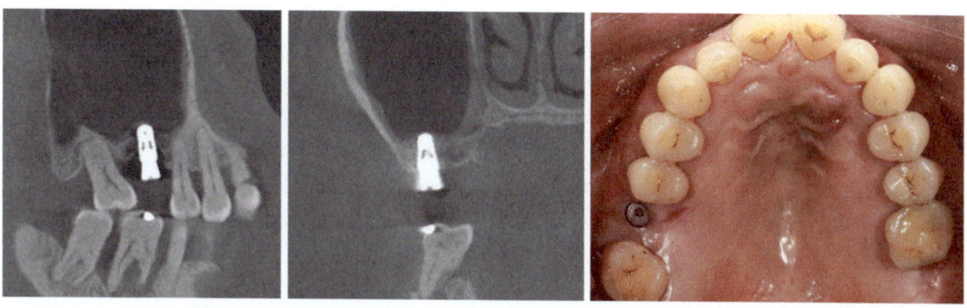

Fig. 11.14 CBCT taken after implant: sagittal (left) and coronal (middle) images, as well as clinical view of the implant placed with healing abutment (right)

Regarding postoperative care, antibiotics, analgesics, and mouth rinse solutions were prescribed, and the sutures were removed after 7 days. Posteriorly, another CBCT scan that was taken after the surgery was imported to the software to determine the position of the implant. The postoperative CBCT images showed that the implant was well positioned (Fig. 11.14), with no maxillary sinus membrane perforation. The elevated height of the maxillary sinus floor was 2 mm. Commencing from the initial drill entry into the oral cavity during the implantation procedure as the baseline time point, the immediate beginning of the postoperative phase following the placement of the dental implant was designated as the surgical endpoint for time calculation. The total operating time was 20 min.

The application of ADIR in transcrestal sinus floor elevation procedures addresses important challenges of traditional surgery by integrating advanced sensing and robotic control technologies. This integration not only enhances the precision of implant placement but also provides a more predictable surgical environment, which is particularly crucial for patients with complex anatomical conditions in the posterior maxilla. The real-time force monitoring and visual feedback capabilities of the robotic system allow for immediate adjustments during surgery, further reducing the risk of intraoperative complications such as sinus membrane perforation.

An analysis of the force variation on the drill at the end of the implant motor during robot-assisted maxillary sinus elevation surgery showed that the force increased sharply at the moment that the tip of the drill touched the cortical bone of the sinus floor and decreased abruptly at the moment that it penetrated the sinus. Based on this mechanical change, two force threshold parameters were established, namely, the sinus floor contact force threshold and the sinus penetration force threshold. During the grinding of the sinus floor cortical bone, it is necessary to simultaneously reduce the speed of the implant machine and the moving speed of the robotic arm to avoid accidental penetration of the drill into the maxillary sinus cavity due to inertia, thereby reducing the risk of maxillary sinus membrane injury. The software module for maxillary sinus internal elevation surgery of the autonomous oral implant robot has successfully been developed, based on in vitro tests on anatomical models.

Robotic systems are expected to address the inefficiency and drawbacks of current and future manual operational tasks. However, clinicians and staff require time to undergo professional training and accumulate experience in using these devices. In the digital workflow, accurate data collection and standardized execution of preoperative steps are crucial for the optimal performance of robotic systems. In the reported sinus elevation case, the robotic system assisted the doctors to overcome the lack of tactile sensation and experience by providing adequate visual data with professional supervision during the surgical procedure. It is suggested that these workflows might become more commonly performed with the evolution of the technology used.

11.1.2.3 Case Study: AI-Driven Robotic Full-Arch Implant Placement

A 66-year-old male patient presented with a chief complaint of mandibular tooth loss for 2 years, accompanied by discomfort associated with the use of a removable prosthesis, and requested implant-supported rehabilitation. The patient's medical history revealed that, 2 years earlier, all mandibular teeth and several maxillary teeth had been sequentially extracted due to chronic periodontitis. The maxilla had subsequently been rehabilitated with a removable partial denture, while the mandible was restored with a complete edentulous denture adapted from a removable partial denture. The patient reported persistent discomfort when wearing the mandibular prosthesis. He was otherwise in good general health, reported light smoking, and denied any history of systemic disease.

Intraoral examination revealed complete edentulism of the mandible. The overall height of the alveolar ridge was relatively well preserved, with no evident bony prominences. A localized depression of the alveolar ridge was observed in the right anterior mandibular region, along with resorption of the keratinized mucosa in the posterior regions.

In the maxilla, teeth 17–15, 23, and 24 were missing; tooth 22 was restored with a metal-ceramic crown, and tooth 11 exhibited rotation. Oral hygiene status was assessed as fair. Bilateral temporomandibular joints showed no clicking or pain (Fig. 11.15). Cone-beam computed tomography (CBCT) revealed a flat mandibular alveolar crest with ideal alveolar ridge width and height (Fig. 11.16).

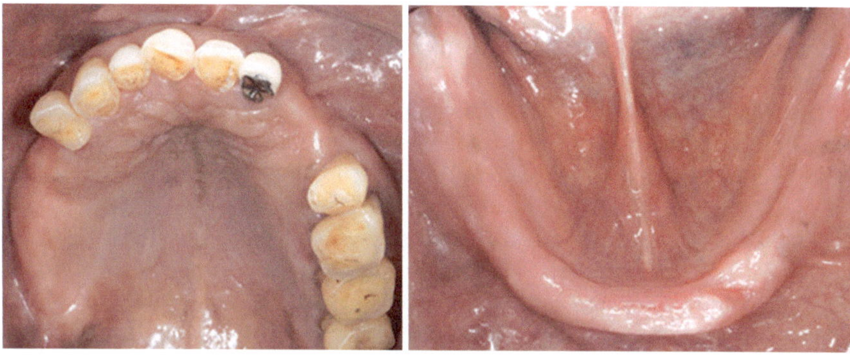

Fig. 11.15 Initial clinical situation of the case

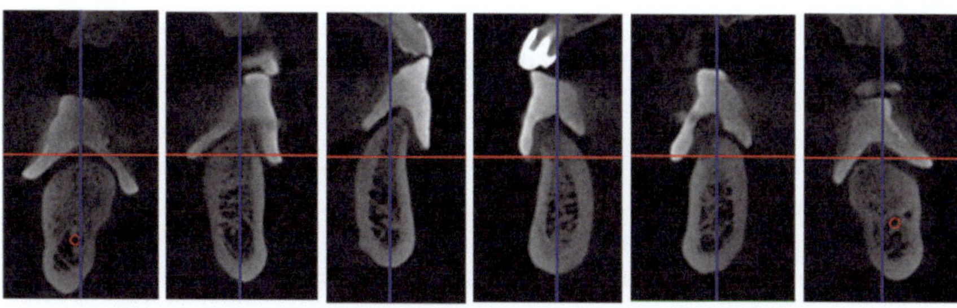

Fig. 11.16 CBCT cross-sectional images of the case

Given the favorable mandibular alveolar ridge conditions, implant-supported prosthetic rehabilitation was planned. To ensure accurate implant placement in accordance with a prosthetically driven preoperative plan and to minimize surgical trauma, an autonomous robotic oral implant system was selected for the procedure. In addition, to shorten the patient's edentulous period, an immediate prosthesis was designed based on the preoperative plan, enabling same-day postoperative restoration.

The autonomous robotic oral implant system integrates both visual servoing (control of the robotic motion using real-time feedback from cameras or vision sensors) and force servoing (robotic control strategy that uses feedback from force/torque sensors) capabilities. Under visual servoing, the robot performs registration and data fusion to accurately map the virtual implant plan generated in the robot-specific software DentalNavi (YakeBot, China) onto the real surgical field. A motion-following mechanism automatically compensates for minor patient movements, ensuring that the robotic system executes the procedure strictly along the predefined trajectory. Under force servoing, the robot continuously monitors the forces acting on the end effector and dynamically adjusts both the robotic arm velocity and drill rotational speed. Previous clinical studies have demonstrated that implant placement deviations in full-arch robotic implant surgery can be controlled within 1 mm, enabling precise, minimally invasive, safe, and efficient surgical outcomes.

Treatment plan consisting implant-supported prosthetic rehabilitation of the edentulous mandible was planned. Six dental implants (Astra EV, Dentsply Sirona, USA) were scheduled for placement in the mandible, followed by immediate loading.

A radiographic guide denture was fabricated prior to surgery, and a double-scan CBCT protocol was performed. The CBCT datasets were imported into the robotic implant planning software DentalNavi. Radiopaque markers were used to register the jawbone anatomy with the radiographic guide denture, enabling accurate data alignment (Fig. 11.17).

Based on the available bone volume and the planned implant emergence profile, appropriate implants were selected from the implant library. Six mandibular implants (Astra EV) were planned. Angular measurements between adjacent implants were performed within the software, with a maximum inter-implant angulation of less than 6° (Fig. 11.18).

The parameters for autonomous robotic implant placement included the drilling sequence, drilling torque and rotational speed, as well as the start and end positions of the drill. These parameters could be adjusted by the operator within a visualized three-dimensional model or more intuitively refined using two-dimensional cross-sectional views. Finally, the spatial orientation of the implant handpiece was optimized to prevent collision with adjacent teeth during drilling (Fig. 11.19).

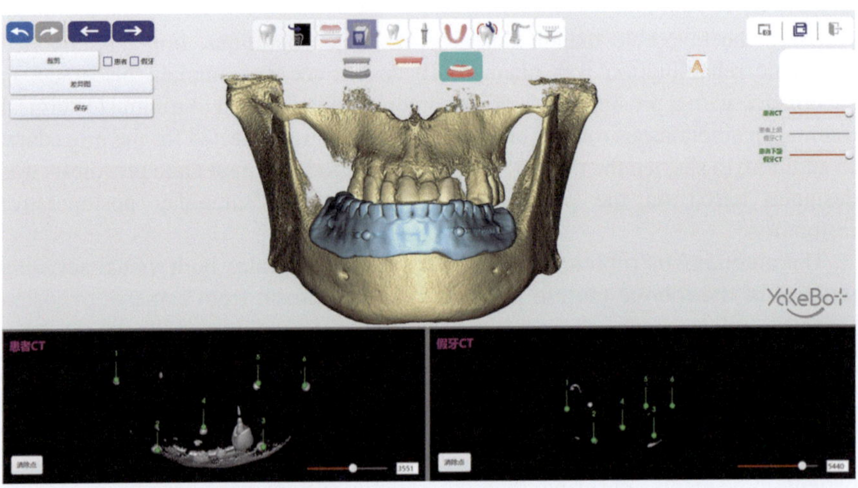

Fig. 11.17 Software-based registration of double-scan data

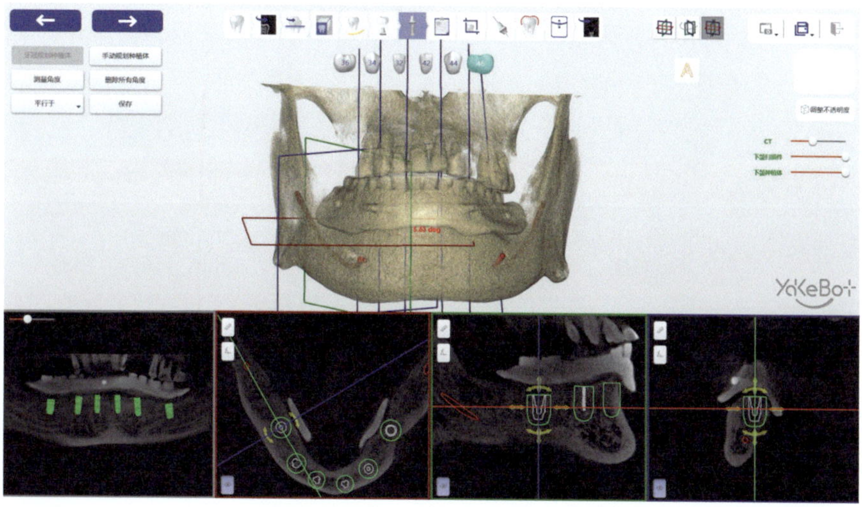

Fig. 11.18 Planning of implant positions

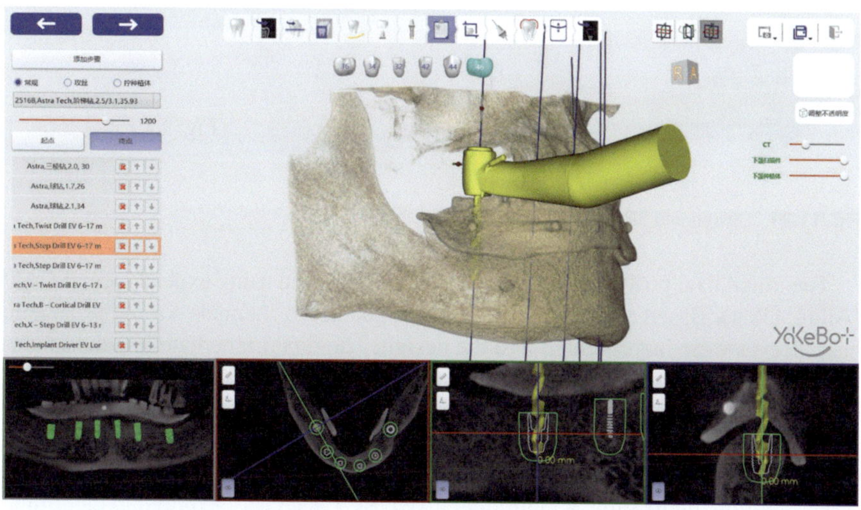

Fig. 11.19 Configuration of autonomous robotic implantation parameters

Using the modular design function of the software, a saliva suction accessory for autonomous robotic implant placement was designed. This accessory also served to assist the patient in maintaining mouth opening during the procedure. Upon completion of the design, the accessory was fabricated as a resin component using three-dimensional printing (Fig. 11.20).

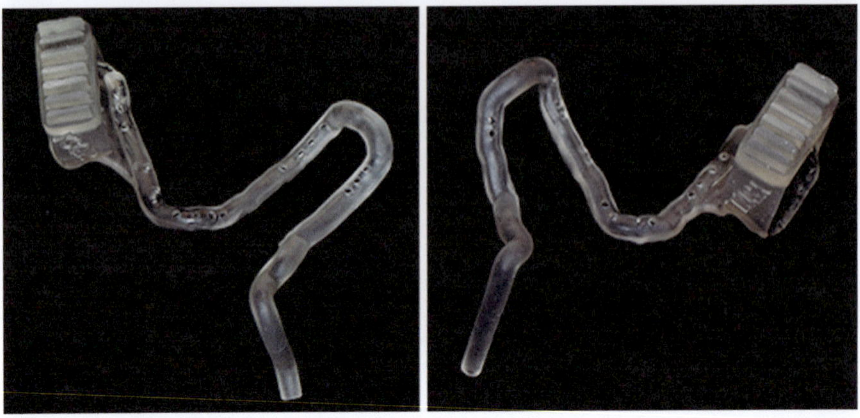

Fig. 11.20 Autonomous saliva suction accessory

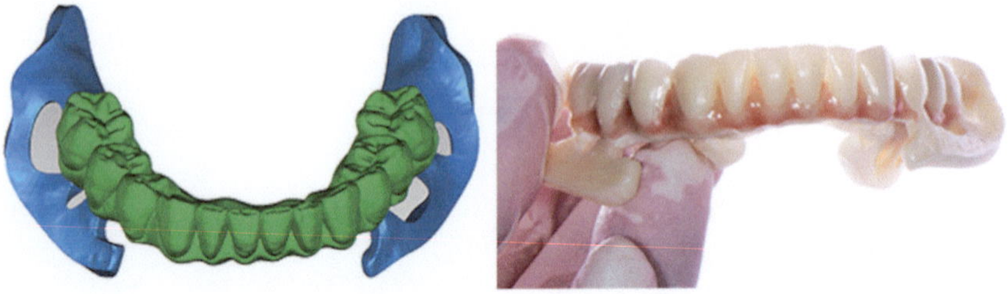

Fig. 11.21 Design and 3D printing of the immediate prosthesis

The immediate postoperative prosthesis was designed using exocad Dental CAD (Align, USA). Based on the planned implant positions, channels for the prosthetic base sleeves were incorporated into the design. The final immediate prosthesis was fabricated using a temporary crown material through three-dimensional printing (Fig. 11.21).

On the day of surgery, under local anesthesia, a visual positioning accessory was secured to the labial vestibule of the anterior mandibular region using cortical bone screws. Following fixation, an intraoperative CBCT scan was acquired to determine the spatial relationship between the jawbone and the positioning accessory.

After patient disinfection and sterile draping, the robotic system was calibrated under visual guidance, and simultaneous spatial registration of the jaw was performed (Fig. 11.22).

The robotic system autonomously prepared the implant osteotomies and placed the dental implants (Fig. 11.23).

Immediate placement of the provisional restoration (Fig. 11.24) and postoperative CBCT evaluation (Fig. 11.25).

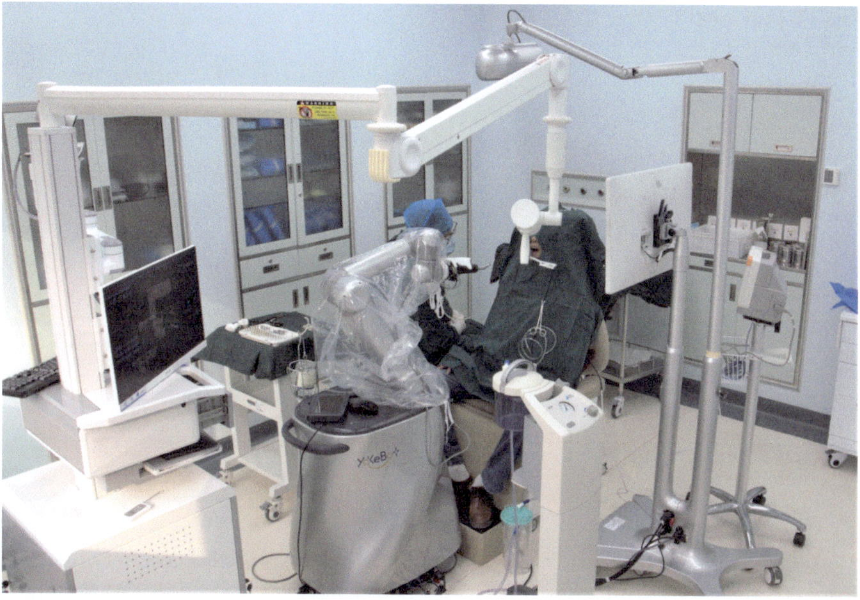

Fig. 11.22 Surgical setup

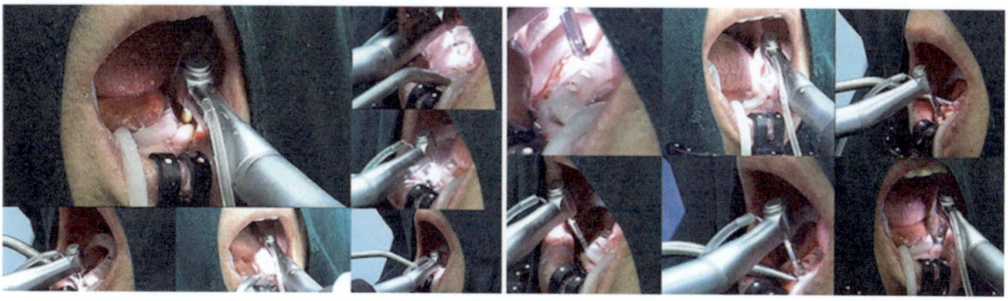

Fig. 11.23 Autonomous robotic preparation of implant osteotomies and implant placement. Immediate postoperative restoration

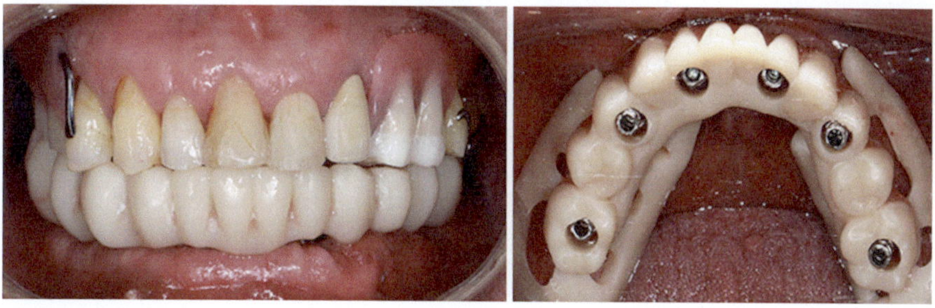

Fig. 11.24 Postoperative placement of the immediate prosthesis

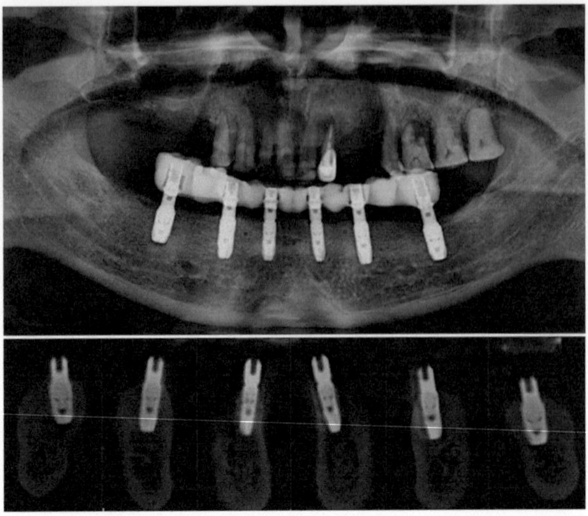

Fig. 11.25 Postoperative CBCT analysis

At the 3-month postoperative follow-up, the implants were successfully osseointegrated, and the peri-implant soft tissues had healed satisfactorily. The definitive prosthetic restoration was performed using a fully digital workflow (Fig. 11.26).

Precise implant placement represents a central challenge in implant rehabilitation of the edentulous jaw, as it requires positioning implants at optimal locations and angulations within a three-dimensional anatomical space. This precision is essential not only to minimize the risk of complications but also to adhere to prosthetically driven principles, ensuring that each implant provides stable and functional support for the definitive restoration.

The autonomous robotic oral implant surgery system integrates visual sensing, force sensing, three-dimensional visualization, and miniaturized modular robotic technologies, enabling the robot to autonomously perform osteotomy preparation and implant placement. The associated software supports preoperative registration, implant position planning and robotic motion trajectory design, accessory fabrication, intraoperative real-time navigation and safety monitoring, as well as postoperative accuracy assessment. In addition, multiple safety strategies are incorporated into the system, including motion-following calibration, force-feedback control, emergency stop mechanisms, and a safety-protective patient chair, collectively ensuring procedural safety during robotic surgery.

In the present case, the autonomous robotic oral implant system enabled prosthetically driven, highly accurate implant placement, demonstrating precision, minimal invasiveness, safety, and procedural efficiency. These findings highlight the clinical applicability and potential value of autonomous robotic systems in implant rehabilitation of the edentulous jaw.

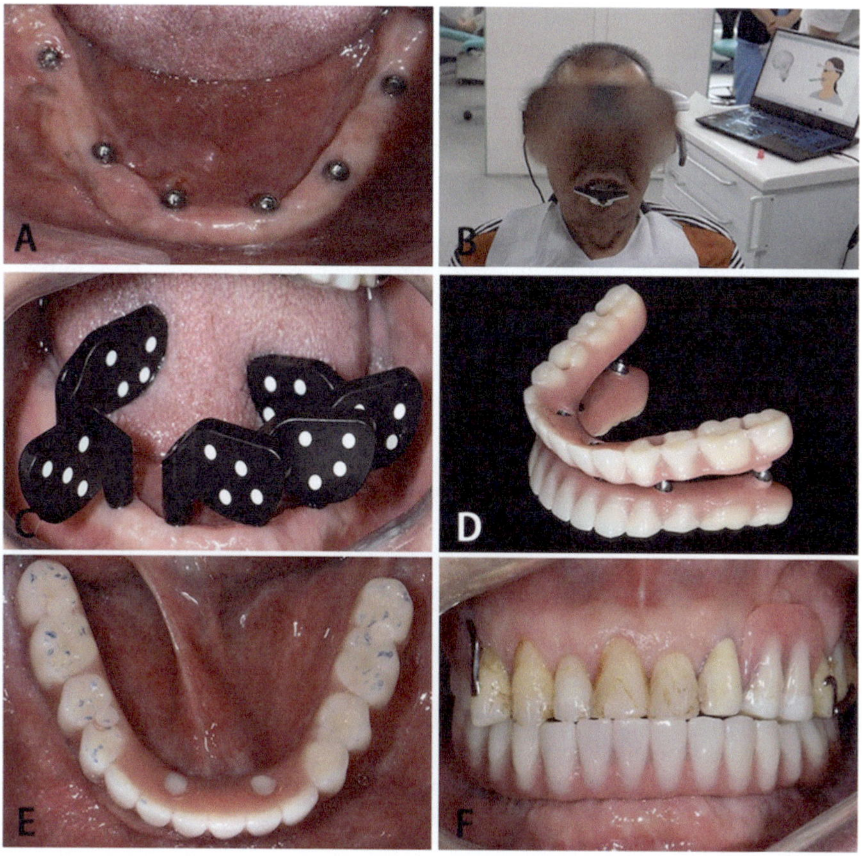

Fig. 11.26 Definitive restoration. (**a**) Intraoral view at 3 months postoperatively. (**b**) Acquisition of the patient's dynamic jaw relationship using an electronic facebow. (**c**) Digital workflow for the definitive restoration. (**d**) Implant position acquisition using an impression positioning device. (**e**) Implant-supported fixed prosthesis. (**f**) Occlusal intraoral view after completion of the restoration

11.2 Research on Comparative Performance Analyses

A recent systematic review and meta-analysis of in vitro studies found that robot-assisted implant surgery demonstrated a statistically significant improvement in accuracy compared to d-CAIS [9]. Robotic systems achieved the following:

- Angular deviation: 1.22 degrees lower
- Coronal deviation: 0.15 mm lower
- Apical deviation: 0.19 mm lower

Specific systems have reported even higher levels of precision in controlled studies. The highest accuracy results reported include the following:

- Lowest entry deviation: 0.59 ± 0.24 mm (Remebot) [21]
- Lowest apical deviation: 0.61 ± 0.23 mm (Remebot) [21]
- Lowest angular deviation: 0.74 ± 0.25° (hybrid robotic system) [13]

Despite the accuracy of robotic execution, a gap remains between AI-driven planning and clinical reality. A study comparing AI-planned implant positions to those placed freehand by experienced clinicians found significant mean deviations of 2.99 ± 1.56 mm coronally, 3.66 ± 1.68 mm apically, and 7.56 ± 4.67° in angulation. These findings suggest that current AI planning tools require significant clinician supervision and are best utilized as decision-support systems rather than fully autonomous planners [22].

The preclinical evaluation of the robot-guided laser osteotomy system highlights the developmental stage of this novel technology. It demonstrated comparatively larger deviations: 2.50 ± 1.30 mm at the base, 2.80 ± 1.00 mm at the tip, and 6.60 ± 3.10° in angulation. It is important to note that these mean 3D offsets exceed the clinically accepted 2 mm safety margin recommended by the International Team for Implantology (ITI). This indicates that further technological maturation is required before this approach is ready for clinical use [20].

AI demonstrates a clear impact on improving workflow efficiency. A study comparing planning times for single-tooth implants found that AI-assisted planning required an average of 11.84 ± 3.22 min. This was statistically significantly faster than the 21.50 ± 4.87 min needed for manual planning by a senior implantologist, showcasing AI's potential to reduce the time burden of presurgical preparation [23].

11.3 Robotic Tooth Autotransplantation

Autonomous robotics is being applied to complex procedures like tooth autotransplantation, where a patient's own tooth is moved to replace a non-restorable one. In this workflow, the robot prepares the recipient socket with high precision based on a preoperative plan. A 3D-printed replica of the donor tooth is used for a trial fitting to ensure a perfect match. The primary clinical benefit of this automated approach is minimizing the critical extra-alveolar time for the donor tooth, a key determinant of the procedure's success. Postoperative follow-ups in documented cases have revealed favorable outcomes, with stable fixation of the transplanted tooth and progressive bone healing [18].

11.4 Robotics in Oral and Maxillofacial Surgery

The precision of r-CAIS is being extended to oral surgery, exemplified by its use in mandibular angle osteotomy. This procedure is challenging due to the limited intraoral line of sight. Robotic systems that utilize electromagnetic tracking offer a distinct advantage by enabling precise navigation in constrained surgical fields, allowing for smaller exposures, reduced operative trauma, and improved patient safety [17].

11.5 Robotics in Restorative Dentistry

Robotics is also showing signs of progress in restorative dentistry with systems like the semiautomated robotic preparation system (SARP) for crowns. This system features a unique design where the robot clamps directly to the patient's dentition, allowing it to compensate for minor head movements while maintaining exceptional sub-50 μm accuracy. This enables the robot to execute a preplanned preparation precisely, facilitating a same-day treatment workflow and improving clinic efficiency [24].

11.6 Robotics in Oral Hygiene Education

A previous scoping review assessed how artificial intelligence is being used to support oral hygiene education across different populations and settings [25]. By screening more than 3000 publications, the authors identified 20 studies published between 2008 and 2022 that applied AI to improve daily oral hygiene practices. These studies varied widely in design, ranging from randomized controlled trials to case series, surveys, and research protocols. The AI tools described included smartphone applications using deep learning to detect dental plaque, smart toothbrushes equipped with sensors, augmented-reality feedback systems, and even humanoid robots delivering oral hygiene instructions. Despite the diversity of approaches, most interventions aimed to provide personalized, real-time or near-real-time feedback to help users improve brushing technique and biofilm control.

Across the included studies, the abovementioned review found promising but inconsistent evidence that AI-assisted tools can enhance oral hygiene behaviors [25]. Some trials reported reductions in plaque levels or improved brushing performance, while others showed minimal or no added benefit compared to traditional instruction. A recurring challenge was the quality of intraoral images captured by users, which often limited the accuracy of AI-based plaque detection. Ethical considerations such as privacy, data transparency, and user autonomy were rarely addressed in depth. Overall, the authors conclude that AI has significant potential to support personalized oral hygiene education, but higher-quality research, better imaging methods, and more thoughtful integration of ethical principles are needed to advance the field.

Another study used an in vitro design to investigate whether a collaborative tactile robot equipped with integrated artificial intelligence could remove interproximal artificial plaque as effectively as a human operator [26]. Using maxillary and mandibular phantom models coated with occlusion spray, the researchers compared two conditions: a dental student manually performing interdental cleaning with appropriately sized interdental brushes and the same student programming a seven-degree-of-freedom tactile robot to execute an identical cleaning protocol. Cleaning outcomes were quantified by means of standardized photography, HSV-based image processing, and binary surface analysis to determine the percentage of remaining plaque. Across 60 total cleaning procedures, no statistically significant differences were detected between robotic and manual cleaning, with mean residual plaque values of 0.41% and 0.42%, respectively. These findings suggest that modern tactile robots can reliably navigate and clean unknown interproximal surfaces, achieving plaque removal comparable to that of a trained human operator. This proof-of-concept research highlights the potential of tactile robotics to support oral hygiene in populations with limited motor or cognitive abilities, such as elderly individuals or those requiring assisted care. The authors emphasize that future research should extend to real plaque models, expert-level robot programming, and eventual clinical testing. The study also mentions broader potential implications for dentistry, including robotic assistance in hygiene procedures, evaluation of new oral care devices, and enhanced resilience of dental care systems during infectious disease outbreaks.

11.7 Challenges and Future Directions

Despite promising performance data, the transition of AI and robotics from research settings to routine clinical practice is contingent upon overcoming significant practical barriers and capitalizing on future developmental opportunities. The literature identifies several primary challenges that currently hinder the widespread adoption of these technologies, including cost, complexity of procedures, training and workflow disruption, and need for further validation.

The high development, acquisition, and implementation costs of surgical robots remain a major barrier for many clinics. Furthermore, these systems often have a steep learning curve and require disruption of established clinical protocols, necessitating a significant perceived benefit to justify their adoption [9, 18, 27]. It is also noteworthy that current systems can involve complex calibration processes and may still require manual refinements by the surgeon to correct for imprecise robotic work [18, 20]. Finally, there is a broad consensus on the need for large-scale research including long-term clinical trials to rigorously validate the safety, efficacy, and cost-effectiveness of these systems compared to existing standards of care [9, 23, 24].

11.8 Future Trajectory of Development

Ongoing research points toward several important directions for the future of AI and robotics in dentistry. First, the field is expected to progress toward higher levels of automation (Level 3–4 autonomy) for specific, repeatable tasks like bone drilling, thereby offloading more of the surgical workload from the clinician [2]. Moreover, there is significant potential in combining robotics with advanced imaging modalities like optical coherence tomography (OCT) to enable the automated detection of caries and selective, robot-guided removal of only diseased tissue, thereby maximizing the preservation of healthy tooth structure [24]. Therefore, AI could be able to revolutionize surgical training by analyzing surgical video and instrument data to recognize specific surgical gestures and provide automated performance metrics (APMs), delivering objective, targeted feedback to trainees [2]. Finally, as AI tools become more autonomous, it is essential to develop robust ethical frameworks to address issues such as patient data privacy, model transparency, algorithmic bias, and clinical accountability [2].

11.9 Conclusion

The scientific review of this chapter and the case studies support that the integration of AI and robotics has the potential to significantly enhance precision, efficiency, and standardization and reduce operator fatigue in dental surgery. Promising applications have been demonstrated across implantology, autotransplantation, and restorative dentistry, showcasing the versatility of these emerging technologies. However, performance exists on a maturity spectrum. On one hand, robot-assisted mechanical osteotomy for implant placement has demonstrated validated, superior accuracy over other methods in controlled settings. On the other hand, nascent technologies like robot-guided laser osteotomy, while biologically promising, still exhibit considerable deviation from planned outcomes and require further refinement.

The challenges related to cost, complexity, and the need for further clinical validation indicate that robotic systems are not yet positioned to fully replace established static and dynamic computer-assisted methods. While AI-driven robotics aims to establish a new paradigm in precision oral surgery, its widespread clinical adoption is not yet at hand. The full realization of its potential will depend on overcoming significant technical and economic challenges by means of continued research, iterative development, and rigorous validation in large-scale clinical trials.

References

1. Peres MA, Macpherson LMD, Weyant RJ, Daly B, Venturelli R, Mathur MR, et al. Oral diseases: a global public health challenge. Lancet. 2019;394(10194):249–60.
2. Knudsen P, Hauberg S, Matzen ME, Bardow A. Generative artificial intelligence in dental robotic surgery. J Robot Surg. 2024;18(1):102.
3. Mahardawi B, Jiaranuchart S, Arunjaroensuk S, Dhanesuan K, Mattheos N, Pimkhaokham A. The accuracy of dental implant placement with different methods of computer-assisted implant surgery: a network meta-analysis of clinical studies. Clin Oral Implants Res. 2025;36(1):1–16.
4. Block MS, Emery RW, Cullum DR, Sheikh A. Implant placement is more accurate using dynamic navigation. J Oral Maxillofac Surg. 2017;75(7):1377–86.

5. Sun X, McKenzie FD, Bawab S, et al. Automated dental implantation using image-guided robotics: registration results. Int J CARS. 2011;6:627–34.
6. Chen J, Bai X, Ding Y, Shen L, Sun X, Cao R, et al. Comparison the accuracy of a novel implant robot surgery and dynamic navigation system in dental implant surgery: an in vitro pilot study. BMC Oral Health. 2023;23(1):179.
7. Tao B, Feng Y, Fan X, Zhuang M, Chen X, Wang F, et al. Accuracy of dental implant surgery using dynamic navigation and robotic systems: an in vitro study. J Dent. 2022;123:104170.
8. Cao Z, Qin C, Fan S, Yu D, Wu Y, Qin J, et al. Pilot study of a surgical robot system for zygomatic implant placement. Med Eng Phys. 2020;75:72–8.
9. Jain S, Sayed ME, Ibraheem WI, Ageeli AA, Gandhi S, Jokhadar HF, et al. Accuracy comparison between robot-assisted dental implant placement and static/dynamic computer-assisted implant surgery: a systematic review and meta-analysis of in vitro studies. Medicina (Kaunas). 2024;60(1):11.
10. Xia J, Tang Q, Liu H, et al. Evaluation of the accuracy of semi-autonomous robotic system versus dynamic navigation in completely edentulous implant surgery: an in vitro study. BMC Oral Health. 2025;25:1751.
11. Wu Y, Wang F, Fan S, Chow JK. Robotics in dental implantology. Oral Maxillofac Surg Clin North Am. 2019;31(3):513–9.
12. Li Y, Hu J, Tao B, Yu D, Shen Y, Fan S, et al. Automatic robot-world calibration in an optical-navigated surgical robot system and its application for oral implant placement. Int J Comput Assist Radiol Surg. 2020;15(10):1685–92.
13. Feng Y, Fan J, Tao B, Wang S, Mo J, Wu Y, et al. An image-guided hybrid robot system for dental implant surgery. Int J Comput Assist Radiol Surg. 2022;17(1):15–26.
14. Tao B, Feng Y, Fan X, Lan K, Zhuang M, Wang S, et al. The accuracy of a novel image-guided hybrid robotic system for dental implant placement: an in vitro study. Int J Med Robot. 2023;19(1):e2452.
15. Kan TS, Cheng KJ, Liu YF, Wang R, Zhu WD, Zhu FD, et al. Evaluation of a custom-designed human-robot collaboration control system for dental implant robot. Int J Med Robot. 2022;18:e2346.
16. Gao Y, Qin C, Tao B, Hu J, Wu Y, Chen X. An electromagnetic tracking implantation navigation system in dentistry with virtual calibration. Int J Med Robot. 2021;17:e2215.
17. Sun M, Lin L, Chen X, Xu C, Zin MA, Han W, et al. Robot-assisted mandibular angle osteotomy using electromagnetic navigation. Ann Transl Med. 2021;9(7):567.
18. Liu Y, Song J, Chen X, Zhang C, Yang Y, Liu D, et al. Robot-assisted autotransplantation of third molars in the maxilla: two case reports. Front Oral Health. 2025;6:1661873.
19. Wang W, Xu H, Mei D, Zhou C, Li X, Han Z, et al. Accuracy of the Yakebot dental implant robotic system versus fully guided static computer-assisted implant surgery template in edentulous jaw implantation: a preliminary clinical study. Clin Implant Dent Relat Res. 2024;26(2):309–16.
20. Thieringer FM, Walher R, Halbeisen FS, Garnier Q, Dragu A, Msallem B. Accuracy evaluation of robot-guided laser osteotomy for dental implant bed preparation—a digital high-tech procedure. Front Robot AI. 2025;12:1614659.
21. Yang S, Chen J, Li A, Li P, Xu S. Autonomous robotic surgery for immediately loaded implant-supported maxillary full-arch prosthesis: a case report. J Clin Med. 2022;11(21):6594.
22. Che SA, Yang BE, Park SY, On SW, Lim HK, Lee CU, et al. Clinical evaluation of AI-based three-dimensional dental implant planning: a multicenter study. J Dent. 2025;162:106066.
23. Ma H, Wu Y, Bai H, Xu Z, Ding P, Deng X, et al. Preclinical investigation of artificial intelligence-assisted implant surgery planning for single tooth defects: a case series study. J Oral Rehabil. 2025; https://doi.org/10.1111/joor.14009.
24. Ciriello C, Gallucci G, Getto P, Doeringer J, Rosen J, Pala K. First in-human intervention using a semi-automated robot for tooth restorative treatment. 2025. https://doi.org/10.21203/rs.3.rs-6455412/v1. [Preprint].

25. Tay JRH, Ng E, Chow DY, Sim CPC. The use of artificial intelligence to aid in oral hygiene education: a scoping review. J Dent. 2023;135:104564. https://doi.org/10.1016/j.jdent.2023.104564.
26. Pieper L, Stiesch M, Eich L, Haddadin S, Grischke J. Interproximal tooth cleaning operated by a tactile robot. An in vitro analysis. Int J Comput Dent. 2024;27(3):251–8. https://doi.org/10.3290/j.ijcd.b4224851.
27. Lawrie L, Gillies K, Duncan E, Davies L, Beard D, Campbell MK. Barriers and enablers to the effective implementation of robotic assisted surgery. PLoS One. 2022;17(8):e0273696.

MIX
Papier aus verantwortungsvollen Quellen
Paper from responsible sources
FSC® C105338

If you have any concerns about our products,
you can contact us on
ProductSafety@springernature.com

In case Publisher is established outside the EU,
the EU authorized representative is:
Springer Nature Customer Service Center GmbH
Europaplatz 3, 69115 Heidelberg, Germany

Printed by Libri Plureos GmbH
in Hamburg, Germany